# Conscious Will and Responsibility

**Series in Neuroscience, Law, and Philosophy**

Series editors
Lynn Nadel, Frederick Schauer, and Walter Sinnott-Armstrong

*Conscious Will and Responsibility*
Edited by Walter Sinnott-Armstrong and Lynn Nadel

# Conscious Will and Responsibility

*Edited by*

Walter Sinnott-Armstrong and

Lynn Nadel

OXFORD
UNIVERSITY PRESS
2011

OXFORD
UNIVERSITY PRESS

Oxford University Press, Inc., publishes works that further
Oxford University's objective of excellence
in research, scholarship, and education.

Oxford New York
Auckland Cape Town Dar es Salaam Hong Kong Karachi
Kuala Lumpur Madrid Melbourne Mexico City Nairobi
New Delhi Shanghai Taipei Toronto

With offices in
Argentina Austria Brazil Chile Czech Republic France Greece
Guatemala Hungary Italy Japan Poland Portugal Singapore
South Korea Switzerland Thailand Turkey Ukraine Vietnam



Published by Oxford University Press, Inc.
198 Madison Avenue, New York, New York 10016

www.oup.com



Library of Congress Cataloging-in-Publication Data
Conscious will and responsibility : a tribute to Benjamin Libet / edited by
Walter Sinnott-Armstrong and Lynn Nadel.—1st ed.
p. cm.
ISBN 978-0-19-538164-1 1. Will. 2. Responsibility.
3. Consciousness. I. Libet, Benjamin, 1916- II. Sinnott-Armstrong,
Walter, 1955- III. Nadel, Lynn.
BF611.C64 2010
153.8—dc22

2010007431

9 8 7 6 5 4 3 2 1
Printed in the USA
on acid-free paper

# PREFACE

The work of Benjamin Libet on the consciousness of intentions has implications for psychologists, philosophers, neuroscientists, and lawyers. When Walter Sinnott-Armstrong suggested the notion of holding a workshop in Libet's honor that would bring an interdisciplinary group of scholars together to consider these implications, I quickly agreed. We decided right away to hold the meeting in Tucson, and the idea emerged to connect it to the Tucson Consciousness meeting—a natural link.

We are grateful to the organizers of the Consciousness meeting, in particular Uriah Kriegel and Stuart Hameroff, for making this possibility a reality. The workshop was supported by the MacArthur Law and Neuroscience Program at UC Santa Barbara, and by a number of sources at the University of Arizona: the College of Law, the Eller College of Business and Public Administration, the College of Social and Behavioral Sciences, the Program in Cognitive Science, and the Office of the Vice President for Research. We thank these various contributors for their support. In addition, Catherine Carlin of Oxford University Press quickly saw the virtues of this workshop and provided both financial backing and a contract for this book. We thank her for this support, and for helping us initiate what we hope will be an exciting series of volumes at the interdisciplinary interface represented in this collection.

Lynn Nadel and Walter Sinnott-Armstrong

# CONTENTS

# CONTRIBUTORS

**Larry Alexander**
Warren Distinguished Professor
University of San Diego School of Law
San Diego, CA

**William P. Banks**
Professor, Department of Psychology
Pomona College
Claremont, CA

**Francesca Carota**
Postdoctoral Fellow
Center for Cognitive Neuroscience
CNRS
Bron, France

**Michel Desmurget**
Assistant Professor
Centre de Neurosciences Cognitives
CNRS
Bron, France

**Jeffrey P. Ebert**
Postdoctoral Fellow
Department of Psychology
Harvard University
Cambridge, MA

**Chris D. Frith**
Wellcome Trust Centre for Neuroimaging
University College London
London, UK

**Tashina L. Graves**
Research Assistant
Department of Psychology
Columbia University
New York, NY

**Patrick Haggard**
Professor of Cognitive Neuroscience
Institute of Cognitive Neuroscience
University College London
London, UK

**Mark Hallett**
Chief, Human Motor Control Section
National Institute of Neurological Disorders and Stroke
National Institutes of Health
Bethesda, MD

**John-Dylan Haynes**
Professor for Theory and Analysis of Large-Scale Brain Signals
Bernstein Center for Computational Neuroscience
Charité–Universitätsmedizin Berlin
Berlin, Germany

**Terry Horgan**
Professor
Department of Philosophy
University of Arizona
Tucson, AZ

**Eve A. Isham**
Postdoctoral fellow
Center for Mind and Brain
University of California
Davis, CA

**Hakwan Lau**
Assistant Professor
Department of Psychology
Columbia University
New York, NY

**Christine E. Looser**
Psychological and Brain Sciences
Dartmouth College
Hanover, NH

**Brian Maniscalco**
PhD Candidate
Department of Psychology
Columbia University
New York, NY

**Alfred R. Mele**
William H. and Lucyle T. Werkmeister
Professor of Philosophy
Department of Philosophy
Florida State University
Tallahassee, FL

**Michael S. Moore**
Walgreen University Chair, Professor of Law
Professor of Philosophy
Professor in the Center for Advanced Study
Co-Director, Program in Law and Philosophy
University of Illinois
Champaign, IL

**Lynn Nadel**
Regents Professor
Department of Psychology
University of Arizona
Tuscon, AZ

**Thomas Nadelhoffer**
Assistant Professor
Department of Philosophy
Dickinson College
Carlisle, PA

**Elisabeth Pacherie**
Senior Researcher
Institut Jean Nicod
ENS, EHESS, CNRS
Paris, France

**Susan Pockett**
Honorary Research Fellow
Department of Physics
University of Auckland
New Zealand

**Suzanne C. Purdy**
Associate Professor
Department of Psychology
University of Auckland
Auckland, New Zealand

**Adina L. Roskies**
Department of Philosophy
Dartmouth College
Hanover, NH

**Walter Sinnott-Armstrong**
Chauncey Stillman Professor of Practical Ethics
Philosophy Department
Kenan Institute for Ethics
Duke University
Durham, NC

**Angela Sirigu**
Research Director
Center for Cognitive Neuroscience
CNRS
Bron, France

**Deborah Talmi**
Lecturer
School of Psychological Sciences
University of Manchester
Manchester, UK

**Daniel M. Wegner**
Professor
Department of Psychology
Harvard University
Cambridge, MA

**Thalia Wheatley**
Assistant Professor
Psychological and Brain Sciences
Dartmouth College
Hanover, NH

**Gideon Yaffe**
Associate Professor of Philosophy and Law
University of Southern California
Los Angeles, CA

# Introduction

*Walter Sinnott-Armstrong, Duke University*
*Lynn Nadel, University of Arizona*

Traditional philosophers often assume that the main challenge to moral and legal responsibility in general comes from determinism: If our choices and actions are determined, we cannot do otherwise, so we are not free, and then how could we be responsible? In reply to this challenge, compatibilists claim that we can have it all: complete and universal determinism as well as total freedom and responsibility.[1] According to common versions of compatibilism, responsibility does not require freedom from causation. Instead, responsibility and freedom require only that agents be responsive to reasons for and against their actions and/or that agents act on desires that fit with their values or second-order desires. Understood in these ways, freedom and responsibility are compatible with determinism. Moreover, modern legal systems nowhere explicitly mention determinism or presuppose that people and their acts are not caused or determined or that they have free will of any kind that excludes determinism.[2] Courts do not and need not settle the issue of determinism before they put criminals in jail. That's lucky, because it is doubtful that courts could settle that perennial issue, especially within the temporal and evidential limits of trials. Of course, some moral philosophers and legal scholars still argue that determinism does or would undermine moral and legal responsibility,[3] but many contemporaries think that they know at least roughly how to answer this traditional challenge to moral and legal responsibility.

Even if so, a separate challenge still needs to be met. Unlike the old issue of determinism, this new challenge concerns not whether anything causes our wills but, instead, whether our wills cause anything. This question is about the effects rather than the causes of our wills. It does not ask whether our wills are free but, rather, whether our wills are efficacious. The answer affects whether or how we can control what we do (that is, our actions) instead of whether we control what we choose to do (that is, our wills).

If our wills lack the power to cause the willed actions, this impotence is supposed to raise doubts about whether we are morally or legally responsible for those actions. These doubts arise from the assumption that causation by will or conscious will is necessary for complete moral or legal responsibility. This requirement seems enshrined in the voluntary act requirement, which is present in almost all modern systems of criminal law. For example, the Model Penal Code Section 2.01 says, "a bodily movement that otherwise is not a product of the effort or determination of the actor, either conscious or habitual" is not a voluntary act and, hence, cannot alone be the basis for criminal liability or guilt. If "a product of" means "caused by," and "effort or determination" means "will," then non-habitual actions cannot alone be the basis for legal guilt under this voluntary act requirement unless they are caused by conscious will.

The fact that this legal requirement is so widespread suggests that it is based on common sense. This suggestion receives additional support from moral intuitions. Consider normal reflective actions. When I choose to bet rather than fold in a poker game, I normally go through a conscious process of deliberation and then consciously choose to bet or fold by moving my mouth and hands in a certain way and at a certain time rather than earlier or later. Acts that result from such conscious processes are seen as paradigms of acts for which agents are responsible. That seems to be why people are required to pay their poker debts, at least normally.

In contrast, when a person with Tourette's syndrome yells or moves his or her body as a result of brain mechanisms that do not involve such conscious processes, then we do not and should not hold that person responsible for the act. Just imagine a person with Tourette's syndrome playing poker and yelling "all in." Even if the person was thinking about moving all in (that is, betting all of his chips), and even if he had decided to do so and was just waiting for the right moment, if this particular act of saying "all in" was a result of the Tourette's syndrome and not a result of the conscious will to make that bet, then we would and should not hold him responsible for making the bet.

Similarly, people with alien hand syndrome also would and should not be held responsible for what their alien hand does, when that bodily movement was not produced by any conscious choice. If a poker player with alien hand syndrome moves her chips into the pot and then tells us that what pushed the chips was her alien hand and not what she really chose to do, then (if we believe her) we would and should let her take back the chips, even though people are not normally allowed to take back such bets. People with Tourette's or alien hand syndrome might be held responsible for not avoiding situations where their neural maladies would be misinterpreted or cause harm, but they are not and should not usually be held responsible for the acts themselves.

What removes or reduces responsibility in such cases seems to be the fact that the agent's conscious will does not cause these bodily movements. Other interpretations are possible, of course, but cases like these suggest to many people that we cannot be responsible for actions unless those actions are caused by a conscious will.

A problem arises when people deny that conscious will causes action in normal people. If responsibility requires causation by conscious will, but conscious will never causes actions, then even normal agents are never responsible for their actions. The critical question, then, is whether we should deny that conscious will causes action in normal people.

Some philosophers deny that any mental event or state can cause any bodily movement, such as an action. One form of this problem arises from *dualism*, which is the view that mind and body are distinct and separable substances.[4] Most dualists, including Descartes, held that body affects mind and mind affects body. This view was labeled *interactionism*. Critics argued, however, that mind and body differ so much in their natures that we cannot make sense of causal relations between mind and body. How can changes in a substance without any spatial properties, such as mind, cause or be caused by changes in a substance with spatial properties, such as body? These critics were led to strange positions like *parallelism* (the view that neither mind nor body causes changes in the other, although they change in parallel because of a preestablished harmony that God created), *occasionalism* (the view that, on those occasions when humans will physical motions, God detects the will and causes the movement),[5] and *epiphenomenalism* (the view that physical events cause mental events but mental events never cause physical events).[6] These views are general theories that apply as much to pain and perception as to will. Still, the last three views—parallelism, occasionalism, and epiphenomenalism—all imply that conscious wills, which are a kind of mental event, never cause bodily movements, which are a type of physical event.

Although these old positions all assume dualism, some materialists or physicalists in the nineteenth century adopted a variation on epiphenomenalism. Even if a mental event is always also a physical event, it is still a special kind of physical event. Some physical events or states (such as some brain states) are also mental events, whereas other physical events or states (such as rain states) are not mental. Indeed, many brain events, such as blood flow in the brain stem, seem to have no mental properties at all. Thus, even physicalists can hold that changes in physical properties can cause changes in mental properties, but changes in mental properties cannot ever cause changes in physical properties. This position amounts to a physicalist version of epiphenomenalism.

Since epiphenomenalism (whether dualist or physicalist) is about all mental events and states, it does not apply only to will. Other philosophers, in contrast, restrict their claim to the particular mental event of willing. They deny that willing to move ever causes any bodily movement. Nietzsche, for example, says, "The 'inner world' is full of phantoms and will-o'-the-wisps: the will is one of them. The will no longer moves anything, hence does not explain anything either—it merely accompanies events; it can also be absent."[7] This claim applies not only to conscious will but to all will.

This broad claim is hard to evaluate scientifically, because it applies to unconscious wills, and unconscious wills are hard to detect. A person who has an unconscious will cannot detect it, because it is unconscious. Observers (such as scientists) also cannot detect it without reports or some telling effect. Moreover, many theorists hold that wills, choices, intentions, and related mental events or states are necessarily conscious, so the notion of an unconscious will is an oxymoron. For such reasons, most scientists and philosophers have focused on conscious will in this debate.

This new challenge is still not about consciousness in general. Even if consciousness does have some kinds of effects, such as through perception, that does not show that conscious will causes action. The issue is also not about whether conscious will has any effects at all. Consciousness of willing an act might affect how much guilt an agent feels after doing that act, for example. Still, such later effects show only that conscious will can have side-effects, not that it has effects on the act that is willed. The real question, then, is whether conscious will causes that act that is willed.

A negative answer to this question can be reached through a general claim about consciousness, namely, that consciousness and conscious mental states or events never cause physical states or events. Thomas Huxley seems to have held something like this position.[8] It can be called epiphenomenalism about consciousness, and it implies epiphenomenalism about conscious will.

This position needs to be distinguished from the claim that unconscious forces affect our decisions and our lives. Building on predecessors, Sigmund Freud emphasized the role of unconscious mental states, especially unconscious desires. More recently, psychologists[9] have shown how choices that seem to be based on conscious reasons are affected by unconscious factors. A well-known example is that people named Ken are more likely than chance to move to Kentucky, people named Denis or Dennis are more likely than chance to become dentists, and so on. This suggests that unconscious connections influence choices. However, that claim is compatible with conscious reasons also having a lot of influence on choices. After all, choices might be influenced by both conscious and unconscious causes. Moreover, the claim that unconscious forces influence choices is about what causes the will rather than about what the will causes. Hence, this common claim is distinct from epiphenomenalism about consciousness or about conscious will.

Another body of evidence might seem to support the view that conscious wills never cause the willed actions. Some relevant experiments were performed by Benjamin Libet and others who used methods derived from Libet. Additional experiments, using different paradigms, were performed later by Dan Wegner and his followers. Most recently, John-Dylan Haynes has reported striking results that have led some commentators to endorse related views. Of course, more scientists have been involved in this tradition. Many of these experiments are described in various chapters in this volume, so there is no need to summarize them here. The point for now is just that these scientific findings are often seen as suggesting that conscious wills never cause the willed acts.

Although this challenge is usually presented universally about all acts, it could instead be restricted to a subset of actions. This restriction would not rob the thesis of interest if the acts that are not caused by conscious will are ones whose agents seem responsible or where responsibility is controversial. Even if epiphenomenalism about conscious will holds only for some but not for all acts, this new challenge can still undermine common ascriptions of responsibility in special cases and, hence, can challenge common standards of responsibility.

Even if these challenges can be met, their value should be clear. Libet's experiments along with later research in the same tradition have raised new questions about common assumptions regarding action, freedom, and responsibility. Even if we retain those assumptions in the end, rethinking them can increase our confidence in them as well as our understanding of why they are true. Libet's work, thus, contributes a lot even to those who reject his claims. That is why the contributors all pay tribute to him in this collection.

The best tribute to any thinker is careful attention to his ideas, even when this attention leads to rejection. Libet's views include descriptive claims about the role of conscious will in action as well as philosophical and normative conclusions that are supposed to follow from his descriptive premises given additional normative assumptions.[10] Whether those claims, assumptions, and conclusions are defensible—and whether those conclusions follow from his premises or from later work in this tradition—are the issues addressed in the essays in this volume.

This volume opens with a classic essay in which Libet lays out his basic experimental results and draws philosophical lessons regarding free will and responsibility. This chapter raises the issues to be discussed in the rest of the volume.

One crucial issue concerns the interpretation of the readiness potential (RP). In Chapter 2, Roskies questions the relation between the RP and movement initiation as well as the importance of the timing of the initial rise of the RP. In Chapter 3, Mele argues that the RP is better seen as an urge that causes a decision than as a decision itself and also that the RP has not been shown to be sufficient for action. In Chapter 4, Pockett and Purdy then present new experimental evidence that the RP is not sufficient for action and begins significantly later than Libet suggested when subjects make decisions rather than merely act on urges. Pockett and Purdy conclude that movements resulting from conscious decisions are unlikely to be initiated preconsciously. They, along with Roskies, also raise the issue of whether and, if so, how the sorts of phenomena that Libet explores bear upon freedom and responsibility.

Another important problem for Libet's method concerns the meaning and reliability of his subjects' reports of the time when they became conscious of choosing or willing to move (W). In Chapter 5, Banks and Isham describe a new series of experiments suggesting that the moment of decision is not introspected but is, instead, inferred from the action. In line with Libet, Banks and Isham conclude that conscious will is not involved in the cause of the action. In Chapter 6, Mark Hallett describes an experiment designed to time the thought (T) of movement without relying on introspective data or retrospective reconstruction. Hallett's experiment found that T occurred later than observable brain events linked to action. His results also suggest that there is not enough time to veto action after willing becomes conscious, contrary to Libet's way of saving free will.

Some critics have charged that Libet conflates different mental states. In Chapter 7, Pacherie and Haggard distinguish immediate intentions from prospective intentions as well as what-decisions and how-decisions from when-decisions. They use their framework to clarify which mental states Libet's experiments were about. In Chapter 8, Haynes reports experiments using fMRI and pattern classifiers to explore less immediate intentions and choices than Libet studied. Haynes found signals from unconscious brain activity that predict, above chance, decisions 7–10 seconds in advance, and he was also able to separate the "what" from the "when" in a decision.

These results raise important questions about when and why our wills become conscious. The issue of consciousness is addressed in Chapter 9, where Carota, Desmurget, and Sirigu present evidence that the motor system is mainly aware of its intention but not of the details of the ongoing movements, as long as the goal is achieved. In Chapter 10, Graves, Maniscalco, and Lau discuss evidence that complex actions can be performed without consciousness or can be directly influenced by unconscious information. They question whether the function of consciousness is to enable us to deliberate about our actions, and they suggest an experiment to demonstrate the true function of consciousness.

In Chapter 11, Talmi and Frith place these issues of consciousness in a larger context by reinterpreting Libet's results in light of a distinction between Type 1 and Type 2 mental processing. They use this framework to explain why we have a conscious experience of our own free will, and they discuss potential moral consequences of seeing apparent free will as an illusion. The sense of freedom is closely allied with a sense of agency, which is the topic of the next two chapters. In Chapter 12, Ebert and Wegner argue that we determine whether we are authors of actions through a variety of clues, including temporal proximity between thoughts, actions, and events. When authorship is inferred, we then bind the action and subsequent events together by perceiving the action and events as closer than they otherwise would seem to be. In Chapter 13, Wheatley and Looser cite cases where the feeling of will is imputed, manipulated, and taken away inappropriately and independent of action. These cases are supposed to show that our sense of will, intentionality, and agency is inferred retrospectively and might well be illusory.

In Chapter 14, Horgan argues that the work of Libet and others is fully compatible with the phenomenal character and content of the experience of initiating an act. In his view, conscious agentive experience is not illusory. In contrast, Nadelhoffer argues in Chapter 15 that recent advances in psychology and neuroscience have the potential to radically transform traditional views of human agency and free will.

The ultimate issue in these debates concerns moral and legal responsibility. In Chapter 16, Yaffe explains the meaning and explores the historical sources of the voluntary act requirement in law, and then he argues that Libet probably has not shown that our acts are not voluntary in the sense that is relevant to law. In Chapter 17, Alexander suggests that the gatekeeper role for conscious will, which Libet allows, does not require any revision of traditional notions of moral and criminal responsibility. In Chapter 18, Moore then distinguishes three challenges to responsibility and proposes a novel model of how conscious will causes bodily movement and, hence, of how we can be morally responsible for our voluntary actions. Finally, in Chapter 19, Sinnott-Armstrong argues that the empirical findings of Libet and his followers do not undermine moral or legal responsibility in general but do raise profound issues for some kinds of minimal action.

These all-too brief descriptions of the chapters do not do justice to their complexity, subtlety, and richness. To appreciate those qualities, the essays simply have to be read. Taken together, these essays show how fruitful and important Libet's research has been. Whether or not we agree with Libet's claims, he clearly sets the stage for a great deal of fascinating research and discussion.

## NOTES

1. See http://plato.stanford.edu/entries/compatibilism/
2. See Stephen Morse, "The Non-problem of Free Will in Forensic Psychiatry and Psychology," *Behavioral Sciences and the Law* 25 (2007): 203–220.
3. See the chapters by van Inwagen, O'Connor, Clarke, Ginet, Kane, Strawson, and Pereboom in Kane, *Oxford Handbook of Free Will* (New York: Oxford University Press, 2001).
4. See http://plato.stanford.edu/entries/dualism/
5. See http://plato.stanford.edu/entries/occasionalism/
6. See http://plato.stanford.edu/entries/epiphenomenalism/
7. Friedrich Nietzsche, *Twilight of the Idols* in *The Portable Nietzsche*, translated and edited by Walter Kaufmann (New York: Viking, 1954), pp. 494–495.
8. T. H Huxley, "On the Hypothesis That Animals Are Automata, and Its History," *The Fortnightly Review*, n.s. 16 (1874): 555–580. Reprinted in *Method and Results: Essays by Thomas H. Huxley* (New York: D. Appleton & Company, 1898). Huxley reported the case of Sergeant F., who was hit by a bullet around his parietal lobe and later sometimes exhibited complex behavior

(e.g., singing, writing a letter, "reloading," "aiming," and "firing" his cane with motions appropriate to a rifle) while he seemed unconscious (because he was not sensitive to pins and shocks, as well as sounds, smells, tastes, and much vision). This case is supposed to suggest the possibility that consciousness is not necessary for complex and purposeful movements, but it cannot show that conscious will is never necessary for any bodily movement in normal humans.

9. Such as those collected in R. R. Hassin, J. S. Uleman, and J. Bargh, *The New Unconscious* (New York; Oxford University Press, 2005).
10. This argument need not derive "ought" from "is" or commit any "naturalistic fallacy," because the science need not settle any normative issue without additional normative premises that also need to be defended.

# CHAPTER 1

## Do We Have Free Will?

*Benjamin Libet*

### ABSTRACT

*I have taken an experimental approach to this question. Freely voluntary acts are preceded by a specific electrical change in the brain (the "readiness potential," RP) that begins 550 ms before the act. Human subjects became aware of intention to act 350–400 ms* ***after*** *RP starts, but 200 ms before the motor act. The volitional process is therefore* ***initiated*** *unconsciously. But the conscious function could still control the outcome; it can veto the act. Free will is therefore not excluded. These findings put constraints on views of how free will may operate; it would not initiate a voluntary act but it could* ***control*** *performance of the act. The findings also affect views of guilt and responsibility.*

*But the deeper question still remains: Are freely voluntary acts subject to macrodeterministic laws or can they appear without such constraints, non-determined by natural laws and "truly free?" I shall present an experimentalist view about these fundamental philosophical opposites.*

The question of free will goes to the root of our views about human nature and how we relate to the universe and to natural laws. Are we completely defined by the deterministic nature of physical laws? Theologically imposed fateful destiny ironically produces a similar end-effect. In either case, we would be essentially sophisticated automatons, with our conscious feelings and intentions tacked on as epiphenomena with no causal power. Or, do we have some independence in making choices and actions, not completely determined by the known physical laws?

I have taken an experimental approach to at least some aspects of the question. The operational definition of free will in these experiments was in accord with common views. First, there should be no external control or cues to affect the occurrence or emergence of the voluntary act under study; i.e., it should be endogenous. Second, the subject should feel that he/she wanted to do it, on her/his own initiative, and feel he could control what is being done, when to do it or not to do it. Many actions lack this second attribute. For example, when the primary motor area of the cerebral cortex is stimulated, muscle contractions can be produced in certain sites in the body. However, the subject (a neurosurgical patient) reports that these actions were imposed by the stimulator, i.e., that he did not will these acts. And there are numerous clinical disorders in which a similar discrepancy between actions and will occurs.

These include the involuntary actions in cerebral palsy, Parkinsonism, Huntington's chorea, Tourette's syndrome, and even obsessive compulsions to act. A striking example is the "alien hand syndrome." Patients with a lesion in a fronto-medial portion of premotor area may find that the hand and arm on the affected side performs curious purposeful actions, such as undoing a buttoned shirt when the subject is trying to button it up; all this occurs without or even against the subject's intention and will (cf. Spence & Frith, 1999, p. 23).

### TIMING OF BRAIN PROCESSES AND CONSCIOUS WILL

Performance of "self-paced" voluntary acts had, surprisingly, been found to be preceded by a slow electrical change recordable on the scalp at the vertex (Kornhuber & Deecke, 1965). The onset of this electrical indication of certain brain activities preceded the actual movement by up to 1 s or more. It was termed the "Bereitschaftpotential" or "readiness potential" (RP). To obtain the RP required averaging the recordings in many self-paced acts. Subjects were therefore asked to perform their acts within time intervals of 30 s to make the total study manageable. In our experiments, however, we removed this constraint on freedom of action; subjects performed a simple flick or flexion of the wrist at any time they felt the urge or wish to do so. These voluntary acts were to be performed capriciously, free of any external limitations or restrictions (Libet, Wright, & Gleason, 1982). RPs in these acts began with onsets averaging 550 ms before activation of the involved muscle (Fig. 1.1).

The brain was evidently beginning the volitional process in this voluntary act well before the activation of the muscle that produced the movement. My question then became: *when* does the *conscious* wish or intention (to perform the act) appear? In the traditional view of conscious will and free will, one would expect conscious will to appear before, or at the onset of, the RP, and thus command the brain to perform the intended act. But an appearance of conscious will 550 ms or more before the act seemed intuitively unlikely. It was clearly important to establish the time of the conscious will relative to the onset of the brain process (RP); if conscious will were to *follow* the onset of RP, that would have a fundamental impact on how we could view free will.

To establish this temporal relation required a method for measuring the time of appearance of the conscious will in each such act. Initially, that seemed to me an impossible goal. But after some time it occurred to me to try having the subject report a "clock-time" at which he/she was *first aware* of the wish or urge to act (Fig. 1.2) (Libet, Gleason, Wright, & Pearl, 1983). The clock had to be much faster than the usual clock, in order to accommodate time differences in the hundreds of ms. For our clock, the spot of light of a cathode ray oscilloscope was made to revolve around the face of the scope like the sweep-second hand of an ordinary clock, but at a speed approximately 25 times as fast. Each of the marked off "seconds" around the periphery was thus equivalent to about 40 ms. When we tried out this method we were actually surprised to find that each subject reported times for *first awareness of wish to act* (W) with a reliability of 20 ms, for each group of 40 such trials. A test for the accuracy of such reports was also encouraging. In this, the subject remained relaxed and did *not* perform any voluntary act. Instead, a weak electrical stimulus was delivered to the skin of the same hand. The stimulus was applied at random times in the different trials.

The experimental observers knew the actual time for each stimulus. The subject did not know this actual time but was asked to report the clock-time at which he felt each such stimulus. Subjects accomplished this with an error of only −50 ms.

### The Experiment

In the actual experiment, then, each RP was obtained from an averaged electrical recording in 40 trials. In each of these trials the subject performed the sudden flick of the wrist whenever he/she freely wanted to do so. After each of these trials, the subject reported W, the clock-time associated with the first awareness of the wish to move (Libet, Gleason, et al., 1983).

### Brain Initiates Voluntary Act Unconsciously

The results of many such groups of trials are diagrammed in Figure 1.3. For groups in which all the voluntary acts were freely spontaneous, with no reports of rough preplanning of when to act, the onset of RP averaged −550 ms (before the muscle was activated). The W times for first awareness of wish to act averaged about −200 ms., for all groups.

This value was the same even when subjects reported having preplanned roughly when to act! If we correct W for the −50 ms error in the subjects' reports of timings of the skin stimuli, we have an average corrected W of about −150 ms. Clearly, the brain process (RP) to prepare for this voluntary act began about 400 ms. before the appearance of the conscious will to act (W). This relationship was true for every group of 40 trials and in every one of the nine subjects studied.

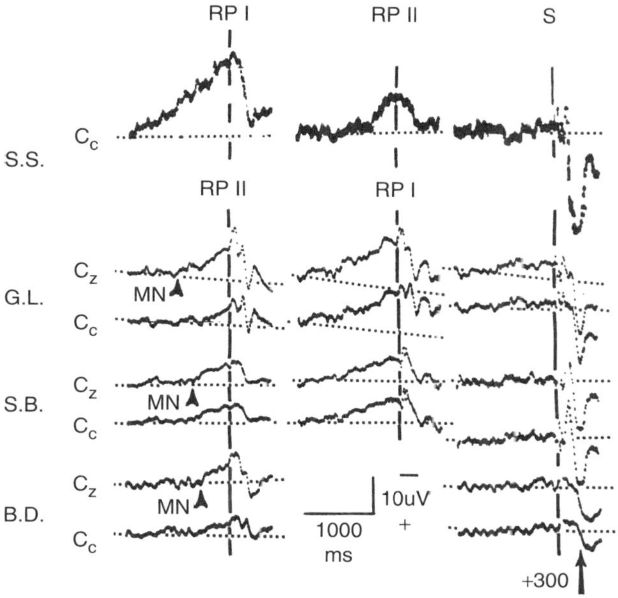


**Figure 1.1 Readiness Potentials (RP) Preceding Self-Initiated Voluntary Acts.** Each horizontal row is the computer-averaged potential for 40 trials, recorded by a DC system with an active electrode on the scalp, either at the midline-vertex (Cz) or on the left side (contralateral to the performing right hand) approximately over the motor/premotor cortical area that controls the hand (Cc). When every self-initiated quick flexion of the right hand (fingers or wrist) in the series of 40 trials was (reported as having been) subjectively experienced to originate spontaneously and with no preplanning by the subject, RPs labeled type II were found in association. (Arrowheads labeled MN indicate onset of the "main negative" phase of the vertex recorded type II RPs in this figure; see Libet et al., 1982.) Onsets were also measured for 90% of the total area of RP). When an awareness of a general intention or preplanning to act some time within the next second or so was reported to have occurred before some of the 40 acts in the series, type I RPs were recorded (Libet et al., 1982). In the last column, labeled S, a near-threshold skin stimulus was applied in each of the 40 trials at a randomized time unknown to the subject, with no motor act performed; the subject was asked to recall and report the time when he became aware of each stimulus in the same way he reported the time of awareness of wanting to move in the case of self-initiated motor acts. The solid vertical line through each column represents 0 time, at which the electromyogram (EMG) of the activated muscle begins in the case of RP series, or at which the stimulus was actually delivered in the case of S series. The dashed horizontal line represents the DC baseline drift. For subject S.S., the first RP (type I) was recorded before the instruction "to let the urge come on its own, spontaneously" was introduced; the second RP (type II) was obtained after giving this instruction in the same session as the first. For subjects G.L., S.B., and B.D., this instruction was given at the start of all sessions. Nevertheless, each of these subjects reported some experiences of loose preplanning in some of the 40-trial series; those series exhibited type I RPs rather than type II. Note that the slow negative shift in scalp potential that precedes EMGs of self-initiated acts (RP) does not precede the skin stimulus in S series. However, evoked potentials following the stimulus are seen regularly to exhibit a large positive component with a peak close to +300 ms (arrow indicates this time); this P300 event-related potential had been shown by others to be associated with decisions about uncertain events (in this case, the time of the randomly delivered stimulus), and it also indicates that the subject is attending well to the experimental conditions.

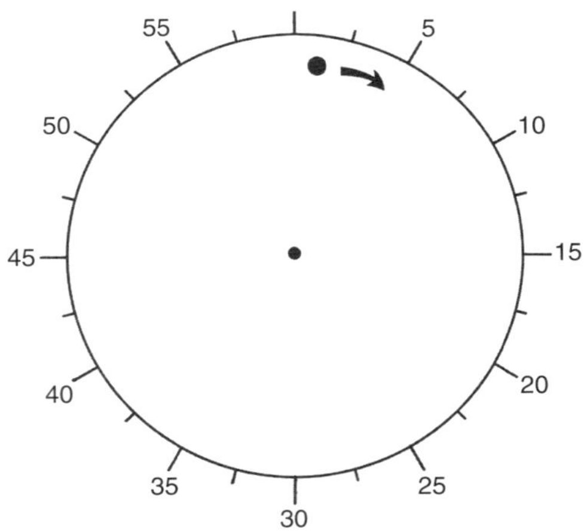


**Figure 1.2 Oscilloscope "Clock."** Spot of light revolves around periphery of screen, once in 2.56 s (instead of 60 s for a sweep-second hand of a regular clock). Each marked-off "second" (in the total of 60 markings) represents 43 ms of actual time here. The subject holds his gaze to the center of the screen. For each performed quick flexion of the wrist, at any freely chosen time, the subject was asked to note the position of the clock spot when he/she first became aware of the wish or intention to act. This associated clock time is reported by the subject later, after the trial is completed.

It should also be noted that the actual difference in times is probably greater than the 400 ms; the actual initiating process in the brain probably starts before our recorded RP, in an unknown area that then activates the supplementary motor area in the cerebral cortex. The supplementary motor area is located in the midline near the vertex and is thought to be the source of our recorded RP.

## ANY ROLE FOR CONSCIOUS WILL?

The initiation of the freely voluntary act appears to begin in the brain unconsciously, well before the person consciously knows he wants to act! Is there, then, any role for conscious will in the performance of a voluntary act? (see Libet, 1985) To answer this it must be recognized that conscious will (W) does appear about 150 ms before the muscle is activated, even though it follows onset of the RP. An interval of 150 ms would allow enough time in which the conscious function might affect the final outcome of the volitional process. (Actually, only 100 ms is available for any such effect. The final 50 ms before the muscle is activated is the time for the primary motor cortex to

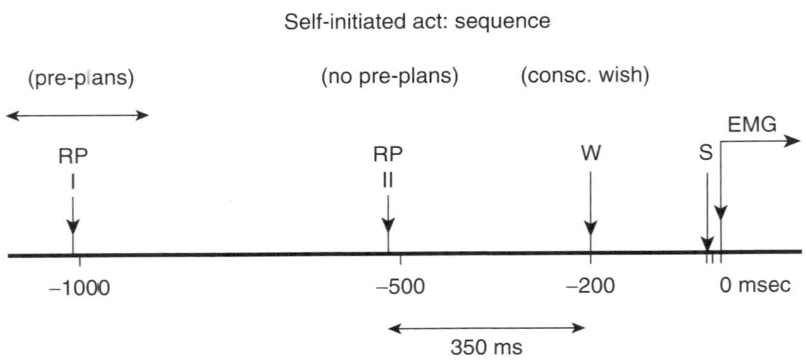


**Figure 1.3 Diagram of Sequence of Events, Cerebral and Subjective, That Precede a Fully Self-Initiated Voluntary Act.** Relative to 0 time, detected in the electromyogram (EMG) of the suddenly activated muscle, the readiness potential (RP, an indicator of related cerebral neuronal activities) begins first, at about −1050 ms when some preplanning is reported (type I RP) or about −550 ms with spontaneous acts lacking immediate preplanning (type II RP). Subjective awareness of the wish to move (W) appears at about −200 ms, some 350 ms after onset even of type II RP; however, W does appear well before the act (EMG). Subjective timings reported for awareness of the randomly delivered S (skin) stimulus average about −50 ms relative to actual delivery time. (From Libet, 1989.)

activate the spinal motor nerve cells. During this time the act goes to completion with no possibility of stopping it by the rest of the cerebral cortex.)

Potentially available to the conscious function is the possibility of stopping or vetoing the final progress of the volitional process, so that no actual muscle action ensues. *Conscious-will could thus affect the outcome* of the volitional process even though the latter was initiated by unconscious cerebral processes. Conscious-will might block or veto the process, so that no act occurs.

The existence of a veto possibility is not in doubt. The subjects in our experiments at times reported that a conscious wish or urge to act appeared but that they suppressed or vetoed that. In the absence of the muscle's electrical signal when being activated, there was no trigger to initiate the computer's recording of any RP that may have preceded the veto; thus, there were no *recorded* RPs with a vetoed intention to act. We were, however, able to show that subjects could veto an act planned for performance at a prearranged time. They were able to exert the veto within the interval of 100 to 200 ms before the preset time to act (Libet, Wright, & Gleason, 1983). A large RP preceded the veto, signifying that the subject was indeed *preparing* to act, even though the action was aborted by the subject. All of us, not just experimental subjects, have experienced our vetoing a spontaneous urge to perform some act. This often occurs when the urge to act involves some socially unacceptable consequence, like an urge to shout some obscenity at the professor. (Incidentally, in the disorder called Tourette's syndrome, subjects do spontaneously shout obscenities. These acts should not be regarded as freely voluntary. No RP appears before such an act. A quick reaction to an unwarned stimulus also lacks a preceding RP, and it is not a freely voluntary act.)

Another hypothetical function for conscious will could be to serve as a "trigger" that is required to enable the volitional process to proceed to final action. However, there is no evidence for this, such as there is for a veto function, and the "trigger" possibility also seems unlikely on other grounds. For example, voluntary acts that become somewhat "automatic" can be performed with no reportable conscious wish to do so; the RP is rather minimal in amplitude and duration before such automatic acts. Automatic acts clearly go to completion without any conscious trigger available.

### Does the Conscious Veto Have a Preceding Unconscious Origin?

One should, at this point, consider the possibility that the conscious veto itself may have its origin in preceding unconscious processes, just as is the case for the development and appearance of the conscious will. If the veto itself were to be initiated and developed unconsciously, the choice to veto would then become an unconscious choice of which we *become* conscious, rather than a consciously causal event. Our own previous evidence had shown that the brain "produces" an awareness of something only after about a 0.5 s period of appropriate neuronal activations (see reviews by Libet, 1993, 1996).

Some have proposed that even an unconscious initiation of a veto choice would nevertheless be a genuine choice made by the individual and could still be viewed as a free will process (e.g., Velmans, 1991). I find such a proposed view of free will to be unacceptable. In such a view, the individual would not consciously control his actions; he would only become aware of an unconsciously initiated choice. He would have no direct conscious control over the nature of any preceding unconscious processes. But, a free will process implies one could be held consciously responsible for one's choice to act or not to act. We do not hold people responsible for actions performed unconsciously, without the possibility of conscious control. For example, actions by a person during a psychomotor epileptic seizure, or by one with Tourette's syndrome, etc., are not regarded as actions of free will. Why then should an act unconsciously developed by a normal individual, a process over which he also has no conscious control, be regarded as an act of free will?

I propose, instead, that the conscious veto may *not* require or be the direct result of preceding unconscious processes. The conscious veto is a *control* function, different from simply becoming aware of the wish to act. There is no logical imperative in any mind-brain theory, even identity theory, that requires specific neural activity to precede and determine the nature of a conscious control function. And, there is no experimental evidence against the possibility that the control process may appear without development by prior unconscious processes.

Admittedly, to be conscious of the decision to veto does mean one is aware of the event. How may one reconcile this with my proposal? Perhaps we should revisit the concept of awareness, its relation to the content of awareness, and the cerebral processes that develop both awareness and its contents. Our own previous studies have indicated that *awareness* is a unique phenomenon in itself, distinguished from the contents of which one may become aware. For example, awareness of a sensory stimulus can require similar durations of stimulus trains for somatosensory cortex and for medial lemniscus. But the *content* of those awarenesses in these two cases is different, in the subjective timings of sensations (Libet, Wright, Feinstein, & Pearl, 1979). The content of an unconscious mental process (e.g., correct detection of a signal in the brain *without any awareness* of the signal) may be the same as the content *with awareness* of the signal. But to become aware of that same content required that stimulus duration be increased by about 400 ms (see Libet et al., 1991).

In an endogenous, freely voluntary act, awareness of the intention to act is delayed for about 400 ms after brain processes initiate the process unconsciously (Libet, Gleason, et al., 1983; Libet, 1985). Awareness developed here may be thought of as applying to the whole volitional process; that would include the content of the conscious urge to act and the content of factors that may affect a conscious veto. One need not think of awareness of an event as restricted to one detailed item of content in the whole event.

The possibility is not excluded that factors, on which the decision to veto (control) is *based*, do develop by unconscious processes that precede the veto. However, the *conscious decision to veto* could still be made without direct specification for that decision by the preceding unconscious processes. That is, one could consciously accept or reject the program offered up by the whole array of preceding brain processes. The *awareness* of the decision to veto could be thought to require preceding unconscious processes, but the *content* of that awareness (the actual decision to veto) is a separate feature that need not have the same requirement.

## WHAT SIGNIFICANCE DO OUR FINDINGS HAVE FOR VOLUNTARY ACTS IN GENERAL?

Can we assume that voluntary acts other than the simple one studied by us also have the same temporal relations between unconscious brain processes and the appearance of the conscious wish/will to act? It is common in scientific researches to be limited technically to studying a process in a simple system; and then to find that the fundamental behavior discovered with the simple system does indeed represent a phenomenon that appears or governs in other related and more complicated systems. For example, the charge on a single electron was measured by Milliken in one isolated system, but it is valid for electrons in all systems. It should also be noted that RPs have been found by other investigators to precede other more complex volitional acts, such as beginning to speak or to write; they did not, however, study the time of appearance of the conscious wish to begin such acts. We may, therefore, allow ourselves to consider what general implications may follow from our experimental findings, while recognizing that an extrapolation to encompass voluntary acts in general has been adopted.

We should also distinguish between *deliberations* about what choice of action to adopt (including preplanning of when to act on such a choice) and the final intention actually "to act now." One may, after all, deliberate all day about a choice but never act; there is *no voluntary act* in that case. In our experimental studies we found that in some trials subjects engaged in some conscious preplanning of roughly when to act (in the next second or so). But even in those cases, the subjects reported times of the conscious wish to actually act to be about −200 ms; this value was very close to the values reported for fully spontaneous voluntary acts with no preplanning.

The onset of the unconscious brain process (RP) for preparing to act was well before the final conscious intention "to act now" in all cases. These findings indicated that the sequence of the volitional processes "to act now" may apply to all volitional acts, regardless of their spontaneity or prior history of conscious deliberations.

## ETHICAL IMPLICATIONS OF HOW FREE WILL OPERATES

The role of conscious free will would be, then, not to initiate a voluntary act, but rather to *control* whether the act takes place. We may view the unconscious initiatives for voluntary actions as "bubbling up" in the brain. The conscious-will then selects which of these initiatives may go forward to an action or which ones to veto and abort, with no act appearing.

This kind of role for free will is actually in accord with religious and ethical strictures. These commonly advocate that you "control yourself." Most of the Ten Commandments are "do not" orders.

How do our findings relate to the questions of when one may be regarded as guilty or sinful, in various religious and philosophical systems? If one experiences a conscious wish or urge to perform a socially unacceptable act, should that be regarded as a sinful event even if the urge has been vetoed and no act has occurred? Some religious systems answer "yes." President Jimmy Carter admitted to having had urges to perform a lustful act. Although he did not act, he apparently still felt sinful for having experienced a lustful urge.[1] But any such urges would be initiated and developed in the brain unconsciously, according to our findings. The mere appearance of an intention to act could not be controlled consciously; only its final consummation in a motor act could be consciously controlled. Therefore, a religious system that castigates an individual for simply having a mental intention or impulse to do something unacceptable, even when this is not acted out, would create a physiologically insurmountable moral and psychological difficulty.

Indeed, insistence on regarding an unacceptable urge to act as sinful, even when no act ensues, would make virtually all individuals sinners. In that sense such a view could provide a physiological basis for "original sin"! Of course, the concept of "original sin" can be based on other views of what is regarded as sinful.

Ethical systems deal with moral codes or conventions that govern how one behaves toward or interacts with other individuals; they are presumably dealing with actions, not simply with urges or intentions. Only a motor act by one person can directly impinge on the welfare of another. Since it is the performance of an act that can be consciously controlled, it should be legitimate to hold individuals guilty of and responsible for their acts.

## DETERMINISM AND FREE WILL

There remains a deeper question about free will that the foregoing considerations have not addressed. What we have achieved experimentally is some knowledge of how free will may operate. But we have not answered the question of whether our consciously willed acts are fully determined by natural laws that govern the activities of nerve cells in the brain, or whether acts and the conscious decisions to perform them can proceed to some degree independently of natural determinism. The first of these options would make free will illusory. The conscious feeling of exerting one's will would then be regarded as an epiphenomenon, simply a by-product of the brain's activities but with no causal powers of its own.

First, it may be pointed out that free choices or acts are *not predictable*, even if they should be completely determined. The "uncertainty principle" of Heisenberg precludes our having a complete knowledge of the underlying molecular activities. Quantum mechanics forces us to deal with probabilities rather than with certainties of events. And, in chaos theory, a random event may shift the behavior of a whole system, in a way that was not predictable. However, even if events are not predictable in practice, they might nevertheless be in accord with natural laws and therefore determined.

Let us rephrase our basic question as follows: *Must* we accept determinism? Is nondeterminism a viable option? We should recognize that both of these alternative views (natural law determinism vs. nondeterminism) are unproven theories, i.e., unproven in relation to the existence of free will. Determinism has on the whole, worked well for the physical observable world. That has led many scientists and philosophers to regard any deviation from determinism as absurd and witless, and unworthy of consideration. But there has been no evidence, or even a proposed experimental test design, that definitively or convincingly demonstrates the validity of natural law determinism as the mediator or instrument of free will.

There is an unexplained gap between the category of physical phenomena and the category of subjective phenomena. As far back as Leibniz it was pointed out that if one looked into the brain with a full knowledge of its physical makeup and nerve cell activities, one would see nothing that describes subjective experience. The whole foundation of our own experimental studies of the physiology of conscious experience (beginning in the late 1950s) was that externally observable and manipulable brain processes and the related reportable subjective introspective experiences must be studied simultaneously, as independent categories, to understand their relationship. The assumption that a deterministic nature of the physically observable world (to the extent that may be true) can account for subjective conscious functions and events is a speculative *belief*, not a scientifically proven proposition.

Nondeterminism, the view that conscious-will may, at times, exert effects not in accord with known physical laws, is of course also a non-proven speculative belief. The view that conscious will can affect brain function in violation of known physical laws, takes two forms. In one it is held that the violations are not detectable, because the actions of the mind may be at a level below that of the uncertainty allowed by quantum mechanics. (Whether this last proviso can in fact be tenable is a matter yet to be resolved). This view would thus allow for a nondeterministic free will without a perceptible violation of physical laws. In a second view it may be held that violations of known physical laws are large enough to be detectable, at least in principle. But, it can be argued, detectability in actual practice may be impossible. That difficulty for detection would be especially true if the conscious will is able to exert its influence by minimal actions at relatively few nerve elements; these actions could serve as triggers for amplified nerve cell patterns of activity in the brain. In any case, we do not have a scientific answer to the question of which theory (determinism or nondeterminism) may describe the nature of free will.

However, we must recognize that the almost universal experience that we can act with a free, independent choice provides a kind of prima facie evidence that conscious mental processes can causatively control some brain processes (Libet, 1994). As an experimental scientist, this creates more difficulty for a determinist than for a nondeterminist option. The phenomenal fact is that most of us feel that we do have free will, at least for some of our actions and within certain limits that may be imposed by our brain's status and by our environment. The intuitive feelings about the phenomenon of free will form a fundamental basis for views of our human nature, and great care should be taken not to believe allegedly scientific conclusions about them which actually depend upon hidden ad hoc assumptions. A theory that simply interprets the phenomenon of free will as illusory and denies the validity of this phenomenal fact is less attractive than a theory that accepts or accommodates the phenomenal fact.

In an issue so fundamentally important to our view of who we are, a claim for illusory nature should be based on fairly direct evidence. Such evidence is not available; nor do determinists propose even a potential experimental design to test the theory. Actually, I myself proposed an experimental design that could test whether conscious will could influence nerve cell activities in the brain, doing so via a putative "conscious mental field" that could act without any neuronal connections as the mediators (Libet, 1994). This difficult though feasible experiment has, unfortunately, still to be carried out. If it should turn out to confirm the prediction of that field theory, there would be a radical transformation in our views of mind-brain interaction.

My conclusion about free will, one genuinely free in the nondetermined sense, is then that its existence is at least as good, if not a better, scientific option than is its denial by determinist theory. Given the speculative nature of both determinist and nondeterminist theories, why not adopt the view that we do have free will (until some real contradictory evidence may appear, if it ever does). Such a view would at least allow us to proceed in a way that accepts and accommodates our own deep feeling that we do have free will. We would not need to view ourselves as machines that act in a manner completely controlled by the known physical laws. Such a permissive option has also been advocated by the neurobiologist Roger Sperry (see Doty, 1998).[2]

I close, then, with a quotation from the great novelist Isaac Bashevis Singer that relates to the foregoing views. Singer stated his strong belief in our having free will. In an interview (Singer, 1981/1968) he volunteered that "The greatest gift which humanity has received is free choice. It is true that we are limited in our use of free choice. But the little free choice we have is such a great gift and is potentially worth so much that for this itself life is worthwhile living."

## NOTES

1. President Carter was drawing on a Christian tradition deriving from the following two verses in the Sermon on the Mount: "[Jesus said], "Ye have heard that it was said by them of old time, Thou shalt not commit adultery: But I say unto you, That whosoever looketh on a woman to lust after her hath committed adultery with her already in his heart"' (Matthew 5.27–28).
2. The belief by many people that one's fate is determined by some mystical reality or by divine intervention produces a difficult paradox for those who also believe we have free will and are to be held responsible for our actions. Such a paradox can arise in the Judeo-Christian view that (a) God is omnipotent, knows in advance what you are going to do, and controls your fate, while (b) also strongly advocating that we can freely determine our actions and are accountable and responsible for our behavior. This difficulty has led to some theological attempts to resolve the paradox. For example, the Kabbalists proposed that God voluntarily gave up his power to know what man was going to do, in order to allow man to choose freely and responsibly, and to possess free will.

## REFERENCES

Doty, R. W. (1998) Five mysteries of the mind, and their consequences. In A. Puente (Ed.), *Views of the brain: A tribute to Roger W. Sperry.* Washington, DC: American Psychological Association.

Kornhuber, H., & Deecke, L. (1965). Hirnpotentialanderungen bei Willkurbewegungen und passiven Bewegungen des Menschen: Bereitschaftspotential und reafferente Potentiale. *Pfluegers Arch Gesamte Physiol Menschen Tiere, 284,* 1–17.

Libet, B. (1985). Unconscious cerebral initiative and the role of conscious will in voluntary action. *Behavioral and Brain Sciences, 8,* 529–566.

Libet, B (1989). Conscious subjective experience vs. unconscious mental functions: A theory of the cerebral processes involved. In R. M. J. Cotterill (Ed.), *Models of Brain Function.* New York: Cambridge University Press.

Libet, B. (1993). The neural time factor in conscious and unconscious mental events. In Ciba Foundation, *Experimental and Theoretical Studies of Consciousness.* Ciba Foundation Symposium 174. Chichester: Wiley.

Libet, B. (1994) A testable field theory of mind-brain interaction. *Journal of Consciousness Studies, 1*(1), 119–126.

Libet, B. (1996). Neural time factors in conscious and unconscious mental function. In S. R. Hameroff, A. Kaszniak, & A. Scott (Eds.), *Toward a Science of Consciousness.* Cambridge, MA: MIT Press.

Libet, B., Gleason, C. A., Wright, E. W., & Pearl, D. K. (1983). Time of conscious intention to act in relation to onset of cerebral activity (readiness potential): The unconscious initiation of a freely voluntary act. *Brain, 106,* 623–642.

Libet, B., Pearl, D. K., Morledge, D. E., Gleason, C. A., Hosobuchi, Y., & Barbaro, N. M. (1991). Control of the transition from sensory detection to sensory awareness in man by the duration of a thalamic stimulus: The cerebral time-on factor. *Brain, 114,* 1731–1757.

Libet, B., Wright, E. W., & Gleason, C. A. (1982). Readiness potentials preceding unrestricted spontaneous pre-planned voluntary acts. *Electroencephalography and Clinical Neurophysiology, 54,* 322–325.

Libet, B.,Wright, E. W., & Gleason, C. A. (1983). Preparation—or intention-to-act, in relation to pre-event potentials recorded at the vertex. *Electroencephalography and Clinical Neurophysiology, 56,* 367–372.

Libet, B., Wright, E. W., Jr., Feinstein, B., & Pearl, D. K. (1979). Subjective referral of the timing for a conscious sensory experience: A functional role for the somatosensory specific projection system in man. *Brain, 102,* 191–222.

Singer, I. B. (1981/1968). Interview by H. Flender. In G. Plimpton (Ed.), *Writers at Work.* New York: Penguin Books.

Spence, S. A., & Frith, C. D. (1999). Towards a functional anatomy of volition. *Journal of Consciousness Studies, 6*(8–9), 11–29.

Velmans, M. (1991). Is human information processing conscious? *Behavioral and Brain Sciences, 3,* 651–669.

# CHAPTER 2

## Why Libet's Studies Don't Pose a Threat to Free Will

*Adina L. Roskies*

Benjamin Libet's controversial papers on the neural basis of action and the relation between action and conscious intention have dominated discussions of the effects that neuroscientific understanding can have on our conception of ourselves as free and responsible agents. In a collection of studies spanning almost 40 years, Libet developed a series of claims that purport to undermine our common conceptions of ourselves as agents who act because of conscious volition. Instead, Libet paints a picture of ourselves as beings hijacked by automatic, non-conscious brain processes that initiate actions prior to our awareness of our own intentions to act. Consciousness of intention follows, rather than precedes, the initiation of action, and our perception that we consciously initiate our actions is merely illusion. Although Libet attempted to "save the phenomenon" of freedom by postulating that we nonetheless have veto power over our automatically generated actions (i.e., that we have "free won't"), if his primary claims stand they pose a real challenge to our commonsense intuitions about our own autonomy.

In this paper, I will review Libet's main claims, and the implications he drew from them about free will and responsibility. Then I'll consider first whether, on the supposition that the claims are correct, the empirical interpretations that Libet and many since have gleaned from his data really are warranted (hint: the answer is probably not). In the second part of the discussion I address whether his empirical claims really have the implications he thinks they have for free will. In sum, I argue that neither Libet's data nor the reasoning that follows strongly support the fairly radical claims about free will that many have supposed.

### I. LIBET'S RESULTS AND TECHNICAL COMMENTARY

#### 1. Summary of Libet's Empirical Results

Libet's main empirical findings are the following:

E1) Direct stimulation of somatosensory cortex (central stimulus presentation) with trains of electrical pulses at liminal levels of intensity leads to a conscious perception of sensation only after a significant period of time, usually 500 ms or more (Libet et al., 1964). Stimulation at liminal levels for less than that duration produced no conscious experience (Libet et al., 1964). Direct stimulation at supraliminal levels shortened the time required for a conscious perception (Libet et al., 1964).

E2) Subjects report consciousness of somatosensory stimuli delivered to the peripheral nervous system with a much shorter latency than the direct cortical stimuli reported in (E1). In fact, subjects can accurately report the time at which they become conscious of a peripheral stimulus to within approximately 50–100 ms of when the stimulus actually occurred (Libet, Wright,

Feinstein, & Pearl, 1979; Libet, Wright Jr., & Gleason, 1982).

E3) In cases in which subjects are asked to judge which of two paired stimuli is experienced first, the peripheral or the central, subject's judgments are consistent with a long time lag for central stimuli (as in E1) and a perceived shorter lag for peripheral stimuli (E2) (Libet et al., 1979).

E4) In cases in which subjects are asked to spontaneously will a basic action (movement of the wrist or finger), an evoked potential measured at the scalp surface (the readiness potential, or RP) precedes the movement by approximately 500–600 ms (Libet et al., 1982). This is what Libet calls the type II RP. In cases in which such action is preplanned, the RP (a type I RP) is seen even earlier, about 1000 ms before the motor activity (Libet et al., 1982).

E5) When subjects are asked to report the time of their conscious intention to act (W) by indexing it to a moving spot on a clock face, the time of intention (W) typically precedes the movement by approximately 200 ms (Libet, Gleason, Wright, & Pearl, 1983; Libet, 1985).

## 2. Libet's Interpretation of the Empirical Results

### C1) Neuronal Adequacy

*For a neural signal to reach consciousness, approximately 500 ms of central activity is necessary. For example, neurons in the somatosensory cortex representing the hand must be active for approximately 500 ms before one can report awareness of a tactile sensation in the hand.*

Libet derives C1 from E1, the fact that shorter periods of direct liminal stimulation of somatosensory cortex do not result in any conscious awareness of sensation (Libet et al., 1964), and from experiments that show that the experience of peripheral stimulation can be affected (suppressed or enhanced) by cortical stimulation occurring up to several hundred milliseconds after the peripheral stimulus (Libet, 1992; Libet, Alberts, Wright Jr., & Feinstein, 1972). Libet hypothesizes that late components of cortical processing are present whenever stimuli elicit conscious awareness, and absent in cases in which awareness is lacking (Libet, Alberts, Wright Jr., & Feinstein, 1967). The implication is that these late components are related to awareness.

*Critique of C1* C1 seems to rest on rather shaky footing. Stimulating cortex with a surface electrode is a highly biologically unrealistic stimulus, and it is not clear what can be concluded about normal sensory innervation and consciousness from such data. Normal activation of cortex from peripheral stimulation first innervates cortical cells by synapses of sensory afferents from the dorsal horn on cells of layer IV of somatosensory cortex. Somatosensory cortex is highly structured, and although the local circuits in cortex are not extremely well understood, it is clear that information is processed in a highly organized fashion, from inputs in layer IV to other cells in both deep and superficial layers of the same cortical column, as well as via lateral connections, before synapsing on efferents in layer V. In contrast, the direct activation of cortical neurons from stimulation on the surface of the brain requires a much higher level of stimulation than does normal peripheral somatosensory activation (Libet et al., 1964). Moreover, direct stimulation indiscriminately affects a relatively broad region of cortex rather than a restricted network of cells, and it presumably affects the superficial layer(s) of cortex before or concurrently with stimulation of the layer normally receiving afferents from the peripheral nervous system (Libet, 1973). In all likelihood, direct cortical stimulation plays functional havoc with the complex and highly structured functional-anatomical organization of cortex, activating neurons antidromically (i.e., in the opposite direction as normal stimulation) and in haphazard order. Inferring something about normal processing from such an artificial method is like inferring normal features about the transportation system of a city from the movements of its inhabitants during a terrorist attack.

Beyond these general worries about suitability of the methods used to make inferences about normal function, there are a number of specific reasons to doubt that the finding regarding neuronal adequacy can illuminate much about normal somatosensory processing. First, we are exquisitely aware of somatosensory experiences from single electrical pulses delivered to the periphery, even weak ones that elicit relatively weak cortical responses (Libet, 1973). In contrast, single pulses administered centrally are unable to elicit any conscious awareness (Libet, 1973; Libet et al., 1967; Libet, Alberts, Wright Jr., Lewis, & Feinstein, 1975).

Second, the physiologically unrealistic inputs often do not result in the same sorts of somatosensory sensations that normal (peripheral) stimulation do (Libet et al., 1964; Libet, 1973; Libet et al., 1975). The fact that the sensations, though conscious, are reported as strange suggests that we cannot infer much about how normal signals are temporally processed from this data.

Third, supraliminal stimuli reach consciousness much earlier than the liminal stimuli Libet concentrates on. For example, he writes that "repetitive activations lasting much less than 0.5 sec may if intense enough be effective for eliciting conscious sensory experience" (Libet et al., 1972, p. 159). He reports that stimuli as brief as 50 ms lead to conscious experiences.

Libet argues that the ability to alter the (report of) the subjective experience of a peripheral stimulus by stimulating cortex 200–500 ms after the skin stimulus is delivered is further proof of neuronal adequacy. This may provide some evidence for the claim, but it should be noted that some retroactive effects suppressed and others enhanced the experience, and the reasons for this are not clear. Since reports always occur at least that long after stimulation (Libet 1992, 1973), it is unclear whether what is being altered is the initial sensation, or aspects processed later, or the recollection/assessment of the experience.

One additional reason to doubt that Libet's claims may generalize to conscious experience writ large is the following. Libet has based his claim for this requirement for conscious experience upon experiments that are purely somatosensory, but it is conceivable that other modalities work differently. This possibility is made more salient when one considers that the brain has to solve a problem that arises for the somatosensory system that does not arise for other sensory systems (at least not to the same degree)—to wit, it must make temporal judgments about events that occur at radically different distances from the central processor, and because nerve conduction takes time, different distances involve different time lags. So, for instance, a stimulus from the toe must travel approximately two meters in order to reach the brain, whereas a stimulus to the ear must travel only a few inches. Given the conduction velocity of somatosensory nerve fibers, this difference in distance could give rise to timing discrepancies of approximately 30–50 ms. If we assume that there has been evolutionary pressure to be able to accurately reflect simultaneity or relative timing of somatosensory stimuli (for example, in determining which direction to flee from noxious stimuli or predators), then it will have had to come up with a strategy for taking into account the larger time lag from more distal stimuli. One way to do this is to delay the processing of proximal stimuli; another is to backward-refer (to different degrees) the subjective experience of more distal stimuli. Since there may be more cost to the former, it is not wholly surprising if the brain has adopted the latter in the case of the somatosensory system. It is unclear, however, whether the same argument can be made for backward referral of stimuli in other modalities. So although there may be a rationale for backward referral in the case of somatosensation, I doubt whether such a rationale exists for other modalities, since the disparity in conduction times are much reduced in these other domains. Moreover, we do not have evidence for an analogous argument in other domains. As far as I know it is not known, for instance, whether direct stimulation of the visual cortex also requires 500 ms or more of pulses in order to reach neuronal adequacy. Thus, even if backward referral occurs for somatosensation, whether it occurs for other sensory systems remains dubious.

### C2) Backward Referral of Subjective Timing

*People backward-refer in time their conscious experiences (of peripheral stimuli), taking them to have occurred at a time earlier than they were in fact conscious of them.*

Libet argues that subjects refer their conscious experiences to a time that is prior to the actual time at which they become conscious of them (Libet et al., 1979). Libet's reasoning is based largely on C1, the claim that cortex must be active for approximately 500 ms before stimuli reach awareness. Thus, backward referral is inferred from empirical claims E1 and E2. The reasoning behind this conclusion is as follows: If it takes 500+ ms in order for a supraliminal stimulus to reach conscious awareness (E1) and if subjects report the time of their conscious peripheral stimuli accurately (E2), then they must actually report the time of their awareness of such a peripheral stimulus as before the time at which they actually became conscious of the event in question.

Further experiments are consistent with this interpretation. If C2 is true, one would predict that if presented with simultaneous central and peripheral stimuli, subjects will perceive the latter to occur prior to the former. This is confirmed by E3. Libet's experiments showed that when central and peripheral stimuli were both presented at the same time, subjects judged the peripheral stimulus to have occurred first (Libet et al., 1979). Delaying presentation of the peripheral stimulus relative to the central by approximately 500 ms led to a reversal of the order judgment (Libet et al., 1979).

How does backward referral work? Libet hypothesizes that timing of external stimulation is referred back to the time of the initial arrival of the afferent activity from sensory stimulation to cortex. Stimulation of periphery or the ascending pyramidal tract elicits a fast evoked potential in cortex (the primary EP), followed by further cortical activity, whereas stimulation by a single pulse centrally at the cortical surface, in the white matter, and in ventral posterior lateral nucleus of the thalamus by central electrodes fails to elicit a primary EP, though it does engender cortical activity (Libet et al., 1972). Libet hypothesizes that the primary EP provides a "time-stamp" to which later experiences are backward referred. He surmises that cortical or other central stimulation is not backward referred, because it does not elicit a primary EP. These factors could account for the discrepancy between temporal judgments of centrally and peripherally generated stimulation.

*Critique of C2* Neural processes are physical processes, and physical processes take time; the same is true for neural processes that lead to conscious awareness of external or internal events. It is clear that we can detect stimuli of very short duration, but less clear how to determine how long it takes for stimuli to reach consciousness, since not all responses are conscious responses, and conscious responses take time to execute.

Since neuronal conduction and processing takes time, then to the extent that people accurately report the time of peripheral stimulation, some sort of backward referral occurs. It seems that people's reports are accurate to within 100 ms. A lot of neural processing can occur within that time. Thus, it is not clear that backward referral is necessary, nor that the effect is nearly as great as Libet supposes. Recall that Libet's reasoning is based largely on C1, the claim that cortex must be active for approximately 500 ms before stimuli reach awareness. If C1 is mistaken, there is little reason to believe C2. For if it does not take very long for a peripheral stimulus to reach consciousness, there is not much need to refer one's experiences backward in time. The effect he found is consistent with the falsity of the neuronal adequacy claim and little to no backward referral in ordinary contexts. The order effects he found can be explained away by considering again the unecological nature of the central stimulation techniques.

### C3) We Do Not Consciously Initiate Our Spontaneous Voluntary Actions

*Neural signatures of intention to move are evident well before we are conscious of willing to move. Thus, conscious intentions occur only after actions are already initiated, and so are not the causes of our actions.*

This conclusion is implied from a series of studies that follow upon and from his work on neuronal adequacy and backward referral. These studies explore the timing of motor activity relative to evoked potentials recorded at the scalp, and relative to reports of volitional acts or intentions to move. Libet claims things like, "Since onset of RP regularly begins at least several hundreds of milliseconds before the appearance of a reportable time for awareness of any subjective intention or wish to act, it would appear that some neuronal activity associated with the eventual performance of the act has started well before any (recallable) conscious initiation or intervention could be possible," and "These considerations would appear to introduce certain constraints on the potential of the individual for exerting conscious initiation and control over his voluntary acts" (Libet et al., 1983, p. 641). Thus, although C3 is never stated clearly as such, it is the conclusion we are meant to draw from this work.

The experiments upon which this claim is based employ scalp recordings and relate the timing of deflections from baseline to subjective reports of timing of intentions or urges. E4 demonstrates that when scalp recordings are triggered by a motor action (in this case, a finger movement), and when the prior EEG signals are averaged time-locked to that motor action, there is a ramplike change in the EEG that precedes the motor action (Libet et al., 1982). This ramp, or "readiness potential" (RP) begins approximately 500 ms prior to spontaneous movement, peaking just before motor activity begins, and falls to baseline afterward (Libet et al., 1983). The RP begins even earlier for planned movements (Libet et al., 1982).

E5 provides evidence that the subject's experience of willing an action occurs after the initial rise of the RP, approximately 200 ms prior to the time of the movement (Libet, 1985; Libet et al., 1983). From E4 and E5 emerges the claim that conscious will follows, rather than precedes, the initiation of action. The lag between unconscious initiation of action and the experience of conscious will is presumed to be even greater than measured if the conscious experience of willing is thought to be subject to backward referral. For if experiences of conscious will are backward referred, as Libet claims experiences of external events are, and if the timing is similar to the timing in the case of sensation (approximately 500 ms), then those experiences actually occur some time after the movement occurs.

*Critique of C3* All neural processes take time. Moreover, we proceed from the basic assumption that all mental processes are or are the result of brain processes, and brain processes are caused by prior brain processes. Thus, it is expected and not surprising that neural activity should precede any mental event as well as any behavior. It is therefore unsurprising that there will be neural signatures of events that are predictive of behaviors such as finger movements, and unsurprising if we also find neural signatures that are predictive of subjective experiences of will. To expect this not to be the case is to refuse to accept basic commitments of physicalism. The fact that Libet finds it surprising that there is a neural signature that occurs before consciousness of intention belies a dualistic perspective about conscious experience (see commentaries accompanying Libet, 1985).

The real questions at issue, at least with regard to the interpretation of the experimental results, are whether Libet is correct in causally connecting the RPs with impending motor movements, rather than with intentions to move.

### On the Interpretation of E4

The significance of Libet's data for the efficacy of the will would be undermined if it were shown that the RP reflected processes involved in forming a conscious intention to act, rather than a movement. We cannot presume this to be the case, but neither can Libet presume it is not the case.

The assumption Libet makes is that the RP is causally connected to the motor activity, so that RP generation leads to motor action (barring some sort of intervention, such as Libet's hypothesized "stop" signal, or "free won't" [Libet, 1985; Libet et al., 1983]). There is undoubtedly a correlation between a change in (presumably) motor cortex and subsequent motor activity. However, many circumstances may result in correlations, and not all would justify Libet's interpretation of the data. Here I suggest a few reasons to be suspicious of his interpretation.

We must scrutinize this reported correlation between RP and motor activity more carefully. The RPs that Libet reports are averaged over many trials. Let us call the electrical changes that occur in individual trials, those that are averaged together to produce the RP, "individual-RPs." First, and most critically, Libet's data collection method is triggered by motor activity, so his methods drastically bias the picture, for only epochs in which motor activity occurs are collected, and only these are averaged and time-locked to such a signal. Any individual-RPs that occur but are not followed by a finger movement will be unrecorded. It is possible, however, that individual-RPs frequently occur but do not result in motor activity. Were such epochs present they would drastically change the interpretation of the RP as a causal precursor to motor activity. Because such epochs would never be seen given Libet's methods of investigation, Libet's interpretation of the RP as a signature for subsequent motor action (or unconscious initiation of motor activity) should be called into question.

A perhaps lesser issue is this: because the RPs reported are the average of many trials, we could be subject to a statistical illusion. It is tempting to think that each individual trial will elicit a somewhat noisy individual-RP that shares the same basic shape and time course as the RPs reported. It is also tempting to think that averaging all the individual-RPs together merely cleans up the signal. If this were the case, one could make several predictions about how the RP works. For example, one might think of the RP as a single waveform that is initiated with the deviation from baseline, and that "beginning" of the type II RP is approximately 500 ms before the motor activity. Moreover, the shape of the RP may prompt one to think that motor activity is elicited when the RP reaches some threshold, such as the peak of the RP. While these predictions may be natural, they are probably far from correct. The shape and time course of the individual-RPs could be quite different from those of the RPs reported; the ramplike features of the RP could be an artifact of the averaging procedure. Thus, features such as the time of RP initiation may merely be artifacts that lead us to mistakenly believe the brain had "decided" to move well before our conscious intention of the movement; this interpretation would be mistaken.

Finally, the methods Libet uses are not ideal for localizing the source of the signal. Indeed, it is not clear that the RP signal comes from primary motor cortex, rather than higher-level cortical areas involved in what may be motor planning or motor intention. An alternative hypothesis to Libet's is that the neural processes reflected in the RP are associated with the formation of intention, perhaps ultimately culminating in consciousness of intention, and not with motor activity per se. A more recent study by Haggard and Eimer pursues this possibility, but suggests that a different brain signal, the Lateralized Readiness Potential (LRP), is better correlated with the awareness of timing of motor action (Haggard & Eimer, 1999). Viewing these brain signals as precursors to conscious intention would not lead to the same kind of challenge for free will, at least not given a basic physicalist stance.

The above considerations call into question the link between the RP and movement initiation, as well as the focus on the timing of the initial rise of the RP as a relevant parameter. They thus also call into question the interpretations of the significance of the RP for the question of volition. Further questions could be raised about the validity of methods of using the clock paradigm in order to determine the timing of conscious awareness, but instead I will focus upon more philosophical aspects of his paradigms.

## II. PHILOSOPHICAL OBJECTIONS TO LIBET'S CONCLUSIONS ABOUT FREE WILL

Thus far, I have questioned whether we ought to accept Libet's interpretation of his empirical results. In critical instances, I have concluded that we needn't. In what follows, I will change gears somewhat, and focus upon issues more of concern to philosophers. I begin by summarizing Libet's main philosophical conclusions. Then I focus on two issues. First, if Libet's conclusions are correct, would they show that the conscious will is not efficacious, or that we are in fact not free? I will argue that even if we accept Libet's empirical claims and their direct implications for the generation of motor action, the philosophical implications for free will that people often draw do not follow. Second, I contend that what Libet is actually measuring differs both from what he thinks he is measuring, and from what is relevant to the question of free will.

### 1. Philosophical Implications Libet Draws from His Findings

According to Libet, the previously discussed experiments have dramatic consequences for our understanding of the conscious will and freedom of action. C1 and C2 suggest a dissociation between the timing of brain responses and the timing of subjective experiences. On the basis of C3, Libet argues that our actions are not consciously initiated or controlled. As he puts it, "These considerations would appear to introduce certain constraints on the potential of the individual for exerting conscious initiation and control over his voluntary acts" (Libet et al., 1983, p. 641). What he means by this is that our conscious intentions do not drive or control our actions, but rather arise subsequent to the action that is already underway. These actions are unconsciously initiated, and we have a post-hoc experience as of consciously willing them. It is a suppressed premise that conscious intention must somehow govern free action, and if we do not consciously initiate or control our actions, they are not freely willed (Libet, 1985; Libet et al., 1983). Libet hypothesizes that if there is room for freedom at all, it is not in the conscious initiation of spontaneous action, but instead in the possibility of aborting an action whose neural underpinnings are already set in motion by unconscious processes. This possibility of the freedom of the veto, or "free won't," is Libet's suggestion for how to save freedom in the face of his data (Libet, 1985; Libet et al., 1983). He also concedes that "In those voluntary actions that are not 'spontaneous' and quickly performed, that is, in those in which conscious deliberation (of whether to act or of what alternative choice of action to take) precedes the act, the possibilities for conscious initiation and control would not be excluded by the present evidence" (Libet et al., 1983, p. 641).

### 2. What is the Appropriate Target for Discussions of Freedom?

One reason to doubt the radical conclusion that we lack free will comes from examination of the target of Libet's experiments. Libet focuses on the spontaneous generation of simple motor movements as his paradigm for free action. As he claims, "the simple voluntary motor act studied here has in fact often been regarded as an incontrovertible and ideal example of a fully endogenous and 'freely voluntary' act" (Libet et al., 1983, p. 640). He is joined in this view by many others, for simple arbitrary decisions and movements have long been targeted by philosophers as toy examples of freedom of the will. How many philosophy professors illustrate freedom by asking their students to decide whether or not to raise their hands, and then to raise them if they have so decided? There are reasons for using such examples: perhaps the primary one is to try to boil down the decision-action process into its simplest and least controversial components, and thus to provide a classroom illustration of freedom equivalent to the Moorean proof for knowledge of external objects: "Here is one hand, here is another." To be sure, Libet's own justification for his choice of simple motor action as a paradigm has more to do with the scientific reasons for starting with the simplest and best understood aspects of action in constructing an experiment. But as in Moore's proof, the seemingly self-evident can be misleading, in that in accepting what appears to be unproblematic we unconsciously buy into far more than that.

The first reason we should worry about the choice of finger or wrist movements as a paradigm case of free will is that when we think about freedom, what we care about is that we are free to act for reasons, and for those reasons we judge to be salient and compelling. Freedom matters because it is thought to ground moral responsibility, and the notion of holding someone morally responsible for an action that has no real consequences seems for the most part pointless. However, when we generate actions spontaneously in the context of such an experiment, we do not act for reasons at all, save the reason of complying with the experimenter's demands. As Banks and Pockett have noted (Banks & Pockett, 2007), subjects in the experiment are in one sense compelled to move their fingers, since they have agreed to participate in the experiment and comply with the experiment's demands.

What they are deciding is not whether to move their finger, but rather *when* to. However, there are no reasons that govern their choices to act when they do. It does not matter, for the satisfactory execution of the experimental task, whether the subjects move their finger now . . . or now. . . . (see also Mele, chapter 3 in this volume). The entire time course of experimental evaluation may be a more appropriate unit of analysis in response to those demands, but this is not what Libet's experiments assay.

Arbitrary action is, at best, a degenerate case of freedom of the will, one in which what matters about freedom fails to hold. Suppose, for example, that it turned out that in purely arbitrary cases in the absence of reasons (including foreseeable consequences of those actions), actions were the result of random fluctuations in the nervous system, and suppose further that in all cases in which there are reasons relevant to the decision to act, we responded appropriately to these reasons, deliberating and weighing them, and then regulating our actions so as to bring them in line with our deliberations. Would we conclude on the basis of the random mechanisms that caused actions in cases where our actions had no consequences that we lacked freedom? Of course not, for many of our actions would be free.

Imagine, for instance, that Fred wakes in the morning, gets out of bed in order to get to work on time, and puts on his pants one leg at a time. Whether he puts on the right leg first or the left leg first is an arbitrary choice; which one he actually does today is due to unconscious, subpersonal neural mechanisms. Fred gets into his car in order to drive to work. The traffic is bad. Fred stops at the red light, because one is supposed to stop at red lights, but he glances at his watch and realizes that he'll be late for his morning meeting. Deciding that he cannot be late again, for his boss will probably dock his Christmas bonus, Fred does not stop at the stop sign. Had he not considered this, he would have stopped. In driving through the stop sign, Fred hits a small child crossing the street. Would we consider Fred free or unfree? Despite the fact that we may argue that his "choice" of putting on the right pant leg before the left was not free, we would nonetheless consider his choice of action while driving free, and we'd hold him responsible for it. In this scenario, given what we know about the matter, in the cases in which our choices matter, freedom (and responsibility) are preserved. Libet's experiments are equivalent to probing the choice of priority-of-pant-leg, and so in the absence of an argument for why they should be considered relevant to the other type of reasons-based choice, I would argue that they are irrelevant to the philosophically interesting question of whether we have free will.

The foregoing argument is not demonstrative—just because the timing of the spontaneous finger movements in Libet's experiments is arbitrary does not entail that the neural underpinnings are not reflective of the very same processes that govern choices in other situations that have real consequences and moral import. However, I have offered a reason to think that this kind of choice is not the kind we care about when we think about the importance of freedom, and if this is the case, it is at least conceivable (and I would argue, plausible) that even if the data does suggest that in spontaneously deciding to move our fingers our movements are not governed by our conscious will, this is entirely consistent with the supposition that in other types of cases—those for which we want to hold people morally responsible—awareness of intention does precede our actions. Libet himself acknowledges this, but his circumspection on this point has often been overlooked. The burden of proof, therefore, is on the foe of freedom to argue that spontaneous movement is a good paradigm for free action, and that conclusions from this should carry over to other kinds of more complex, deliberative actions.

The sorts of actions we want to hold people responsible for, and thus the ones for which freedom most matters, are typically far more complex than mere finger movements, either because they involve orchestrated sequential behavior (for example, breaking into a locked house), or because they show a disregard for reasons that we presume are evident to the agent. In other words, we hold people responsible for planned action, and not in general for the individual motor movements they perform. While at first blush it may seem that we hold people responsible for pulling the trigger of a gun, which is not too disanalogous to deciding to move one's finger in this experiment, it is not so clear that their finger movement is all that enters into our calculations of responsibility. In almost all cases of homicide, the pulling of the gun's trigger is the final action in a series of actions that include procuring a firearm, putting it in one's hand, doing so in a situation in which you can use it to inflict harm on someone else, and so on. While the finger motion is necessary for the homicide, it is not sufficient. In the absence of the other elements the finger movement would have no impact.

Having and weighing reasons also comes into play in the assignment of moral responsibility. For instance, people are held less culpable in crimes of passion, where it is presumed that in the heat of the moment it is understandable that reason does not prevail. Thus it seems to me mistaken to think of these simple and arbitrary motor actions as the appropriate ones to focus upon in investigating freedom of the will. In the case of Libet's experiments, the construct that would be more analogous to the type of act we ought to be focusing on if we are concerned about free will, is in the intention to perform the experiment according to the experimenter's dictates. Throughout the experiment, the subject has a certain mental set, namely to execute the plan *move finger at random moments* or some gloss on that. It is this temporally extended intention to act, and one that is formed well in advance of the sorts of measurements that Libet makes, that is more relevant to the notion of freedom than individual motor signals. Libet's experiments do not probe the nature of this intention or the elements of its control. One can safely surmise, however, that the establishment (or choice) of such a plan to act or an alternative one is something that occurs well *before* the RP, even if the RP precedes the motor action itself.[1] Thus, my first main contention is that the sorts of phenomena Libet explores are not the correct ones to focus on if what we are interested in is how awareness and action are related insofar as they bear upon freedom and responsibility.

The friend of Libet may try to defend the choice by arguing that regardless of overarching plans or mental sets, all morally relevant consequences are results of actions, and all actions can be parsed into more and more basic movements. By showing that even at this fundamental level, the level of the basic action, we lack a certain kind of intentional control, the friend of Libet will try to argue that control lacking at the most basic level just entails a similar control lacking at the level of more complex actions. This is a sort of foundationalist view of freedom: free complex action is built up from free simple actions. Although at times even I have felt the force of this response, I think it is flawed. First, it is not clear that our commonsensical way of conceiving of basic action accurately reflects the taxonomy of action in the brain. For example, it was found that individual finger movements involve much more cortical activity than more "complex" movements involving all the fingers in ecologically meaningful gestures. This suggests that what seem to be simple from the folk perspective are actually more neurally demanding. Thus, what we naively consider to be basic may not be basic at all. Second, I believe that the higher-level motor plan is more central to free action, and that this plan is not itself just a combination of simple motor movements, but something established prior to and affecting the release or generation of its more simple components. Higher-level motor programs and plans are realized in Supplementary Motor Area (SMA) and other frontal areas, and not in motor cortex itself. Given this, Libet's experiments may be assaying a phenomenon only tangentially related to freedom of the will.

Assuming we accept all the empirical results that Libet discusses, as well as his interpretations of them, what implications does his body of work have for free will? It seems I can accept that the RP for a finger movement precedes conscious awareness of an intention to move, and still deny that this has much to say about whether or not we are free in the cases and contexts in which freedom really does matter. Libet's subjects may have freely chosen to participate in the experiment, may have freely chosen to comply with the experimenter's instructions, and to have raised their fingers when they felt the urge to do so. The timing of the RP says nothing about any of these matters, yet these are the ones that seem much more salient for assessments of freedom. If so, Libet's studies definitively impact our understanding of only a small number of our actions, and these appear to be the ones that are least likely to matter for discussions of freedom.

### 3. Is Libet Really Asking the Question He Claims to Be Asking?

The preceding discussion calls into question the extent to which we should take Libet's results to bear upon the philosophical question of freedom. Here I consider a question that I think seriously undermines Libet's arguments for unconscious initiation of action. Let us consider again the experiments in which Libet asks subjects to indicate the position of a dot moving around a clock face when they become aware of an intention to move. This is the experiment that he thinks really undermines the idea that conscious will is involved in initiating action, for he shows that RP precedes W (consciousness of intending, willing, wanting).

Let us consider Libet's experiment in closer detail. The subject is asked to do two different tasks: (1) to spontaneously move his or her finger, and (2) to report where a rotating dot was on a clock face at the time he or she became aware of the intention to move it (W). (2) is a complicated task, and it requires (a) recognizing that one has an intention to move; (b) indexing the visual stimulus of the clock face when (a) is satisfied; and (c) reporting the result of (b). It is likely that satisfying (a) requires attention to an internal state, and it is certain that satisfying (b) requires attention to an external stimulus, and it is possible that transitioning between (a) and (b) involves a shift of attention that takes time, causing the indexed visual stimulus of the clock time to be later than the actual time of occurrence of (a). That could explain some of the lag between RP and W. Establishing whether this is the case, and the temporal costs involved, are empirical questions. Libet tries to control for some of these factors by including a condition that probes timing of awareness of a somatosensory stimulus, but for reasons elaborated below, it is not clear that this control condition is adequate.

However, there is a more philosophical objection in the area, concerning the nature and content of the relevant states. Libet claims to be probing the time of conscious intent to move. The relative timing of conscious intent to move and the initiation of movement are the components one would want to assay if one were interested in the efficacy of conscious will. However, a closer look at Libet's experimental design suggests that these are not the states that he is measuring. Instead, Libet's experiment with the clock face probes the relative timing of a meta-state, *consciousness of conscious intent,* and the initiation of movement (assuming the worries above are discounted). There is good reason to think that consciousness of conscious intent may occur some time after conscious intent, and thus the fact that this occurs after the RP has begun is compatible with conscious intent occurring prior to the RP.

It seems likely that our ordinary volitional actions are not preceded by intentions that are consciously available in the same way that many perceptual stimuli are. In ordinary life we don't attend to our intentions and in fact we are largely unaware of them, whereas we ordinarily attend to and are aware of perceptions or sensations, and/or to the objects that cause those perceptions and sensations in us. For instance, I am conscious of driving when I drive, and I consciously steer, accelerate, check my speed, and so on, and I intend to do so. I act volitionally. However, I often am not conscious of intending to steer, accelerate, etc., in the sense that the commands I give to my body are not present to me. What is present to me is the road, the scenery, the cop car on the side of the freeway. However, I by no means think I act unconsciously, and still less do I think I do it unfreely. If our acts that are volitional are accompanied by conscious intentions, they are conscious in that they are *available* for report if attended to, but they do not enter our ordinary experience by being phenomenologically *present* to us. This phenomenological difference suggests that attending to and awareness of intentions differs from attending to and awareness of perceptions. Indeed, many perceptual stimuli exogenously command or draw attention, whereas our attention must be effortfully and endogenously focused on intentional states in order to report on them. Another way to think of it is that willing, and even willing consciously or deliberately, is an executive, and not ordinarily perceptual function, and to perceive it involves additional perceptual operations. If this is so, we have reason to believe that reporting a conscious intention and reporting a conscious perception may be dissimilar in important ways.

If this is right, we must think about Libet's experiments in a different way. In order to perform task (1) (spontaneously but deliberately moving a finger), the subject must form a conscious intention that we may characterize as having the content "move finger" (or perhaps "move finger now"). In order to monitor one's conscious state and report on the timing of one's intention, task (2), one has to effortfully direct attention to one's intentional state, because intentions don't present themselves in the same way as perceptions. The conscious state that one is in when one reports is thus a meta-state that we may describe with the content "I am conscious of having a state with the content 'move finger'". If this is so, then the report Libet is eliciting is not the report of the time of conscious intention, which is what would be required to probe the relative timing of willing and acting, but rather the report of some other state, albeit a state causally and intentionally related to the desired state. If this is so, it invalidates Libet's analysis as an analysis of the causal antecedents of free action, and instead is suitable only as an analysis of the timing of self-conscious action. Self-conscious action may also be important for discussions of freedom, for perhaps it is the case that some sorts of deliberations and weighings of reasons must occur self-consciously. Nevertheless, while our commonsense concept of freedom may require that our actions causally involve conscious intention, it is not clear that it requires self-conscious intention (or consciousness of conscious intention).

Moreover, the above analysis would explain why RP precedes W. Since the state required for the report of conscious intention is about that prior state, it obviously depends upon the existence of the prior state. This would be expected, for instance, if the subsequent state requires an operation on the content of the prior intentional state. Since the states are not identical, and the latter depends upon the former, it is not unreasonable to think that the formation of the latter state will occur after the former, and perhaps some time after (especially if Libet is right in thinking that conscious awareness requires some half-second of processing, although I suggested reasons to doubt this figure). Thus, if the reported time of awareness is dependent upon the conscious apprehension of a conscious state, there is good reason to expect the reported time of awareness to occur relatively late in processing. It wouldn't be particularly surprising, nor diagnostic, if that awareness occurred well after the initiation of the RP. This leaves open the temporal relation between the conscious intention and the action.

I can imagine two different responses to this objection that the friend of Libet could offer: (1) conscious intention is just an intention of which I am conscious at the time; and (2) conscious intention and consciousness of having that intention occur simultaneously. I don't think either of these is compelling. Regarding the first, if we grant that a conscious intention is nothing but consciousness of an intention, then we rarely have conscious intentions at all. Because our intentions are not ordinarily present to us, this type of consciousness seems to be an experimental contrivance that plays little role in ordinary action, or in our conception of freedom.

Regarding the second, one might accept that consciousness of our intentions are indeed meta-intentional states, but yet maintain that consciousness is temporally transparent, so that consciousness-of-intention, if it occurs, occurs simultaneously with intention. I'm not sure what the argument for this would be. Without a theory of consciousness on offer, it seems much more likely that distinct states with an asymmetric dependence (which these would be, if the content of one involves causal operations on the content of the other) do not occur simultaneously, since mental processes take time. In any case, the burden of proof is on the person who thinks consciousness of a state doesn't lag that state's occurrence.

## SUMMARY

In the first part of this paper, I discussed empirical reasons to be skeptical of some of Libet's interpretations of his data for the dissociations between neural and subjective events, and for his studies on volition. However, even if one were to accept Libet's interpretations, his experiments would not necessarily undermine our concept of human freedom. In the second part of this paper, I discussed two philosophical reasons to doubt that his paradigm is appropriate for probing the temporal relation between conscious volition and action. Ultimately, what we conclude about the relation between conscious intent and action will have to take into account a host of other studies, many of them also skeptical about whether we can be free. For now, however, it seems too early to lay to rest the treasured notion that we freely will our actions.

## NOTE

1. And if perchance the neural correlate of the establishment of a plan does occur prior to awareness of such a plan, there is likely plenty of time for plan revision after the awareness and before the action, which again seems to leave room for freedom and responsibility.

## REFERENCES

Banks, W. P., & Pockett, S. (2007). Benjamin Libet's work on the neuroscience of free will. In M. Velmans & S. Schinder (Eds.), *Blackwell companion to consciousness* (pp. 657–670). Malden, MA: Blackwell.

Haggard, P., & Eimer, M. (1999). On the relation between brain potentials and the awareness of voluntary movements. *Experimental Brain Research, 126,* 128–133.

Libet, B. (1973). Electrical stimulation of cortex in human subjects and conscious sensory aspects. In A. Iggo (Ed.), *Handbook of sensory physiology.* Berlin: Springer-Verlag.

Libet, B. (1985). Unconscious cerebral initiative and the role of conscious will in voluntary action. *Behavioral and Brain Sciences, 8,* 529–566.

Libet, B. (1992). Retroactive enhancement of a skin sensation by a delayed cortical stimulus in man: Evidence for delay of a conscious sensory experience. *Consciousness and Cognition, 1,* 367–375.

Libet, B., Alberts, W. W., Wright, E. W., Jr., Delattre, L. D., Levin, G., & Feinstein, B. (1964). Production of threshold levels of conscious sensation by electrical stimulation of human somatosensory cortex. *Journal of Neurophysiology, 27,* 546–578.

Libet, B., Alberts, W. W., Wright, E. W., Jr., & Feinstein, B. (1967). Responses of human somatosensory cortex to stimuli below threshold for conscious sensation. *Science, 158*(3803), 1597–1600.

Libet, B., Alberts, W. W., Wright, E. W., Jr., & Feinstein, B. (1972). Cortical and thalamic activation in conscious sensory experience. In G. G. Somjen (Ed.), *Neurophysiology studied in man.* Amsterdam: Excerpta Medica.

Libet, B., Alberts, W. W., Wright, E. W., Jr., Lewis, M., & Feinstein, B. (1975). Cortical representation of evoked potentials relative to conscious sensory responses, and of somatosensory qualities—in man. In H. H. Kornhuber (Ed.), *The somatosensory system.* Stuttgart: Georg Thieme Verlag.

Libet, B., Gleason, C. A., Wright, E. W., & Pearl, D. K. (1983). Time of conscious intention to act in relation to onset of cerebral activity (readiness-potential): The unconscious initation of a freely voluntry act. *Brain, 106*(3), 623–642.

Libet, B., Wright, E. W., Jr., Feinstein, B., & Pearl, D. K. (1979). Subjective referral of the timing for a conscious sensory experience: A functional role for the somatosensory specific projection system in man. *Brain: A Journal of Neurology, 102,* 193–224.

Libet, B., Wright, E. W., Jr., & Gleason, C. A. (1982). Readiness-potentials preceding unrestricted "spontaneous" vs. pre-planned voluntary acts. *Electroencephalography, Clinical Neurophysiology, 54,* 322–335.

# CHAPTER 3

# Libet on Free Will: Readiness Potentials, Decisions, and Awareness

*Alfred R. Mele*

Scientific work on free will has gained a lot of momentum in recent years. It features some striking claims. For example, Benjamin Libet contends both that "the brain 'decides' to initiate or, at least, prepare to initiate [certain actions] before there is any reportable subjective awareness that such a decision has taken place" (1985, p. 536)[1] and that "if the 'act now' process is initiated unconsciously, then conscious free will is not doing it" (2001, p. 62; see 2004, p. 136). He also contends that once we become conscious of our proximal decisions, we can exercise free will in vetoing them (1985, 1999, 2004, pp. 137–149). Libet has many critics and many supporters. Some people follow him part of the way. They accept the thesis about when and how decisions are made but reject the window of opportunity for free will as an illusion (Hallett, 2007).

Elsewhere, I have argued that these striking claims are not warranted by the data Libet and others offer in support of them (Mele, 2006a, ch. 2; 2006b; 2008b; 2009, chs. 3 and 4). Here, after providing some conceptual and empirical background, I discuss three major problems.

## 1. SOME CONCEPTUAL BACKGROUND: DECISIONS, INTENTIONS, AND WANTING

Some conceptual background is in order. I focus on the concept of deciding: that is, deciding to do something—*practical deciding*—as opposed to deciding that something is true (as in "Ann decided that Bob was lying"). And I briefly discuss its connections to some related concepts. Like many philosophers, I take *deciding* to *A* to be an action.[2] In my view, it is a momentary action of forming an intention to *A* (Mele, 2003, ch. 9). Deliberation about what to do is not momentary, but it must be distinguished from an act of deciding that is based on deliberation.

Not all intentions are formed in acts of deciding. Consider the following: "When I intentionally unlocked my office door this morning, I intended to unlock it. But since I am in the habit of unlocking my door in the morning and conditions . . . were normal, nothing called for a *decision* to unlock it" (Mele, 1992, p. 231). If I had heard a fight in my office, I might have paused to consider whether to unlock the door or walk away, and I might have decided to unlock it. But given the routine nature of my conduct, there is no need to posit an action of intention formation in this case. My intention to unlock the door may have been acquired without having been actively formed. If, as I believe, all decisions about what to do are prompted partly by uncertainty about what to do (Mele, 2003, ch. 9), in situations in which there is no such uncertainty, no decisions will be made. This is not to say that, in such situations, no intentions will be acquired.

Some decisions and intentions are about things to do straightaway. They are *proximal* decisions and intentions. Others—*distal* decisions and intentions—are about things to do later. A shy student who has been thinking about when to raise his hand to attract his teacher's attention decides to raise it now. This is a proximal decision. Later, after thinking about when to start writing a term paper, he decides to start it next Tuesday. This is a distal decision. Although Libet focuses on proximal decisions and intentions, some other scientists study their distal counterparts (Gollwitzer & Sheeran, 2006).

Deciding to do something should be distinguished from wanting (or having an urge) to do it. Sometimes people want to do things that they decide not to do. And often, when people want to do each of two incompatible things—for example, meet some friends for dinner at 7:00 and attend a lecture at 7:00—they settle matters by deciding which one to do. Just as deciding should be distinguished from wanting, so should intending. Intending to do something is more tightly connected to action than is merely wanting to do it (Mele, 1992, 2003).

The account of practical deciding sketched here is not the only account of it. For critical discussion of alternative accounts, see Mele 2003, chapter 9. For the purposes of this article, a virtue of the account just sketched is that it is consonant with Libet's apparent conception of deciding.

## 2. SOME EMPIRICAL BACKGROUND: LIBET'S STUDIES

In some of Libet's studies, subjects are regularly encouraged to flex their right wrists whenever they wish. In such subjects who do not report any "preplanning" of flexings, electrical readings from the scalp (EEGs)—averaged over at least 40 flexings for each subject—show a shift in "readiness potentials" (RPs) that begins about 550 milliseconds (ms) before the time at which an electromyogram (EMG) shows relevant muscular motion to begin (1985, pp. 529–530). These are "type II RPs" (p. 531). Subjects who are not regularly encouraged to act spontaneously or who report some preplanning produce RPs that begin about half a second earlier—"type I RPs." The same is true of subjects instructed to flex at a "preset" time (Libet, Wright, & Gleason, 1982, p. 325).[3]

Subjects are also instructed to "recall . . . the spatial clock position of a revolving spot at the time of [their] initial awareness" (Libet, 1985, p. 529) of something, *x*, that Libet variously describes as a decision, intention, urge, wanting, will, or wish to move.[4] (The spot makes a complete revolution in less than three seconds.) On average, in the case of type II RPs, "RP onset" precedes what the subjects report to be the time of their initial awareness of *x* (time W) by 350 ms. Reported time W, then, precedes the beginning of muscle motion by about 200 ms. The results may be represented as follows:

**Libet's results for type II RPs**

| −550 ms | −200 ms | 0 ms |
|---|---|---|
| RP onset | reported time W | muscle begins to move |

(Libet finds independent evidence of what he regards as an error in subjects' recall of the times at which they first become aware of sensations. Correcting for it, time W is −150 ms.)

Again, in Libet's view, consciousness opens a tiny window of opportunity for free will in his subjects. If a subject, Wilma, becomes conscious of her intention at −150 ms, and if by −50 ms her condition is such that "the act goes to completion with no possibility of its being stopped by the rest of the cerebral cortex" (Libet, 2004, p. 138), her window is open for 100 ms. Libet writes: "The role of conscious free will [is] not to initiate a voluntary act, but rather to control whether the act takes place. We may view the unconscious initiatives as 'bubbling up' in the brain. The conscious-will then selects which of these initiatives may go forward to an action or which ones to veto and abort" (1999, p. 54).

Libet mentions what he regards as two sources of evidence for veto power. The first is an experiment in which subjects are instructed to prepare to flex at a prearranged clock time and "to veto the developing intention/preparation to act . . . about 100 to 200 ms before [that] time" (1985, p. 538). Subjects receive both instructions at the same time. Libet writes:

> a ramplike pre-event potential was still recorded . . . resembl[ing] the RP of self-initiated acts when preplanning is present. . . . The form of the "veto" RP differed (in most but not all cases) from those "preset" RPs that were followed by actual

> movements [in another experiment]; the main negative potential tended to alter in direction (flattening or reversing) at about 150–250 ms before the preset time. . . . This difference suggests that the conscious veto interfered with the final development of RP processes leading to action. . . . The preparatory cerebral processes associated with an RP can and do develop even when intended motor action is vetoed at approximately the time that conscious intention would normally appear before a voluntary act. (1985, p. 538)[5]

Subjects' reports about unsolicited vetoing are Libet's second source of evidence for veto power. Subjects encouraged to flex spontaneously (in non-veto experiments) "reported that during some of the trials a recallable conscious urge to act appeared but was "aborted" or somehow suppressed before any actual movement occurred; in such cases the subject simply waited for another urge to appear, which, when consummated, constituted the actual event whose RP was recorded" (Libet, 1985, p. 538). Libet says that his subjects were "free *not* to act out any given urge or initial decision to act; and each subject indeed reported frequent instances of such aborted intentions" (p. 530).

## 3. PROBLEM 1: WHAT HAPPENS AT –550 MS?

Libet contends that in subjects who are regularly encouraged to flex spontaneously and who report no preplanning, proximal decisions to flex are made (or proximal intentions to flex are acquired) around −550 ms on average. His apparent line of reasoning here is straightforward: (1) all overt intentional actions are caused by decisions (or intentions); (2) the type II RPs, which begin on average around −550 ms, are correlated with causes of the flexing actions (because they regularly precede the onset of muscle motion); so (3) these RPs indicate that decisions are made (or intentions acquired) on average at –550 ms.[6] Elsewhere I have argued—on empirical grounds—that it is much more likely that what emerges around −550 ms is a *potential cause* of a proximal intention or decision than a proximal intention or decision itself (Mele, 2006a, ch. 2; 2009, ch. 3). In this section I focus on just one kind of relevant evidence.

If makings of proximal decisions to flex or acquisitions of proximal intentions to flex (or the physical correlates of these events) cause muscle motion, how long does it take them to do that?[7] Does it take about 550 ms? Might reaction time experiments show that 550 ms is too long a time for this? Some caution is in order here. In typical reaction time experiments, subjects have decided in advance to perform an assigned task—to "*A*," for short—whenever they detect the relevant signal. When they detect the signal, there is no need for a proximal *decision* to *A*.[8] (If all decisions are responses to uncertainty about what to do and subjects are not uncertain about what to do when they detect the signal, there is no place here for proximal decisions to *A*.)[9] However, it is plausible that after they detect the signal, they acquire a proximal *intention* to *A*. That is, it is plausible that the combination of their conditional intention to *A* when they detect the signal and their detection of the signal produces a proximal intention to *A*. The acquisition of this intention would then initiate the *A*-ing. And in a reaction time experiment (described shortly) in which subjects are watching a Libet clock, the time between the go signal and the onset of muscle motion is much shorter than 550 ms. This is evidence that proximal intentions to flex—as opposed to potential causes of such intentions—emerge much closer to the time of the onset of muscle motion than 550 ms. There is no reason, in principle, that it should take people any longer to start flexing their wrists when executing a proximal intention to flex in Libet's studies than it takes them to do this when executing such an intention in a reaction time study. More precisely, there is no reason, in principle, that the interval between proximal intention acquisition and the beginning of muscle motion should be significantly different in the two scenarios.[10]

The line of reasoning that I have just sketched depends on the assumption that, in reaction time studies, proximal intentions to *A* are at work. An alternative possibility is that the combination of subjects' conditional intentions to *A* when they detect the signal and their detection of the signal initiates the *A*-ing without there being any proximal intention to *A*. Of course, if this is possible, then there is a parallel possibility in the case of Libet's subjects. Perhaps, on many occasions, the combination of their conditional intentions to flex when they next feel like it—conscious intentions, presumably—together with relevant feelings (for example, felt urges to flex soon) initiates a flexing without there being any proximal intentions to flex. (They may treat their initial consciousness of the urge as a go signal, as suggested in Keller & Heckhausen, 1990, p. 352.) If that possibility is an actuality, then, on these occasions, Libet's thesis is false, of course: there is no intention to flex "now" on these occasions and, therefore, no such intention is produced by the brain before the mind is aware of it.

The reaction time study I mentioned is reported in Haggard and Magno (1999):

> Subjects sat at a computer watching a clock hand . . . whose rotation period was 2.56 s. . . . After an unpredictable delay, varying from 2.56 to 8 s, a high-frequency tone . . . was played over a loudspeaker. This served as a warning stimulus for the subsequent reaction. 900 ms after the warning stimulus onset, a second tone . . . was played. [It] served as the go signal. Subjects were instructed to respond as rapidly as possible to the go signal with a right-key press on a computer mouse button. Subjects were instructed not to anticipate the go stimulus and were reprimanded if they responded on catch trials. (p. 103).

The endpoints of reaction times, as calculated in this study, are the sounding of the go signal and "the EMG signal for the onset of the first sustained burst of muscle activity occurring after the go signal" (p. 104). "Reaction time" here, then, starts *before* any intention to press "now" is acquired: obviously, it takes some time to detect the signal, and if detection of the signal helps to produce a proximal intention, that takes some time too. The mean of the subjects' median reaction times in the control trials was 231 ms (p. 104). If a proximal intention to press was acquired, that happened, on average, nearer to the time of muscle motion than 231 ms and, therefore, much nearer than the 550 ms that Libet claims is the time proximal intentions to flex are unconsciously acquired in his studies. Notice also how close we are getting to Libet's subjects' average reported time of their initial awareness of something he variously describes as an "intention," "urge," "wanting," "decision," "will," or "wish" to move (reported time W: −200 ms). If proximal intentions to flex are acquired in Libet's studies, Haggard and Magno's results make it look like a better bet that they are acquired, on average, around reported time W than around −550 ms.[11] (How seriously we should take Libet's subjects' reports of the time of their initial awareness of the urge, intention, or whatever, is a controversial question. I reserve discussion of it for section 5.)

Someone might claim that even if Libet's subjects do not have proximal intentions to flex before they have conscious intentions of this kind, these conscious intentions cannot be among the causes of their flexing actions because the intentions are "initiated" by something else. This assertion is badly misguided, as attention to the following analogous assertion shows: Burnings of fuses cannot be among the causes of explosions of firecrackers because burnings of fuses are initiated by something else—lightings of fuses. Obviously, both the lighting of its fuse and the burning of its fuse are among the causes of a firecracker's exploding in normal scenarios. Other things being equal, if the fuse had not been lit—or if the lit fuse had stopped burning early—there would have been no explosion. There is no reason to believe that the more proximal causes of firecracker explosions cannot themselves have causes. Analogously, there is no reason to believe that a relatively proximal cause of a flexing action—a conscious proximal intention, perhaps—cannot itself have causes.

Another claim to consider is that even if Libet's subjects' flexing actions do have conscious proximal intentions to flex among their causes, they cannot be *free* actions because the intentions have unconscious causes. If someone who makes this claim is presupposing that free actions must proceed from *uncaused* intentions, I would like to see an argument for the presupposition. (If, at bottom, a magical conception of free will is at work, an argument for the presupposition might bring that fact to the surface.) Is it being presupposed instead that an action is free only if it proceeds from an intention that has no causes of which the agent is not conscious? What recommends this idea? If intentions are caused, neural events of which we are not conscious are among their causes. Why should that be thought to prevent actions that proceed from caused intentions from being free? Perhaps the presupposition is that an action is free only if some of its causes are items of which the agent is conscious; and it may be thought that no conscious items are among the causes of conscious proximal intentions to flex in Libet's subjects. But if these subjects had lacked a conscious understanding of their instructions, they would not have formed or acquired the conscious proximal intentions at issue. Given a respectable conception of causation, a conscious understanding of their task does seem to be among the causes of their conscious proximal intentions.

## 4. PROBLEM 2: HOW IS WHAT HAPPENS AT –550 MS RELATED TO WHAT HAPPENS AT 0 MS?

Daniel Dennett echoes a common judgment when he asserts that the type II RP is "a highly reliable predictor" of flexing (2003, p. 229). Even if this is so, is the brain activity associated with, say, the first 300 ms of this RP—call it *type 300 activity*—a highly reliable predictor of a flexing action or even a muscle burst? In fact, this is not known. In the experiments that yield Libet's type II RPs, it is the muscle burst that triggers a computer to make a record of the preceding brain activity for the purposes of averaging. In the absence of a muscle burst, no such record is made of that activity. So, for all anyone knows, there were many occasions on which type 300 activity occurred in Libet's subjects and there was no associated muscle burst. Type 300 activity may raise the probability that a muscle burst will occur at about 0 ms without raising it anywhere near 1, and it may be at most a potential cause of such a muscle burst. Recall the subjects who reported spontaneously vetoing conscious urges to flex. Libet points out that "in the absence of the muscle's electrical signal when being activated, there was no trigger to initiate the computer's recording of any RP that may have preceded the veto" (2004, p. 141). For all anyone knows, type 300 activity was present before the urges were suppressed. And what is vetoed, rather than being a decision that was unconsciously made or an intention that was unconsciously acquired, might have been a conscious urge. ("Urge" was the spontaneous vetoers' preferred term [see n. 4].)

Some of Libet's subjects may interpret their instructions as including an instruction to wait until they experience an urge to flex before they flex and to flex in response to that experience. Another possibility is that some subjects treat the conscious urge as what may be called a "decide signal"—a signal calling for them consciously to decide right then whether to flex right away or to wait a while. It may be claimed that by the time the conscious urge emerges it is too late for the subject to refrain from acting on it (something that Libet denies) and that is why the conscious urge should not be seen as part of the action-causing process, even if subjects think they are treating the urge as a go or decide signal. One way to get evidence about this is to conduct an experiment in which subjects are instructed to flex at time *t* *unless* they detect a stop signal. (For a users' guide on stop-signal experiments, see Logan, 1994.) In this way, by varying the interval between the stop signal and *t*, experimenters can try to ascertain when subjects reach the point of no return. (Naturally, in most trials there should be no stop signal.) Perhaps it will be discovered that that point is reached significantly later than time W.

Time *t* can be a designated point on a Libet clock, and brain activity can be measured backward from *t*. My guess is that in trials in which there is no stop signal, subjects will produce something resembling a type I RP. In trials in which subjects react to the stop signal by refraining from flexing at *t*, they might produce averaged EEGs that resemble what Libet calls "the 'veto' RP" (1985, p. 538). Although there is a large literature on stop signal studies, I have found no reports on experiments of the sort just sketched. If I had a neuroscience lab, I would conduct the experiment.

Libet asserts that his "discovery that the brain unconsciously initiates the volitional process well before the person becomes aware of an intention or wish to act voluntarily . . . clearly has a profound impact on how we view the nature of free will" (2004, p. 201). Unfortunately, the bearing of Libet's results on the question whether people ever exercise free will has been seriously misunderstood. A striking illustration of this is provided by V. S. Ramachandran, who proposes the following thought experiment:

> I'm monitoring your EEG while you wiggle your finger . . . I will see a readiness potential a second before you act. But suppose I display the signal on a screen in front of you so that you can *see* your free will. Every time you are about to wiggle your finger, supposedly using your own free will, the machine will tell you a second in advance! (2004, p. 87).

Ramachandran asks what you would experience, and he offers the following answer:

> There are three logical possibilities. (1) You might experience a sudden loss of will, feeling that the machine is controlling you, that you are a mere puppet and that free will is just an illusion. . . . (2) You might think that it does not change your sense of free will one iota, preferring to believe that the machine has some sort of spooky paranormal precognition by which it is able to predict your movements accurately. (3) You might . . . deny the evidence of your eyes and maintain that your sensation of will preceded the machine's signal.

This list of possibilities is not exhaustive. Here is another. You might experience an urge to test the machine's powers; and you might wonder whether you can watch for the signal to appear on the screen and intentionally refrain from wiggling your finger for a minute or two after you see it. Libet's data definitely leave it open that you can do this. You might even display an EEG that resembles the EEG displayed by Libet's subjects in the veto experiment. Perhaps you hit on the imagined test because it occurs to you that (1) "Whenever you wiggle your finger, signal *S* appears a second before you wiggle it" does not entail (2) "Whenever signal *S* appears, you wiggle your finger a second later." (A brain event signified by signal *S* may be causally necessary for your wiggling your finger without causally ensuring that you will wiggle it. Incidentally, whenever Lydia wins a lottery prize, she buys a lottery ticket before she wins; but, to her dismay, it is false that whenever she buys a lottery ticket, she wins a lottery prize.) If you succeed in your watch-and-refrain attempt, you might have the further thought that *S* is a sign of the presence of a potential cause of a proximal intention or decision to wiggle your finger and that, even when that potential cause is present, you may decide not to wiggle your finger and you may behave accordingly. But if this is how you are thinking, then, provided that you are thinking clearly, you will not see the machine as controlling you. And, clear thinker that you are, you will neither be tempted to believe that the machine has paranormal predictive powers nor moved to "deny the evidence of your eyes."

I move from Ramachandran's thought experiment back to real-life experiments. Recall that EEGs (what Libet calls "the 'veto' RP") were recorded for subjects instructed to prepare to flex at *t* but not to flex then. The EEGs were back-averaged from *t*, and they resembled type I RPs until "about 150–250 ms before" *t* (Libet, 1985, p. 538)—until *time v*, for short. This is evidence that the brain events indicated by the segment of the type I RPs that precedes time *v* are not sufficient for producing a flexing—and, more precisely, that they are not sufficient for producing events that are sufficient for producing a flexing (that is, less distant sufficient causes). If (1) until time *v*, the veto EEGs and the EEGs for type I RPs are produced by neural events of the same kind, then (2) the occurrence of events of that kind is not sufficient for producing (events that are sufficient for producing) a flexing. For if 1 is true and 2 were false, the subjects in the veto experiment would have flexed.

What about type II RPs and what I called type 300 activity? No one has shown (*S1*) that type 300 activity is sufficient to produce (events that are sufficient for producing) a muscle burst around 0 ms. Nor has anyone shown (*S2*) that *S1* would be true if not for the possibility of a conscious veto. Those who believe that one or the other of these propositions has been shown to be true either do not realize that, in the experiments that yield Libet's type II RPs, the "muscle's electrical signal when being activated" is what triggers the computer to make a record of the preceding brain activity for the purposes of averaging (Libet, 2004, p. 141) or do not recognize the implications of this. How can we, on the basis of the data, be justified in believing that type 300 activity has the actual or counterfactual "sufficiency" at issue, if no one has looked to see whether type 300 activity is ever present in cases in which there is no muscle burst around 0 ms? The answer is simple: we cannot.[12]

## 5. PROBLEM 3: HOW ACCURATE ARE SUBJECTS' AWARENESS REPORTS?

Libet contends that subjects in his main experiment become aware of their proximal intentions well after they acquire them. His primary evidence for the average time of the onset of this awareness comes from reports subjects make after each flex—reports about where they believe the spot was on the clock when they first became aware of their decision, intention, urge, or whatever, to flex. How accurate are these reports likely to be?

The following labels facilitate discussion:

*P-time*: The time at which a proximal decision is made or a proximal intention or proximal urge is acquired.

*C-time*: The time of the onset of the subject's consciousness of an item of the kind just specified.

*B-time*: The time the subject believes to be *C*-time when responding to the experimenter's question about *C*-time.

Libet contends that average *P*-time is −550 ms for subjects who are regularly encouraged to flex spontaneously and report no "preplanning." And he arrives at an average *C*-time of −150 ms by adding 50 ms to his average *B*-time (−200 ms) to correct for what he believes to be a 50 ms bias in subjects' reports. (For alleged evidence of the existence of this bias, see Libet, 1985, pp. 534–535; and 2004, p. 128.) One connection in which *C*-time is important to Libet is his position on veto power. Whether subjects in Libet's studies are ever conscious of relevant proximal urges or intentions early enough to veto them, as he claims, depends partly on what their *C*-times are. The same is true of the question whether, on average, his subjects become conscious of proximal intentions to flex about 400 ms after those intentions emerge in them.

There is a lively literature on how accurate *B*-times are likely to be—that is, on how likely it is that they closely approximate *C*-times (for a review, see van de Grind, 2002). This is not surprising. Reading the position of a rapidly revolving spot at a given time is a difficult task, as Wim van de Grind observes (2002, p. 251). The same is true of relating the position of the spot to such an event as the onset of one's consciousness of a proximal intention to flex a wrist. Patrick Haggard notes that "the large number of biases inherent in cross-modal synchronization tasks means that the perceived time of a stimulus may differ dramatically from its actual onset time. There is every reason to believe that purely internal events, such as conscious intentions, are at least as subject to this bias as perceptions of external events" (2006, p. 82).

One fact that has not received sufficient attention in the literature on accuracy is that individuals display great variability of *B*-times across trials. Patrick Haggard and Martin Eimer (1999) provide some relevant data. For each of their eight subjects, they locate the median *B*-time and then calculate the mean of the premedian (i.e., "early") *B*-times and the mean of the postmedian (i.e., "late") *B*-times. At the low end of variability by this measure, one subject had mean early and late *B*-times of −231 ms and −80 ms and another had means of −542 ms and −351 ms (p. 132). At the high end, one subject's figures were −940 ms and −4 ms and another's were −984 ms and −253 ms. Bear in mind that these figures are for means, not extremes. These results do not inspire confidence that *B*-time closely approximates *C*-time. If there were good reason to believe that *C*-times vary enormously across trials for the same subject, we might not find enormous variability in a subject's *B*-times worrisome in this connection. But there is good reason to believe this only if there is good reason to believe that *B*-times closely approximate *C*-times; and given the points made about cross-modal synchronization tasks in general and the cross-modal task of subjects in Libet-style experiments, there is not.

Another factor that may make it difficult for subjects to provide *B*-times that closely approximate *C*-times is their uncertainty about exactly what they are experiencing. As Haggard observes, subjects' reports about their intentions "are easily mediated by cognitive strategies, by the subjects' understanding of the experimental situation, and by their folk psychological beliefs about intentions" (2006, p. 81). He also remarks that "the conscious experience of intending is quite thin and evasive" (2005, p. 291). Even if the latter claim is an overstatement and some conscious experiences of intending are robust, the claim may be true of many of the experiences at issue in Libet-style studies. One can well imagine subjects wondering occasionally whether, for example, what they are experiencing is an intention (or urge) to act or merely a thought about when to act or an anticipation of acting soon. Hakwan Lau and coauthors say that they require their subjects to move a cursor to where they believed the spot on a Libet clock was "when they first felt their *intention* to press the button" (Lau, Rogers, & Passingham, 2007, p. 82; emphasis mine). One should not be surprised if some subjects given such an instruction were occasionally to wonder whether they were experiencing an intention to press or just an *urge* to press, for example. (Presumably, at least some lay folk treat intentions and urges as conceptually distinct, as dictionaries do.) Subjects may also wonder occasionally whether they are actually *feeling* an intention to press or are mistakenly thinking that they feel such an intention.

One way to seek to reduce variability in a subject's *B*-times is to give him or her a way of conceiving of, for example, making a conscious proximal decision that is easily grasped and applied. Subjects in a Libet-style experiment may be given the following instructions:

> One way to think of deciding to flex your right wrist now is as consciously saying "now!" to yourself silently in order to command yourself to flex at once. Consciously say "now!" silently to yourself whenever you feel like it and then immediately flex. Look at the clock and try to determine as closely as possible where the spot is when you say "now!" You'll report that location to us after you flex. (see Mele, 2008a, p. 10).

Subjects can also be regularly reminded to make their decisions "spontaneously"—that is, to make them without thinking in advance about when to flex.

If, as I predict, subjects given these instructions individually show much less variability in *B*-times than subjects given typical Libet-style instructions, we would have grounds for believing that their reports about when they consciously said "now!" involve *less guesswork* and, accordingly, additional grounds for skepticism about the reliability of *B*-times in typical studies.

I asked how accurate subjects' reports about when they first became aware of a proximal intention or urge are likely to have been. *Not very accurate* certainly seems to be a safe answer. But there may be ways to improve accuracy.[13] If such *B*-times as have actually been gathered are unreliable indicators of *C*-times, little weight can be put on them in arguments about whether or not there ever is time enough to veto conscious proximal urges and the like; and the same is true of arguments about whether or not *C*-time is always too late for conscious proximal intentions and the like to play a role in producing corresponding overt actions.

## 6. PARTING REMARKS

Readers will have noticed that I have not offered an account of the concept of free will here. To do so would require more space than I have at my disposal. Readers interested in a full-blown philosophical discussion of the concept of free will and of the likelihood that we sometimes act freely may wish to consult Mele (2006a). Those who would prefer a relatively brief discussion of leading philosophical theories about free will, may consult Mele (2008b, pp. 326–330; or 2009, ch. 8, sec. 2). In my opinion, it is fair to conclude that, on any reasonable conception of free will, the studies and data reviewed here leave it open both that we sometimes exhibit it and that we never do.[14]

## NOTES

1. Elsewhere, Libet writes, "the brain has begun the specific preparatory processes for the voluntary act well before the subject is even aware of any wish or intention to act" (1992, p. 263).
2. For a defense of this conception of deciding and references to others who share it, see Mele (2003, ch. 9).
3. According to a common use of "readiness potential" (RP), it is a measure of activity in the motor cortex that precedes voluntary muscle motion; and, by definition, EEGs generated in situations in which there is no muscle burst do not count as RPs. Libet's use of the term is broader. For example, because there is no muscle burst in the veto experiment described shortly, some scientists would refer to what Libet calls "the 'veto' RP" (Libet, 1985, p. 538) as an "event-related brain potential" (or ERP) rather than an RP.
4. Libet and coauthors report that "the subject was asked to note and later report the time of appearance of his conscious *awareness of 'wanting' to perform* a given self-initiated movement. The experience was also described as an 'urge' or 'intention' or 'decision' to move, though subjects usually settled for the words 'wanting' or 'urge'" (Libet, Gleason, Wright, & Pearl, 1983, p. 627).
5. For a more thorough discussion of the experiment, see Libet et al. (1983). In Mele (2006a, p. 34), I explain that Libet implausibly describes what is vetoed here as "*intended* motor action." The subjects were instructed in advance *not* to flex, but to prepare to flex at the prearranged time and to "veto" this; and they intentionally complied with the request. They intended from the beginning *not* to flex at the appointed time. So what is indicated by the segment of what Libet refers to as "the 'veto' RP" that precedes the change of direction? Presumably, not the presence of an *intention* to flex; for then, at some point in time, the subjects would have both an intention to flex at the prearranged time and an intention not to flex at that time. And how can a normal agent be in this condition? (Can you have an intention to close this book as soon as you finish reading this note while also having an intention not to do that?).
6. Libet is inclined to generalize from his findings. He writes: "our overall findings do suggest some fundamental characteristics of the simpler acts that may be applicable to all consciously intended acts and even to responsibility and free will" (1985, p. 563).
7. Hereafter, the parenthetical clause should be supplied by the reader.
8. It should not be assumed that detecting the signal is a conscious event (see Prinz, 2003).
9. In a reaction time study in which subjects are instructed to *A* or *B* when they detect the signal and not to decide in advance which to do, they may decide between *A* and *B* after detecting the signal.
10. Notice that the interval at issue is distinct from intervals between the time of the occurrence of events that (indirectly or directly) cause proximal intentions and the time of intention acquisition. The instruction to respond to the go signal as quickly as possible, which is normal in reaction time studies, should be expected to produce shorter reaction times than an instruction simply to respond to it; but this has little bearing on the interval at issue. A *proximal* intention to flex a wrist is an intention to flex it *straightaway*.
11. In a study by Day et al. of eight subjects instructed to flex a wrist when they hear a tone, mean reaction time was 125 ms (1989, p. 653). In their study of five subjects instructed to flex both wrists when they hear a tone, mean reaction time was 93 ms (p. 658). The mean reaction times of both groups of subjects—defined as "the interval from auditory tone to onset of the first antagonist EMG burst" (p. 651)—were much shorter than those of Haggard and Magno's subjects. Day's subjects, unlike Haggard and Magno's (and Libet's), were not watching a clock.
12. One who deems a segment of what Libet calls "the 'veto' RP" (1985, p. 538) to match EEGs for type 300 activity may regard the matching as evidence that type 300 activity is not sufficient to produce (events that are sufficient for producing) a muscle burst around 0 ms.
13. Would subjects' conscious, silent "now!"s actually express proximal *decisions*? Perhaps not. To see why, consider an imaginary experiment in which subjects are instructed to count—consciously and silently—from one to three and to flex just after they consciously say "three" to themselves. Presumably, these instructions would be no less effective at eliciting flexings than the "now!" instructions. In this

experiment, the subjects are treating a conscious event—the conscious "three"-saying—as a go signal. (When they say "three," they are not at all uncertain about what to do, and they make no *decision* then to flex.) Possibly, in a study in which subjects are given the "now!" instructions, they would not actually make proximal decisions to flex but would instead consciously simulate deciding and use the conscious simulation event as a go signal. However, the possibility of simulation is not a special problem for studies featuring the "now!"-saying instructions. In Libet's own studies, some subjects may be treating a conscious experience—for example, their initial consciousness of an urge to flex—as a go signal (see Keller & Heckhausen, 1990, p. 352).

14. For a discussion of imaginary experimental results that would show that no one ever acts freely, see Mele (2009, ch. 8). A draft of this article was written during my tenure of a 2007–2008 NEH Fellowship. (Any views, findings, conclusions, or recommendations expressed in this article do not necessarily reflect those of the National Endowment for the Humanities.) Parts of this article derive from Mele (2009). I am grateful to Walter Sinnott-Armstrong for comments on a draft of this article.

## REFERENCES


Day, B., Rothwell, J., Thompson, P., Maertens de Noordhout, A., Nakashima, K., Shannon, K., et al. (1989). Delay in the execution of voluntary movement by electrical or magnetic brain stimulation in intact man. *Brain, 112,* 649–663.

Dennett, D. (2003). *Freedom evolves.* New York: Viking.

Gollwitzer, P., & Sheeran, P. (2006). Implementation intentions and goal achievement: A meta-analysis of effects and processes. *Advances in Experimental Social Psychology, 38,* 69–119.

Haggard, P. (2005). Conscious intention and motor cognition. *Trends in Cognitive Sciences, 9,* 290–295.

Haggard, P. (2006). Conscious intention and the sense of agency. In N. Sebanz & W. Prinz (Eds.), *Disorders of volition.* Cambridge, MA: MIT Press.

Haggard, P., & Eimer, M. (1999). On the relation between brain potentials and the awareness of voluntary movements. *Experimental Brain Research, 126,* 128–133.

Haggard, P., & Magno, E. (1999). Localising awareness of action with transcranial magnetic stimulation. *Experimental Brain Research, 127,* 102–107.

Hallett, M. (2007). Volitional control of movement: The physiology of free will. *Clinical Neurophysiology, 118,* 1179–1192.

Keller, I., & Heckhausen, H. (1990). Readiness potentials preceding spontaneous motor acts: Voluntary vs. involuntary control. *Electroencephalography and Clinical Neurophysiology, 76,* 351–361.

Lau, H., Rogers, R., & Passingham, R. (2007). Manipulating the experienced onset of intention after action execution. *Journal of Cognitive Neuroscience, 19,* 81–90.

Libet, B. (1985). Unconscious cerebral initiative and the role of conscious will in voluntary action. *Behavioral and Brain Sciences, 8,* 529–566.

Libet, B. (1992). The neural time-factor in perception, volition and free will. *Revue de Métaphysique et de Morale, 2,* 255–272.

Libet, B. (1999). Do we have free will? *Journal of Consciousness Studies, 6,* 47–57.

Libet, B. (2001). Consciousness, free action, and the brain. *Journal of Consciousness Studies, 8,* 59–65.

Libet, B. (2004). *Mind time.* Cambridge, MA: Harvard University Press.

Libet, B., Gleason, C., Wright, E., & Pearl, D. (1983). Time of unconscious intention to act in relation to onset of cerebral activity (readiness-potential). *Brain, 106,* 623–642.

Libet, B., Wright, E., & Gleason, C. (1982). Readiness potentials preceding unrestricted "spontaneous" vs. pre-planned voluntary acts. *Electroencephalography and Clinical Neurophysiology, 54,* 322–335.

Logan, G. (1994). On the ability to inhibit thought and action: A users' guide to the stop signal paradigm. In E. Dagenbach & T. Carr (Eds.), *Inhibitory processes in attention, memory, and language.* San Diego: Academic Press.

Mele, A. (1992). *Springs of action: Understanding intentional behavior.* New York: Oxford University Press.

Mele, A. (2003). *Motivation and agency.* Oxford: Oxford University Press.

Mele, A. (2006a). *Free will and luck.* New York: Oxford University Press.

Mele, A. (2006b). Free will: Theories, analysis, and data. In S. Pockett, W. Banks, & S. Gallagher

(Eds.), *Does consciousness cause behavior? An investigation of the nature of volition*. Cambridge, MA: MIT Press.

Mele, A. (2008a). Proximal intentions, intention-reports, and vetoing. *Philosophical Psychology, 21*, 1–14.

Mele, A. (2008b). Psychology and free will: A commentary. In J. Baer, J. C. Kaufman, & R. Baumeister (Eds.), *Are we free? Psychology and free will*. New York: Oxford University Press.

Mele, A. (2009). *Effective intentions: The power of conscious will*. New York: Oxford University Press.

Prinz, W. (2003). How do we know about our own actions? In S. Maasen, W. Prinz, & G. Roth (Eds.), *Voluntary action*. Oxford: Oxford University Press.

Ramachandran, V. (2004). *A brief tour of human consciousness*. New York: Pi Press.

van de Grind, W. (2002). Physical, neural, and mental timing. *Consciousness and Cognition, 11*, 241–264.

# CHAPTER 4

## Are Voluntary Movements Initiated Preconsciously? The Relationships between Readiness Potentials, Urges, and Decisions

*Susan Pockett and Suzanne C. Purdy*

### ABSTRACT

*Libet's data show that EEG readiness potentials begin before the urge to move is consciously felt. This result has been widely interpreted as showing that spontaneous voluntary movements are initiated preconsciously. We now report two new findings relevant to this conclusion.*

*First, the question of whether readiness potentials (RPs) are precursors of movement per se or merely indicators of general readiness has always been moot. On the basis of both new experimental evidence and an inspection of the literature, we claim that Libet's type II RPs*[1] *are neither necessary nor sufficient for spontaneous voluntary movement. Thus type II RPs are likely to be related to general readiness rather than any specific preparation for movement. This raises the possibility that the actual initiation of movements in Libet's experiments may have occurred much later than the start of the RP—in fact at about the time when the urge to move was reported.*

*Secondly, we report further new experiments, which replicate Libet's original findings for movements based on spontaneous urges, but not for movements based on deliberate decisions. We find that RPs often do not occur at all before movements initiated as a result of decisions, as opposed to spontaneous urges. When RPs do occur before decision-based movements, they are much shorter than urge-related RPs, and usually start at the same time as or slightly after the reported decision times. Thus, even if this third, shorter type of RP could be considered to relate specifically to movement rather than to general readiness, movements resulting from conscious decisions (as opposed to spontaneous urges) are unlikely to be initiated preconsciously.*

### 1. INTRODUCTION

In 1983, Benjamin Libet and colleagues reported an experiment (Libet, Gleason, Wright, & Pearl, 1983) whose results have proved so enduringly controversial that a quarter of a century later they are the inspiration for the present book. The experiment itself was relatively simple. Libet asked his subjects to watch a spot rotate around a clock face, while they made a series of spontaneous finger movements. After each movement, the subject was asked to report the position of the spot at [Libet's words and emphasis] "the time of appearance of conscious *awareness of 'wanting' to perform* a given self-initiated movement. The experience was also described as an 'urge' or 'intention' or 'decision' to move, though subjects usually settle for the words 'wanting' or 'urge'" (Libet et al., 1983, p. 627). This method of timing a subjective event, which is now called the Libet clock, was actually a modification of the "komplikationspendl" method invented a century earlier by Wilhelm Wundt (Cairney, 1975). Libet's big conceptual breakthrough was to compare the reported wanting or urge times with the time course of the readiness potential (RP), a slow negative-going event-related potential which had first been reported 20 years earlier by Kornhuber and Deecke (1965), who extracted it by back-averaging EEG off voluntary movements. Libet's now famous finding was that the subjects' reported urges, wantings, or decisions occurred some 350 ms *after* the start of the RP.

Since 1983, Libet and many others have tacitly assumed that (a) RPs represent the neural activity underlying preparation for movement, and (b) subjects are able to report accurately on the timing of their own urges/wantings/decisions to move, and hence have concluded that, because the RP starts before the conscious urge to move, voluntary movements must be initiated by the brain *before the subject is conscious of willing them*. The implications of this conclusion are so far-reaching that they are still being discussed, 25 years after the original experiment.

But is the conclusion itself justified? The experimental result—that RPs start before reported urges—has now been replicated in several independent laboratories (Keller & Heckhausen, 1990; Haggard & Eimer, 1999; Trevena & Miller, 2002). Given the validity of assumptions (a) and (b) above, the logic of the conclusion is impeccable. What remains questionable is whether or not assumptions (a) and (b) are valid.

Sections 2 and 3 of the present paper report some previously unpublished results of our experimental and literature-based approaches to the question of whether or not assumptions (a) and (b) are valid. Section 4 describes and discusses more experiments from our lab, on the question of whether urges are different from decisions. Section 5 puts the results in context with regard to their legal implications.

## 2. ASSUMPTION (A): DO READINESS POTENTIALS REPRESENT MOVEMENT-GENERATING NEURAL ACTIVITY?

Largely because RPs are extracted by back-averaging off voluntary movements, it is generally assumed that these waveforms accurately reflect the neural activity which causes voluntary movements, and no other neural activity. If this is true, then RPs should be both necessary and sufficient for voluntary movements. Section 2 begins by addressing the two-part question of whether RPs are necessary and/or sufficient for voluntary movement. It then considers the question of whether it is reasonable to assume that the start of the RP represents the initiation of a voluntary movement.

### 2.1 Are RPs Necessary for Voluntary Movements?

When one first begins to investigate the event-related potentials arising in the 2 s prior to voluntary movements, it rapidly becomes clear that not all experimental subjects generate RPs. As with many negative findings, the idea of trying to publish this result is soon overtaken by the realization that it would be far too easily rejected on the grounds that everyone can record RPs, so there must have been some technical inadequacy in the recording sessions where none was seen. An alternative approach, which overcomes this objection, is to look at sessions in which a robust RP definitely is seen, and ask whether or not all of the 40-odd premovement EEG epochs that are normally averaged to extract RPs from brain-generated noise actually contain RP waveforms.

We investigated this question by ignoring the dogma that it is impossible to see event-related waveforms in single trials, and scoring by eye 390 epochs of raw EEG recorded between the vertex (Cz) and a reference electrode at site POz, for each of 6 subjects. Each scored epoch preceded and was time-locked to a single finger movement. All movements for each subject were made during a single half-hour recording session.

Robust RPs were evident for all subjects when all 390 trials for that subject were averaged. By-eye scoring of individual trials revealed that for about 75% of trials, the dogma was right and it was impossible to tell whether or not an RP was present in the noise. But RPs are among the largest of event-related potentials (generally in the range 5–20 μV), and in our hands approximately 12% of individual trials definitely did show RPs. More importantly for our initial question, another ~12% of individual trials had low "noise" levels but almost certainly did not show RPs.

To investigate the possibility that the single trials scored as not containing RPs might actually have contained small waveforms buried in the biological noise, for each individual subject we averaged 50 epochs that had been individually scored as not containing RPs (panel A in Fig. 4.1) and 50 epochs scored as definitely containing RPs (panel B in Fig. 4.1).

Figure 4.1 shows that (i) the averaging procedure has reduced the noise to a similar extent in both panels and (ii) the postmovement event-related potentials are of similar shape and amplitude in both panels. However, there is a clear negative-going waveform starting approximately 500 ms before the movement (i.e., a type II RP) in panel B—and no similar waveform in panel A. This demonstrates that a significant subset of finger movements generated in this session by this subject were not preceded by RPs. The existence of these RP-free trials would normally have been obscured by the standard practice of averaging all available epochs.

One possible explanation for the lack of RPs in some trials is that the subject may not have been paying attention during those trials, to the extent that their finger movements could be considered automatisms rather than genuinely voluntary movements. No data are available either to confirm or deny this possibility, but subjects did appear to be paying attention and making voluntary finger movements throughout the experiment.

Alternatively, RPs might be more to do with expectation than movement, and in the RP-free trials the subjects may have been too occupied with some other decision-related process to do any expecting. This possibility is supported by the data in Section 4 below.

Whatever the reason, the overall conclusion from this simple little experiment is that RPs appear not to be necessary for voluntary movements.

## 2.2 Are RPs Sufficient for Voluntary Movements?

If RPs are not necessary for voluntary movements, are they at least sufficient? Again, the answer may well be no. Waveforms that look like RPs have been known for decades to occur before a variety of expected events that are not

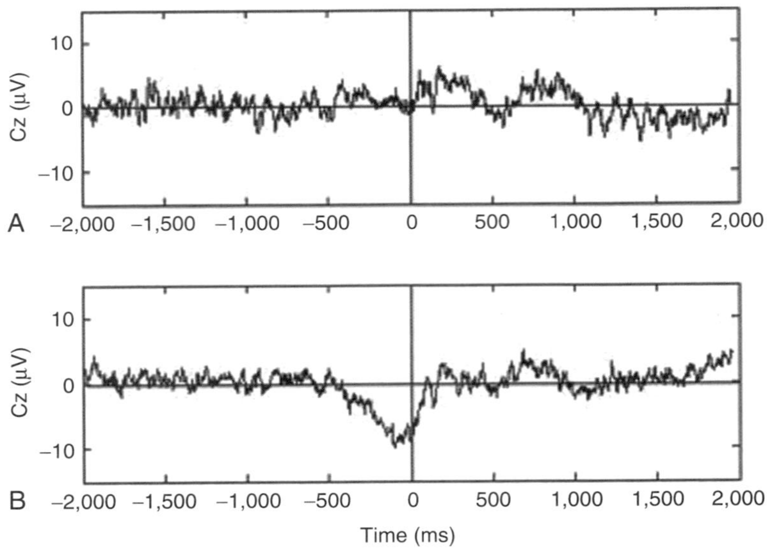


**Figure 4.1 Event-Related Potentials from Two Subsets of Trials in Which a Single Subject Made a Series of Voluntary Finger Movements.** Panel A shows the average of 50 single trials scored as not containing RPs. Panel B shows the average of another 50 single trials from the same recording session, scored as containing RPs. Finger movements occurred at time 0.

movements. Recent examples of the fairly extensive literature on this include papers by Mnatsakanian and Tarkka (2002), Brunia and van Boxtel (2004), Babiloni et al. (2007), and Poli, Sarlo, Bortoletto, Buodo, and Palomba (2007). Of course, such waveforms are not called RPs—that title is reserved for the slow negative-going potentials preceding a voluntary movement. Nonmotor RP-like waveforms are called SPNs (stimulus preceding negativities) or CNVs (contingent negative variations). The relationship between SPNs, CNVs, and RPs was well reviewed 20 years ago by Brunia (1988). One plausible reading of what is undoubtedly a complex situation is that SPNs and CNVs are produced when the subject is expecting or anticipating something, which means that if one is expecting or anticipating making a movement, it is quite likely that at least part of the RP generated before that movement will be essentially the same thing as an SPN or CNV. Hence it is reasonable to conclude that at least some components of the RP (possibly the earlier components, which are of course exactly those at issue in the Libet situation) are not sufficient for movement.

### 2.3 Does the Start of the RP Represent the Initiation of a Movement?

The overall conclusion from the arguments in Sections 2.1 and 2.2 is that RPs are quite likely to be neither necessary nor sufficient for voluntary movements. At best, this would seem to render somewhat insecure the assumption that the start of the RP represents the neural events underlying initiation of movement. But perhaps further light can be thrown on this issue by interrogating the imaging literature to see exactly what neural events are occurring at the time the RP begins. If these neural events occur in brain areas that are known to be specifically movement-related, the idea that the start of the RP represents the start of the movement might be considered to be supported.

In this context, there are two types of RP. What Libet called a type I RP, which appears when movements are preplanned, starts about a second before the movement. It is reasonable to assume that the early parts of this kind of RP might be underpinned by the generation of what have been called willed intentions, in the dorsolateral prefrontal cortex and presupplementary motor area (Pockett, 2006). However, activity in the midline supplementary motor area (SMA) has also been implicated in the early parts of type I RPs (Toro, Matsumoto, Deuschl, Roth, & Hallett, 1993; Praamstra, Schmitz, Freund, & Schnitzler, 1999; Cui, Huter, Egkher, Lang, Lindinger, & Deecke, 2000). What Libet called type II RPs (those exemplified in Fig. 4.1B) occur before spontaneous as opposed to preplanned movements, and start about 500 ms before the movement. Only movements generating type II RPs were studied by Libet, so these are the main target here. What brain areas are active 500 ms before a spontaneous voluntary movement?

Surprisingly, the answer to this question is not clear. Most EEG and MEG measurements put neural activity between −500 ms and the movement as occurring mainly in the contralateral primary sensorimotor area (MI), with some residual activity still going on in the SMA (e.g., Toro et al., 1993; Praamstra et al., 1999; Cui et al., 2000). On the other hand, combined MEG and PET recordings (Pedersen et al., 1998) claim that there is SMA activity in the interval from −300 ms to −100 ms, premotor cortex activity from −100 ms till the onset of the movement, and MI activity only from the onset of the movement till 100 ms after the onset of the movement. Perhaps the real situation more closely resembles that suggested by Pockett, Whalen, McPhail, and Freeman (2007), who conclude on the basis of decomposition of scalp RPs by independent component analysis that the neuroscientific "standard model," in which neural activity occurs sequentially, like billiard balls hitting one another, in a series of discrete local areas each specialized for a particular function, may be less realistic than models in which large areas of brain shift simultaneously into and out of common activity states.

Whatever eventually turns out to be the case, it is clear that the basic reason for the current uncertainty about what neural activity is going on around the start of the RP is related to the technical characteristics of the imaging methods that have been used. In general, methods that measure blood flow have excellent spatial resolution, but are hamstrung by the long (2–3 s) and variable time it takes for blood flow to a particular brain area to increase when that area becomes active. On the other hand, noninvasive electromagnetic measurements have excellent temporal resolution, but spatial resolution on the order of 20 mm, because of the large point spread function due to the distance between site of waveform generation in the brain and sensors on or above the scalp (Pockett et al., 2007). It is not widely appreciated that this distance is 15–20 mm, while the width of cortex generating most waveforms is 2–3 mm.

The spatial resolution of electromagnetic measurements can be greatly increased if the electrodes are placed either in or directly on the surface of the brain. Unfortunately, the few existing accounts of human intracortical recording that could have answered our question definitively have not reported enough detail about the timing of activity in the relevant brain areas to allow any conclusions. Rektor (2002) has recorded intracranial activity in subcortical as well as cortical structures and not unreasonably suggests that scalp-recorded RPs contain contributions from subcortical sources, but his published data do not contain the information needed to determine what brain structures are active specifically at 500 ms premovement. Shibasaki's group (e.g., Satow et al., 2003) have also recorded RPs from inside the skull, but again it is impossible to see from their records exactly what areas are active at 500 ms prior to their subject's movements. Clearly, subdural electrocorticographic (ECoG) measurements specifically aimed at these questions are vital to determination of exactly what brain areas become active (i) at the same time as the start of the scalp RP and (ii) at the same time as reported urges to move.

## 3. ASSUMPTION (B): WHAT ARE SUBJECTS ACTUALLY REPORTING WHEN THEY INDICATE THE TIME OF THEIR "URGES, WANTINGS OR DECISIONS?"

Are subjects able to introspect their urges, wantings or decisions at all? Or do they really infer after the event that, because the experimenter asked about their urge, etc., they must have had one—and it must have occurred a bit before the movement—which puts it probably about . . . there . . .?

Nisbett and Wilson (1977) review a large number of psychological experiments and conclude that, although humans readily answer questions about their thought processes, they are actually extremely bad at knowing how their own cognition operates. Subjects in the experiments described by Nisbet and Wilson were frequently unaware of the influence of external stimuli on what they did, unaware of the very existence of stimuli that influenced what they did, and even unaware of what they did. Their reports on their own cognitive processes tended to be based more on a priori causal theories and judgments than on true introspection.

Bearing these findings in mind, it is possible that Libet's subjects were not actually able to experience their own urges or wantings at all, but rather simply inferred or constructed these supposed events after the movement had happened. Indeed, one of the subjects in our replication of Libet's experiments (reported below) volunteered at the end of the experiment that he didn't think "people" (by which he meant himself) could tell the difference between wanting to move and actually moving. The fact that this particular subject's reports of the times at which he felt the urge to move and the times at which he actually did move were statistically indistinguishable tended to confirm at least his own inability to tell the difference. Others of our subjects did feel they could report accurately the time at which they felt the urge to move, but still produced results that were so variable that they were not significantly different from the time of actual movement. At first blush, this inaccuracy may be inferred to result from our decision to use totally untrained subjects (in marked contrast to the extensive pretraining of Libet's subjects). But Pockett and Miller (2007) report that similarly untrained subjects can use the same method to produce remarkably accurate estimates of when they actually do move. It thus seems to us likely that the variability in the present report may reflect the fact that it is actually not possible to introspect accurately the time of a hypothetical urge to make a spontaneous movement—or indeed the time of a definite decision to move.

In support of this hypothesis, experimenters in other labs (Lau, Rogers, & Passingham, 2007; Banks & Isham, 2009) have found that various experimenter-generated external events occurring after the movement influence reports of the timing of the urge to move. This suggests that subjects may be constructing their reported urge times after the event. However, there are alternative explanations for these findings, as discussed in the relevant papers.

Another relevant datum is that threshold-strength, direct electrical stimulation of the SMA does cause patients to report feeling an urge to move (Fried et al., 1991). However, higher intensity stimulation of the same areas invariably causes actual movement, so it is possible that downstream activation of the primary motor area by the low level stimulation might be the real correlate of the reported urges, or even that very small actual movements might be misinterpreted by the patients as urges.

In summary, it is probably fair to say that the suggestion that reported conscious urges are cognitive constructions rather than actual conscious experiences remains controversial. However, the assumption that subjects are able accurately to introspect their own urges, wantings, and decisions must presently be regarded as less than secure.

## 4. IS AN URGE DIFFERENT FROM A DECISION?

A large part of the importance of Libet's conclusion lies in its implications for the legal system. In most jurisdictions, a conviction for first-degree murder, for example, requires the jury to be sure beyond reasonable doubt of conscious intent on the part of the killer. If all so-called voluntary movements were found to be initiated preconsciously, either the law would have to be changed or nobody could ever be found guilty of first-degree murder.

How do Libet's experiments fit into this context? A priori, it seems clear that a previously mandated "spontaneous" urge to move one finger in a lab setting may not at all be the same thing as a decision to murder one's spouse in real life. Libet's original subjects' choice of word to describe their reports, as quoted in Section 1 of the present paper, tend to reinforce this difference. Given a choice between the words "urge," "wanting" and "decision", Libet's subjects usually opted for "urge" or "wanting." They did not feel that they were making a decision. But urges are ephemeral things, and perhaps of less relevance in most legal situations than definite decisions. We decided to investigate the specific differences between urges and decisions.

To do this, we repeated Libet's experiment, but compared the subjective time reports elicited by Libet's original instructions, which emphasized spontaneity, with those elicited by a new set of instructions, which were designed to eliminate spontaneity and focus all of the subjects' attention in the premovement period on a definite decision about which of two fingers to move. The new instructions required the subject to add two numbers, a different pair for each trial, which appeared in the center of the Libet clock. If the sum was odd they were to press one key. If the sum was even they were to press an adjacent key. After each trial they were asked to report the instant of their decision about which key to press.

In these experiments subjects were not given a choice of whether to report "urges", "wantings" or "decisions." In the trials emphasizing spontaneity, only the word "urge" was used—the words "wanting" or "decision" were not mentioned. In the decision trials the words "urge" and "wanting" were not mentioned: the subject was asked only to report the instant at which they *decided* which key to press. To eliminate any subconscious bias either on the part of the subject or on the part of the experimenter, only completely naïve subjects who had never even heard of Libet's experiments were studied, and no training sessions (where the experimenter might unconsciously have reinforced a desired result) were given. As a further attempt at achieving unbiased accuracy we also inserted an accept/reject step, so that immediately after each trial the subject had the opportunity to reject that trial if they felt they had lost concentration momentarily and had to guess their reported time.

Our hypothesis was that the experiments on spontaneous urges would replicate Libet's result, but in the experiments on definite decisions the reported instant of decision would be shifted back in time to the start of the RP. The results of these experiments are shown in Figures 4.2 and 4.3 and Tables 4.1 to 4.3.

The first problem we encountered is illustrated in Figure 4.2. Particularly for decision trials, the reported times between decision and actual key press usually (a) became markedly shorter as the experiment progressed and (b) included many responses that could best be interpreted as indicating a time *after* the movement had taken place. For some subjects it was not entirely clear where the cut-off should be placed in this latter regard—for example, given that the spot took 2.5 s to complete one rotation, it was not clear how to interpret a response that could either mean the decision was being reported to have occurred 2 s before the key press, or 0.5 s after it. Since our reliance on scalp-recorded RPs meant that at least 40 trials had to be averaged in order to extract a good RP from the noise, it was not possible to compare times and RPs for individual trials. (Again, the greater signal-to-noise ratio of ECoG would allow this experiment to be done much more effectively). We compromised by making three different estimates of urge and decision times: one uncorrected time, one time where any trials reporting a time earlier than 2 s pre-movement were simply ignored, and a third time where such times were rotated, so that a time of −2 s (i.e., 2000 ms premovement) was taken as +0.5 s (500 ms postmovement).

Table 4.1 shows the mean ± standard deviation of all three of these times, for both experiments, for all of the subjects. It can be seen that:

(a) There are substantial differences, in the expected direction, between the corrected and uncorrected times.
(b) The standard deviations are enormous. They do decrease slightly as the trial progresses, suggesting some training effect, but they are still high at the end of the session.
(c) Different subjects give different results. For example, the mean decision times were earlier than the mean urge times (as predicted by our hypothesis) for subjects SP and LF, while the opposite was the case for subjects RP, PS and MS.

The comparison of these reported urge and decision times with the start times of the concomitant RPs is summarized in Tables 4.2 and 4.3. Table 4.2 shows that the urge trials do indeed replicate the essence of Libet's result, in that for all except the first 40 trials of subject RP, the readiness potential starts earlier than the corrected urge times. Thus both Libet's original finding and the first part of our hypothesis (that the experiments on spontaneous urges would replicate Libet's result) are confirmed.

The second part of our hypothesis, that for decision trials the reported instant of conscious decision would be shifted back in time to the start of the RP, is addressed by the data in Table 4.3. Again it is obvious that different subjects give different answers.

Subject PS produced very long RPs (type I RPs in Libet's terms) and reported being unable to tell the difference between his decision times and his actual movements. For the other four subjects, the first 40 decision trials (before the decision was reported to have become automatic) produced either no readiness potentials at all (SP and LF), or readiness potentials that tended to confirm our hypothesis by starting at the same time as or after the reported decision time (RP and MS). However, Figure 4.3 shows that the latter readiness potentials were both smaller and radically shorter than the "normal" RPs recorded during spontaneous movements. Thus our original prediction was not entirely fulfilled.

Probably the most secure conclusion from these experiments is that the ERPs (event-related potentials) associated with decision-related movements are different from the ERPs associated with urge-related movements. This suggests that the early part of a standard RP may, as suggested in Section 2.2, be more related to expectation or readiness than to specific preparation for movement. In the decision trials just described,

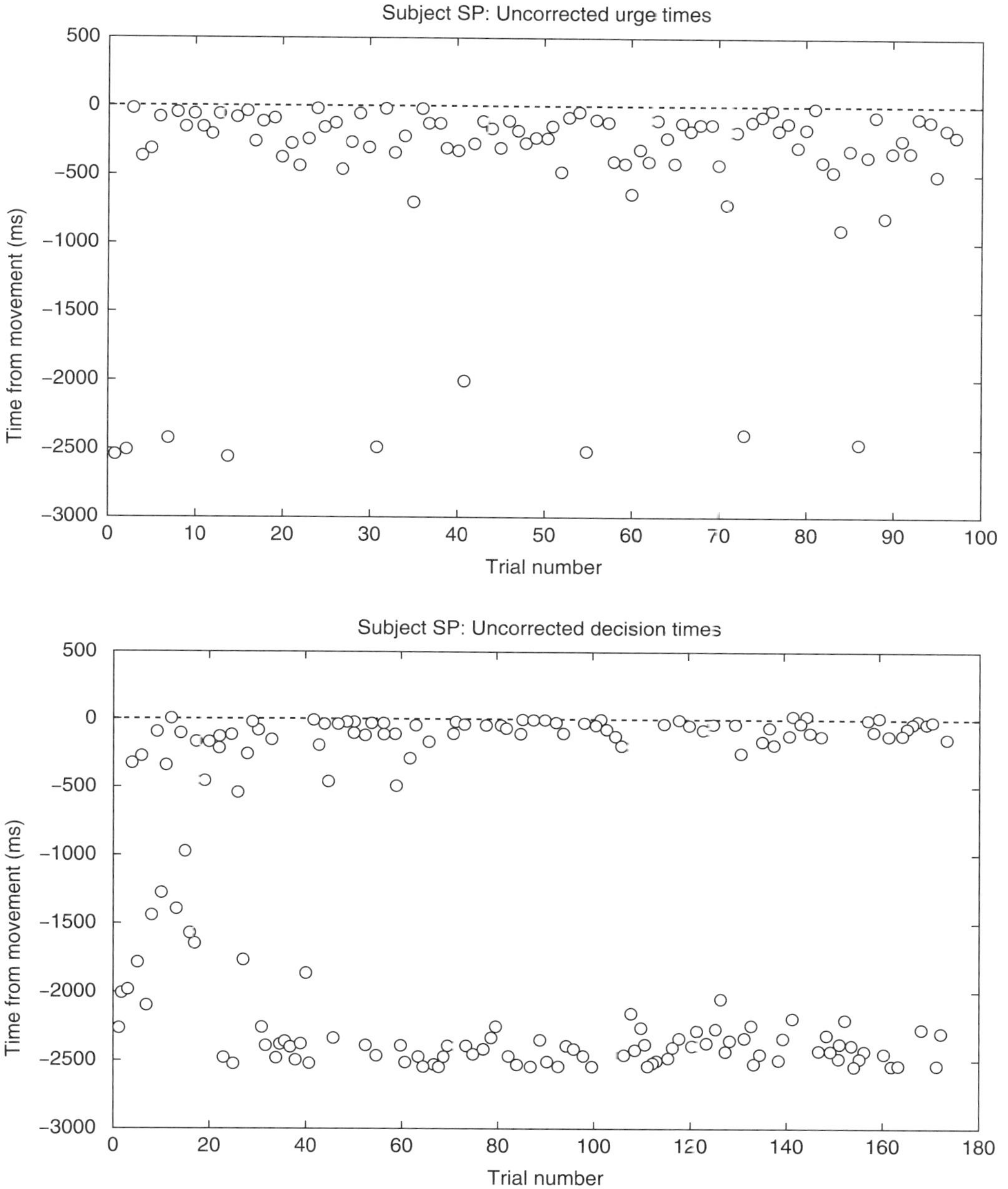


**Figure 4.2 Urge and Decision Times from Successive Individual Trials over the Course of One Experiment.** Top panel shows reported urge times. Bottom panel shows reported decision times. Keypress (movement) is time 0. Experimental conditions as described in section 4 of the text. Subject SP.

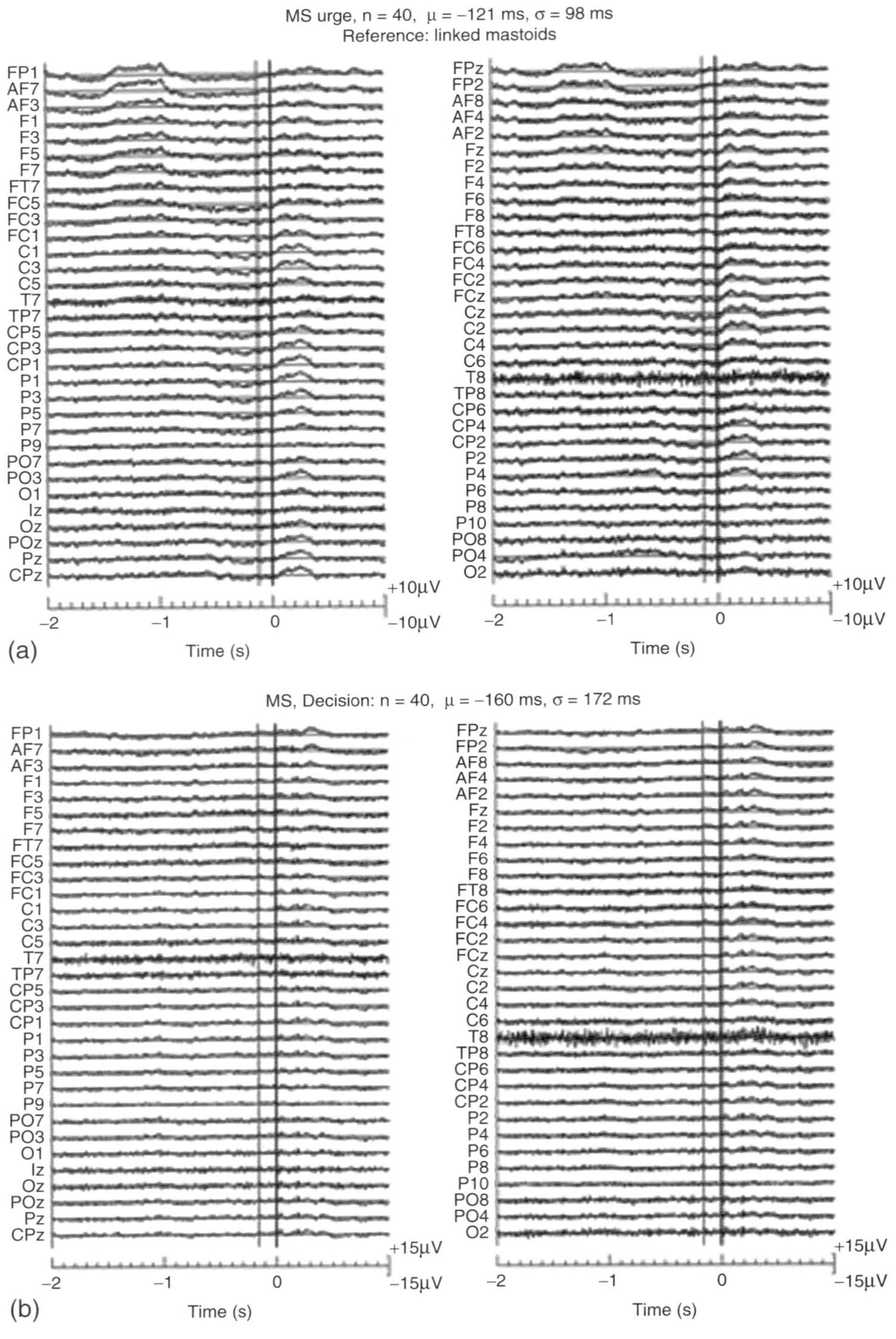


**Figure 4.3 Event-Related Potentials from Urge and Decision Trials.** Top panel shows ERPs averaged off movements for all 64 electrode sites for urge experiments—subject MS. Bottom panel likewise for decision experiments. In both panels, movements occur at time 0 (thick vertical line). Thin vertical line indicates mean urge time (top panel) or mean decision time (bottom panel). μ = mean urge or decision time, σ = standard deviation of mean urge or decision time. n = number of trials included in both the mean urge or decision time, and the averaging procedure generating ERPs. Note that: (a) in the bottom panel (decision experiments) there is no RP at Cz and the RP at $FC_4$ is much smaller and shorter than the RPs at either Cz or $FC_4$ in the top panel (urge experiments); and (b) mean decision time in bottom panel occurs at about the start of the shortened RP.

**Table 4.1** Urge and Decision Times for All Subjects. Raw, Ignore and Rotate are explained in the text.

| Subject | Mean Urge Times (±SD) (ms) | | | Mean Decision Times (±SD) (ms) | | |
|---|---|---|---|---|---|---|
| | Uncorrected (raw) | Ignore times>2s | Rotate times >2s | Uncorrected (raw) | Ignore times >2s | Rotate times >2s |
| SP | −435(±668) | −230 (±183) | −224 (±267) | −1309 (±1128) | −293 (±505) | −484 (±752) |
| RP | −500 (±474) | −427 (±275) | −429(±337) | −1207 (±1128) | −229 (±326) | −72 (±308) |
| LF | −360 (±704) | −126 (±83) | −97 (±131) | −905(±919) | −434 (+417) | −291 (±449) |
| PS | −443 (±822) | −121 (±75) | −96 (±97) | −1678 (±1115) | −106(±124) | +32 (±205) |
| MS | −277(±580) | −165 (±75) | −155 (±84) | −1010 (±1133) | −149(±137) | −63 (±164) |

**Table 4.2** Comparison of Mean Urge Times with Start of Rps at Central Midline and Left Prefrontal Recording Sites. Raw, Ignore and Rotate are explained in the text.

| Subject | RP Start 1st 40 Urge Trials (ms) | 1st 40 Urge Times (ms) | RP Start All Urge Trials (ms) | All Urge Times (ms) |
|---|---|---|---|---|
| SP | Cz −381 | Raw −480 | Cz −389 | Raw −435 |
| | FP-? | Ignore −190 | FP-? | Ignore −230 |
| | | Rotate −160 | | Rotate −224 |
| RP | Cz −356 | Raw −485 | Cz −920 | Raw −500 |
| | FPl -668 | Ignore −377 | FPl −793 | Ignore −427 |
| | | Rotate −357 | | Rotate −429 |
| LF | FCz −145 | Raw −403 | FCz −145 | Raw −360 |
| | FPl −127 | Ignore −130 | FPl −145 | Ignore −126 |
| | | Rotate −83 | | Rotate −97 |
| PS | Cz −1195 | Raw −592 | Cz −1846 | Raw −443 |
| | FP-? | Ignore −113 | FP-? | Ignore −121 |
| | | Rotate −80 | | Rotate −96 |
| MS | Cz −516 | Raw −441 | Cz −535 | Raw −277 |
| | FPl −975 | Ignore −144 | FP1 −967 | Ignore −165 |
| | | Rotate −121 | | Rotate −155 |

**Table 4.3** Comparison of Mean Decision Times with Start of RPs at Central Midline and Left Prefrontal Recording Sites. Raw, Ignore and Rotate are explained in the text.

| Subject | RP Start 1st 40 Decision Trials (ms) | Mean 1st 40 Decision Times (ms) | RP Start All Decision Trials (ms) | Mean All Decision Times (ms) |
|---|---|---|---|---|
| SP | ?? | Raw −1252 | ? Cz −158 | Raw −1309 |
| | | Ignore −517 | FP1 −166 | Ignore −293 |
| | | Rotate −484 | | Rotate −102 |
| RP | Cz −174 | Raw −815 | ? Cz −238 | Raw −1207 |
| | FP-? | Ignore-284 | FP1 −252 | Ignore −229 |
| | | Rotate −175 | | Rotate −72 |
| LF | ?? | Raw −1050 | ?? | Raw −905 |
| | | Ignore −519 | | Ignore −434 |
| | | Rotate −346 | | Rotate −291 |
| PS | Cz −980 | Raw −618 | Cz −1063 | Raw −1678 |
| | FP-? | Ignore −144 | FP-? | Ignore −105 |
| | | Rotate −106 | | Rotate +32 |
| MS | FC4 −135 | Raw −608 | Cz −121 | Raw −1010 |
| | FP1 −125 | Ignore −200 | FP1 −105 | Ignore −149 |
| | | Rotate −150 | | Rotate −63 |

the subject's attention in the time period immediately before the movement is completely taken up by performing the necessary calculations, so that they have no spare capacity to spend on anticipating the arrival of a "spontaneous" urge. In this situation, there were no early RP components—and often no RPs at all.

A second implication of the present results is that, even if one chooses to dispute the conclusion that RPs are associated with general readiness rather than movement per se, it may not be particularly valid to base any conclusions about the conscious or unconscious nature of *decisions*, as opposed to spontaneous urges, on Libet's experimental data. Decisions are different from urges.

## 5. SCIENCE AND LEGAL RESPONSIBILITY

Two different facets of criminal acts are important to the concepts of responsibility and culpability. These relate to the preplanning of the act and to its actual commission. We argue that Libet-type experiments are in principle relevant to only one of these.

### 5.1 Initiation of Criminal Acts

Even if RPs were strictly precursors of movement (which, as argued above, they are probably not) and subjects could reliably report on genuine conscious decisions to move (which, again as argued above, is doubtful), Libet-type experiments would only partly be relevant to criminal responsibility. If subjects are reporting on genuine subjective experiences in Libet-type experiments, the experiences they are reporting are conscious decisions or urges to *initiate* each individual action. All the long-term intentions and decisions, about whether to participate in the experiment at all and what movements to make given that one does choose to participate, have occurred long before the experimental trials are carried out.

Initiation of actions clearly is important in a legal sense, because although many crimes are premeditated, it is only when the preplanned sequence of actions is actually initiated that the crime is committed. It is perfectly possible to plan in great detail what to do (rob a liquor store), how to do it (buy a gun, borrow a mask, steal a getaway car, recruit an accomplice, construct an alibi), even when to do it, in a general sense (next Thursday night, when the takings will be maximal because Thursday is dole day)—but then never actually to get around to carrying the intentions through and committing the crime. When all the long-term planning has been done, there inevitably comes a point at which a criminal (or any other) act needs to be initiated.

If that initiation is the result of a spontaneous urge, Libet's results may be important. Acts predicated on spontaneous urges may well be preconsciously initiated. But if the act is initiated as the result of a definite decision, Libet's results may not be relevant at all. Our present data are less than conclusive, but they tend to show that a conscious decision to act may not occur after the start of the brain activity that is causal for the movement. On the contrary, conscious decisions may occur at about the same time as, or slightly before, the brain activity that initiates a movement. Notwithstanding all the caveats about the meaning of the readiness potential and the doubtful status of subjective reports, the implication here is that a conscious decision (as opposed to a conscious urge) might well be considered to be the immediate cause of a voluntary movement.

### 5.2 Preplanning of Criminal Acts

However, if we are seriously interested in the appropriateness or otherwise of retaining the word "conscious" in the legal requirements for culpable intent, it may be more relevant to consider not Libet-type experiments, but the experiments of Wegner and his many predecessors (Nisbett & Wilson, 1977; Wegner, 2002). There is a long tradition in psychology of evidence that the sort of early, preplanning decision discussed above—the sort of decision that is important for establishing mens rea—is itself far less accessible to conscious introspection than we might have thought.

Nisbett and Wilson (1977) and Wegner (2002) review a great deal of evidence to the effect that introspection of one's long-term motives, intentions, and desires is significantly unreliable. People readily answer questions about why they did things, but as often as not their answers indicate that they are actually inferring rather than experiencing their own motives—and indeed inferring them with little more accuracy than they could infer the motives of other people. Certainly we are sometimes accurately aware of our own intentions and motives—but then we are sometimes accurate about other people's intentions and motives, too. The critical point is that we seem to have little direct introspective access to the thought processes involved in our own evaluations, judgments and problem solving. We often do not know why we do what we do, that we intended to do it, or even whether we did it or somebody else did.

Thus, whatever the eventual verdict on the relevance of Libet's experiments, there may by now be enough data from other sources to render prudent the removal of the word "conscious" from the law relating to intent.

## ACKNOWLEDGMENTS

Thanks are due to Professor R. T. Knight (University of California, Berkeley) and Dr. Grant Searchfield (University of Auckland) for access to the EEG hardware used in the experiments described in Section 2.1 and Section 4 respectively. We thank Mr. A. V. H. McPhail for programming assistance.

## NOTE

1. What Libet called type II RPs start about 500 ms before spontaneous (as opposed to preplanned) movements. Libet concentrated on spontaneous movements, specifically instructing his subjects to avoid preplanning. Preplanned movements are associated with what he called type I RPs, which start about 1000 ms before the movement.

## REFERENCES

Babiloni, C., Brancucci, A., Capotosto, P., Del Percio, C., Luca Romani, G., Arendt-Nielsen, L., et al. (2007). Different modalities of painful somatosensory stimulations affect anticipatory cortical processes: A high-resolution EEG study. *Brain Research Bulletin, 71*, 475–484.

Banks, W. P., Isham, E. A. (2009). We infer rather than perceive the moment we decided to act. *Psychological Science, 20*(1), 17–21.

Brunia, C. H. M. (1988). Movement and stimulus preceding negativity. *Biological Psychology, 26*, 165–178.

Brunia, C. H. M., van Boxtel, G. J. M. (2004). Anticipatory attention to verbal and non-verbal stimuli is reflected in a modality-specific SPN. *Experimental Brain Research, 156*, 231–239.

Cairney, P. T. (1975). The complication experiment uncomplicated. *Perception, 4*(3), 255–265.

Cui, R. Q., Huter, D., Egkher, A., Lang, W., Lindinger, G., & Deecke, L. (2000). High-resolution DC-EEG mapping of the Bereitschaftspotential preceding simple or complex bimanual sequential finger movement. *Experimental Brain Research, 134*, 49–57.

Fried, I., Katz, A., McCarthy, G., Sass, K. J., Williamson, P., Spencer, S. S., et al. (1991). Functional organization of human supplementary motor cortex studied by electrical stimulation. *Journal of Neuroscience, 11*(11), 3656–3666.

Haggard, P., Eimer, M. (1999). On the relation between brain potentials and awareness of voluntary movements. *Experimental Brain Research, 126*, 128–133.

Keller, I., Heckhausen, H. (1990). Readiness potentials preceding spontaneous motor acts: Voluntary vs involuntary control. *Electroencephalography and Clinical Neurophysiology, 76*, 351–361.

Kornhuber, H. H., Deecke, L. (1965). Hirnpotentialänderungen bei Willkürbewegungen und passiven Bewegungen des Menschen: Bereitschaftspotential und reafferente Potentiale. *Pflugers Archiv fur Gesamte Physiologie, 284*, 1–17.

Lau, H. C., Rogers, R. D., & Passingham, R. E. (2007). Manipulating the experienced onset of intention after action execution. *Journal of Cognitive Neuroscience, 19*(1), 81–90.

Libet, B., Gleason, C. A., Wright, E. W., & Pearl, D. K. (1983). Time of conscious intention to act in relation to onset of cerebral activity (readiness-potential): The unconscious initiation of a freely voluntary act. *Brain, 106*, 623–642.

Mnatsakanian, E. V., & Tarkka, I. M. (2002). Task-specific expectation is revealed in scalp-recorded slow potentials. *Brain Topography, 15*(2), 87–94.

Nisbett, R. E., & Wilson, T. D. (1977). Telling more than we can know: Verbal reports on mental processes. *Psychological Review, 84,* 231–259.

Pedersen JR, Johannsen P, Bak CK, Kofoed B, Saermark K and Gjedde A (1998) Origin of human motor readiness field linked to left middle frontal gyrus by MEG and PET. *Neuroimage 8*, 214–220.

Pockett, S. (2006). The neuroscience of movement. In S. Pockett, W. P. Banks, & S. Gallagher (Eds.), *Does consciousness cause behavior?* (pp. 9–24). Cambridge, MA: MIT Press.

Pockett, S., & Miller, A. (2007). The rotating spot method of timing subjective events. *Consciousness and Cognition, 16,* 241–254.

Pockett, S., Whalen, S., McPhail, A. V. H., & Freeman, W. J. (2007). Topography, independent component analysis and dipole source analysis of movement related potentials. *Cognitive Neurodynamics, 1,* 327–340.

Pockett, S., Zhou, Z. Z., Brennan, B. J., & Bold, G. E. J. (2007). Spatial resolution and the neural correlates of sensory experience. *Brain Topography, 20,* 1–6.

Poli, S., Sarlo, M., Bortoletto, M., Buodo, G., & Palomba, D. (2007). Stimulus-preceding negativity and heart rate changes in anticipation of affective pictures. *International Journal of Psychophysiology, 65,* 32–39.

Praamstra, P., Schmitz, F., Freund, H.-J., & Schnitzler, A. (1999). Magneto-encephalographic correlates of the lateralized readiness potential. *Cognitive Brain Research, 8,* 77–85.

Rektor I (2002) Scalp-recorded Bereitschaftspotential is the result of the activity of cortical and subcortical generators – a hypothesis. *Clinical Neurophysiology 113*, 1998–2005.

Satow T, Matsuhashi M, Ikeda A, Yamamoto J, Takayama M, Begum T, Mima T, Nagamine T, Mikuni N, Miyamoto S, Hashimoto N and Shibasaki H (2003) Distinct cortical areas for motor preparation and execution in human identified by Bereitschaftspotential recording and ECoG-EMG coherence analysis. *Clinical Neurophysiology 114*, 1259–1264.

Trevena, J. A., & Miller, J. (2002). Cortical movement preparation before and after a conscious decision to move. *Consciousness and Cognition, 11,* 162–190.

Toro, C., Matsumoto, J., Deuschl, G., Roth, B. J., & Hallett, M. (1993). Source analysis of scalp-recorded movement-related electrical potentials. *Electroencephalography and Clinical Neurophysiology, 86,* 167–175.

Wegner, D. M. (2002). *The illusion of conscious will.* Cambridge, MA: MIT Press.

# CHAPTER 5

# Do We Really Know What We Are Doing? Implications of Reported Time of Decision for Theories of Volition

*William P. Banks and Eve A. Isham*


## ABSTRACT

*Is the moment of conscious decision (known as W), as timed by Benjamin Libet and colleagues, a measure of volition? We begin with an analysis of Banks and Isham (2009), which showed that W is time-locked to an auditory cue presented after the response. This finding implies that W is not based on an intentional move prior to the response but rather is inferred from the apparent time of response. We report a new experiment that shows that the perceived time of response (known as M) is also shifted by the same auditory cue that shifts W. The experiment also showed that the strength of the tactile sensation of pressing the response button does not affect the apparent time of response or the auditory cue. In a second experiment we found that judgments of another person performing in a Libet task show an effect of the delayed cue on M and W. In two final experiments we show that use of a digital clock gives results quite different from the analog clock most often used in these studies. Many inferences drawn from M and W reported from an analog clock need to be recon-sidered. Implications for theories of volition are discussed.*


Benjamin Libet brought the study of volition into neuroscience, when previously it had been the province of philosophy, jurisprudence, and theology. He asked a simple question about a simple act. The act was a free motion of the hand, and the question was, "When did you decide to move?" He knew that electrical activity in the brain would precede the action by 500 ms or more (Kornhuber & Deecke, 1965) and recorded this—potential known as the readiness potential (RP)—as his participants moved at a time of their own choice during a specified interval. They reported the time of decision (termed W) by noting the location of a spot of light moving around a clock face when they decided to move. This experiment provided the first precisely timed measurement of the moment of an act of will.

The results (reported in Libet, Gleason, Wright, & Pearl, 1983) ignited a controversy that has been vigorously debated through the 25 years since they were reported. The participants placed the decision 200 ms before the move. This time of decision was at least 300 ms after the brain potentials signaling an impending move had started. If the action, as indicated by the RP, began 300 ms before the conscious decision, then the act was unconsciously set in motion well before the reported time of the decision. The moment reported as the time of the conscious initiation of the action could not therefore be the cause of the action. While this is a trivial act, it opens many questions about conscious efficacy in volition. If we can be deluded in such an uncomplicated case, in which the decision should be transparent to the actor, we wonder the extent to which our ability to exercise conscious will is an illusion.

Libet's results were bound to draw attention no matter how they had turned out. If the conscious decision had been placed at or before the beginning of the RP, the findings could have been taken as showing that conscious will initiates the brain activity that generates the RP. This finding would have been gladly accepted by anyone hoping for evidence that consciousness does control behavior. Descartes would have been greatly pleased. Such a finding would be perfectly in line with his theory of mind-body interaction. The question this outcome would have aroused is the difficult one of just how mind can control a brain process. Now we know that the joy at this finding would have been short-lived. Subsequent research has put the RP as early as 1200 ms before the action (Trevena & Miller, 2002), and other measures of brain activity predicting the time of the action up to at least 7 s before the action (Soon, Brass, Heinze, & Haynes, 2008).

The same outcome could as well be welcomed by a monist, who believed that the one substance of mind was either all physical or all spiritual. The moment of initiation of the RP would be a single event, with awareness and the RP coordinated as they should be. The finding that the neural preparation for the move extends well before the beginning of the RP would also confound this position.

A third outcome could have been an inconsistent relation between W and the brain activity. An epiphenomenalist would not be surprised at the apparent lack of connection between consciousness and the brain. The moment of W, having roughly the same relationship to the brain mechanisms producing behavior as the smoke of a steam engine has to the motion of the locomotive, would have a coincidental, inconsistent relationship to the real machinery of the action. The resolution we put forward here also entails that W is only indirectly related to brain activity, but not because consciousness is epiphenomenal. Rather it is because we consider that W, for all of its intuitive salience, is theoretically bound to an overly simplistic model of volition and does not mark a significant event in a willed act.

The alternatives are of interest because they reveal assumptions about consciousness. The results normally found in this experiment support Libet's conclusion that the action is initiated unconsciously and not as an act of free will. The consequences of this conclusion for philosophy, where freedom of the will has been a closely argued topic, are clearly important. Consequences go beyond academic fields to the law, where culpability depends on intention. Free will must be assumed to assign blame for intentional acts. If actions are generated unconsciously, and free will is illusory, then it would be illogical to blame anyone for committing a crime.

As a further consequence, because the ability consciously to initiate actions is an essential property of self, the denial of conscious origination of action is a challenge to our sense of selfhood. The possibility opened is that we are not free actors with control over our choices in life. We are only conduits for unconsciously made decisions. Libet's one simple experiment has the potential to slip our entire self-concept from its moorings.

The consequences of Libet's experiment are not confined to free will. Conscious efficacy is also a problem. Even if we acquiesce to the determinist position that our actions are not free in any metaphysical sense, we might hold on to the proposition that they are nevertheless initiated consciously. The finding that W comes after the RP begins indicates that the initiation was not conscious. Our clear sense of conscious control of action also falls by the way.

If it turned out that there is no evidence that W marked a conscious component of the response, we could declare a solution to the problem of conscious efficacy—not a very satisfactory solution, however. It would be that conscious efficacy is illusory, and there is no problem to be solved.

## WHAT DOES W MEASURE?

The question of what W represents neurologically has centered on what brain event takes place at about the time of W. If some neurophysiological marker were discovered that coincided with W we would have found an important connection between conscious volition and brain activity. There have been a number of suggestions as to what W signifies. For a sample of them see the target article and commentary in the issue of *Behavioral and Brain Sciences* (Libet, 1985) covering Libet's findings. There are also suggestions about W in the special issues of the *Journal of Conscious Studies* (1999) and *Consciousness and Cognition* (2002) on volition in terms of the Libet findings.

The most plausible candidate for the origin of W is a cluster of neural events corresponding to W among those generating the RP. Researchers have searched for this cluster (e.g., Eagleman, 2004; Haggard & Clark, 2003; Hallett, 2007; Lau, Rogers, & Passingham, 2007; and Passingham, & Lau, 2006), but no single area or event can be confidently accepted. The supplementary motor area (SMA) seems to be activated when the participant attends to the intention to move rather than to the actual movement (Lau, Rogers, Haggard, & Passingham, 2004), but this effect of "attention to intention" does not directly implicate the SMA as the locus of decision. To draw this conclusion we would need to assume that the BOLD activity consequent to attention accurately identifies the area in which the decision was made. There is evidence that the SMA is active when there is conflict among possible actions (e.g., Nachev, Wydell, O'Neill, Husain, & Kennard, 2007). This activity could imply that the SMA was a decision center of some sort. The fact that the RP begins before activity in the SMA indicates that the SMA is not the initiator of the action but still may modulate it. That is not enough to support the hypothesis that the SMA is the decision center, or that it is the generator of a signal sensed as W.

A number of considerations suggest that there is no single generator of the decision to move, as measured by W. The organization of the act is spread out over time and involves many brain areas. The choice can be predicted up to 7 sec before the action by use of physiological measures (Soon et al., 2008). When W is assessed not by free response but by asking the participant whether he or she has an intention to move at various times before the action (Matsuhashi & Hallett, 2008), it is 1.42 seconds rather than the 200 ms found by Libet. Presumably in the Matsuhashi and Hallett study, if the urge was as yet too weak to be noticed early in the action, the probe would call attention to it. The intention would thereby be found earlier than with an unprompted response. This interpretation implies that, depending on the sensitivity of the measuring technique, the critical time for detecting W could vary over a wide range, and hence the brain area active around the time of W would not be fixed. The Soon et al. research opens the possibility that a decision point could be found within a wider range of time than previously imagined. In that study W was about 600 ms before the response.

Given the large variability in the time of W and the number of brain areas that are candidates for the origin of the choice, we question whether W corresponds to any neural event that is useful in analyzing volition. The origin of the choice of W could be some combination of demand characteristics of the experiment and folk concepts of mental causation. While finding a link between a psychological measure of W and a neural event would be an important scientific breakthrough, the neurophysiological analysis of volition and action can go on without any such link. To put it another way, there is no scientific reason to "save" W as a meaningful measure of volition.

Our own research into the nature of W (Banks & Isham, 2009) arose from questioning the presumption that W is a report of any event or decision that occurred before the response. Our motivation arose in part from the question of whether the idea of an "instant" of decision is coherent, and further, whether there would be a physiological mechanism for monitoring when we made a decision. The concept of an instant of decision seems to be drawn more from folk psychology of action than from neurophysiological considerations. The assumption that we know that instant derives either from the assumption that we have a mechanism to monitor internal brain events or from a Cartesian model by which the decision to act is made in a mind separate from the body and "clear and distinct" to the actor. It seemed more probable that the time of action was based on some observable event, such as the response itself. If there is no neurological signal at all before the response, participants must find some landmark and use it to infer or retrospectively construct W. If for no other reason, they do it to comply with the instructions.

If the time reported as the moment of decision is based on the response, we have a kind of reversed causal direction, but it is only an apparent reversal, because the entire episode is reconstructed after the fact. This reversed causality fits in well with the idea that perception takes place after the event, that is, it lags action, and the perceptual world is constructed from events falling in a period of 80 ms. Eagleman (2004; Eagleman & Sejnowski, 2000) proposed that the critical cue for judgment of intention is perception of the response. Their proposal has a broad range of applications, including the present one of judging W. Hallett (2007) may have been the first to make the explicit suggestion that the choice of W in the Libet paradigm is the result of retrospective inference.

We tested the retrospective inference hypothesis by manipulating the time participants thought they responded. The time of response itself cannot be manipulated, but the participant's perception of when it happened can be. We used a pushbutton as the response modality. When the button made electrical contact the computer emitted a "beep," ostensibly as a signal that the button had been pressed. However, the beep was deceptive. It was delayed to create the illusion that the response was later than it really was. If the perceived time of response is a primary factor in judging one's intention, a delay in the perceived time of the action would result in a delay in the reported time of W.

The alternative hypothesis is that W really does mark a time of decision that took place before the button press. If this is the case, W would be constant no matter what false feedback was presented. Of course, an invariance of W with the delay in feedback could also allow that W was reconstructed, but not from the apparent time of response, or that the false feedback did not fool anyone.

The method is described in Banks and Isham (2009). In brief, we followed the procedure outlined in Libet et al. (1983) to obtain reports of W. The clock was generated by MatLab and on each trial made two full revolutions at 2.6 s each. The participant was to respond at will on the second revolution. The electromyographic potential (EMG) generated when the finger on the button moved downward was also recorded.

Figure 5.1 shows W and the EMG as a function of cue delay. The effect of cue delay on W is strong and reliable, with $F(3,21)=9.05$, $p<.001$. The slope is −.77, that is, for every millisecond the response cue is delayed W is reported as being 0.77 milliseconds later.

If the report of W were exactly based on the beep, the slope relating W to delay of feedback would have been −1.0. If W were based on brain events prior to the response, the function would have had a slope of 0.0, the slope of −.77 might be interpreted as a sum of the illusion created by the beep and a constant W. However, if the beep were added to a response time based on a constant W, the slope would be unaffected. For addition of a hypothetical W to change the slope, it would need to have a different value for each delay. This point shows that the slope of −.77 rather than −1.0 is not evidence for an existing constant W. It is not an argument against it either.

A possible reason for the slope being −.77 is a form of the Stetson effect (Stetson, Cui, Montague, & Eagleman, 2006). This effect is an adaptation to events shortly following a response such that the perception of their temporal placement is shifted apparently closer to the response than it is. The repeated delayed beeps could have induced an adaptation that shifted the slope from −1.0 to −.77.

Further evidence that W is not based on an event that took place before the response is seen in the plot of EMG and W in Figure 5.1. The measure of EMG is taken at the beginning of the increase of the motor potential and marks a time when the response is underway. The response itself in our experiment came about 100 ms after the EMG. The plot of EMG and W in Figure 5.1 shows that for the cue delays of 40 and 60 ms, the response is underway *before* the reported W. There is no way that W, coming after the EMG, could mark an event that precipitated the response.

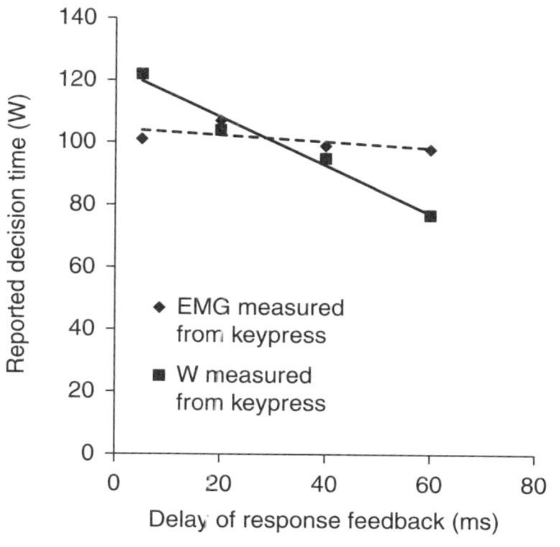


**Figure 5.1** EMG and W measured from keypress response.

A counterargument might be that W is slightly delayed from the real neural event that caused the response. Thus there could be a neural event that took place well before the EMG but was not reported until after it. However, this argument is not consistent with the shift in W with delay of the response cue. The hypothetical neural event invoked by this argument would need to shift with the cue delay, just as W does. Here again we have an impossible causal relationship because the cue delay is known only after the response and obviously cannot affect the prior neural event that led to the response. By contrast, the shift in reported W with the shift in the postresponse beep is not an example of temporally reversed causality. Rather, W is a retrospective construction based on the beep. The construction takes place after the response. If a brain event in real time were responsible for a decision point, that real event could not be moved temporally after the fact.

Another point made by the results in Figure 5.1 is that W is dissociated from the "action." That is the EMG marks the actual initiation of the response, but W is tied to the false feedback, not to the EMG, which is the first evidence for the initiation of action. This observation raises the question of what participants normally use as a landmark for inferring W. Normally there is no beep and the report of W must be related to something. By our hypothesis it is not an internal event. What is it?

One possibility is that kinesthetic or sensory feedback from the act of responding is the reference point for W. The hypothesis that kinesthetic feedback can control action moment-to-moment has been questioned since Lashley (1951) pointed out, among other things, that neural transit time is too slow to control action at the speed needed to account for observed action. In this case the amount of time it would take for the neural message signifying depression of the button to get from the finger to the sensory cortex is long enough to result in a large delay in sensing that a button had been pressed.

While the time for sensory and kinesthetic feedback to get from the hand to the brain is relatively long, some researchers have reported evidence for an effect of feedback on motor action (Obhi, 2007; Obhi, Planetta, & Scantlebury, 2009). To test whether kinesthetic feedback plays a role in control of action we used an experiment in which the button gave a strong, moderate, or weak tactile sensation when pressed. We compared three response buttons, from one almost too soft to feel to a very resistive button with a piece of the sharp side of Velcro glued to it. The intermediate button was the one used in Banks and Isham (2009). The force required to close the soft, medium, and most resistive switches was .022 N, 6.68 N, and 26.7 N, respectively.

Obhi (2007) had a similar manipulation. Rather than using response buttons giving different amounts of tactile stimulation, he had his participants press the button either softly or forcefully. The manipulation by instructions creates a component of explicit planning in addition to whatever feedback may result from the force. However, there is no reason to assume the same component is not present in our participants' anticipation of the button used on a given trial. We used the buttons in blocks of counterbalanced trials, and participants could have prepared themselves for the button used in a given block by planning to use different amounts of force.

We had our participants report M, the time at which they believed they pressed the button.

We used M rather than W because the M judgment is a direct report of the button press, while W may be influenced by other factors. Normally the report of M is between 50 and 100 ms before the response. Libet et al. (1983) and many others since Libet have found an error in M about this size. Why this systematic error? The button has an inherent lag because it makes contact only after they started pushing. This is not likely to be a cause of the misestimation in our experiments because the button made contact when depressed 2.5 mm, and button pressing reached that point well before 50 ms. Given the variety of experiments that have found approximately the same error in M, it seems unlikely that it is a result of physical delays in measurement of the response. Apparently all of the experiments measuring M used the Libet clock, and we will report experiments with a digital clock that give very different results.

Another difference from the Obhi experiment is that we used the same set of beeps as were used in Banks and Isham (2009) and are shown in Figure 5.1. Adding the beeps allowed a comparison of the relative effect of beeps and tactile feedback.

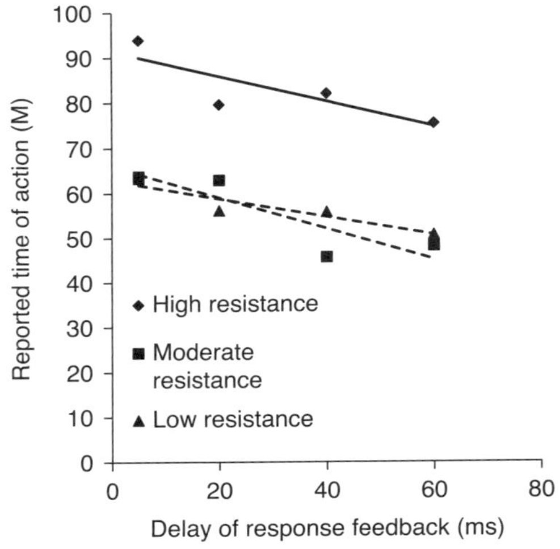


**Figure 5.2** Reported time of response for three different response buttons, plotted as a function of cue delay.

As is seen in Figure 5.2, the effect on M of the three buttons is weaker than the effect of the auditory feedback. The slopes for the three buttons were −.20 for the low resistance button, −.35 for the moderate button, and −.28 for the high resistance button. The intercepts, which estimate what M would be without any delay, were 63 ms, 66 ms, and 91 ms, for the low, medium, and high resistance buttons. The effect of the auditory cue delay was reliable, with $F(3,21)=7.39$, $p=.001$. On the other hand, the difference between the three buttons was unreliable, with $F(2,14)=2.48$, $p=.12$, and the beep delay functions for the three buttons were statistically parallel, $F<1.0$. The same conclusion we earlier made for W applies here. The dependence of M on an auditory signal that comes after the response indicates that M is retrospectively inferred. The additivity of the response signal and the type of response button could simply be a result of the lack of effect of the response button.

If the basis for retrospectively inferring W were the feel of the response button we would expect a reliable difference between the three buttons. It is possible that auditory cues were so much more effective than tactile feedback that the differences between the three buttons were overwhelmed. To be sure that tactile cues are not normally the basis for inferring M or W it would be necessary to compare the three buttons without any auditory cues. Obhi (2007) did find a reliable effect of force of response, with the soft response having an M of −136 ms and the forceful response −81 ms. However, his experiment had the participant push the same response button softly or forcefully, and ours had buttons with different resistances.

The effect of the auditory cue, while stronger than the tactile effect of the buttons, does not support the hypothesis that M is the sole basis for inference of W. If the report of W were based entirely on the perceived M, the slope of W plotted against the beep delay would be around −.35 (the slope for the middle button, which is the one we used) rather than the −.77 we found. Some measure other than M would have to be the landmark on which W is based. While this experiment does not resolve the question of the origin of W, it does show that M as well as W are affected by the auditory feedback and, further, that the tactile feel of the response button is weaker than the auditory cue.

Obhi (2007) found passive movements, those in which the participants had their finger moved by the experimenter, to have the same M as active movements made by the participant. He noted that this was consistent with M being retrospectively inferred from observation of the response, rather than from an internally generated neural signal prior to the response. The results we obtained with delayed auditory signals are supportive of the same hypothesis.

## OBSERVING RESPONSES OF OTHERS: "SHAM" EXPERIMENTS

We took a different approach to understanding the basis for the reported W in a series of "sham" Libet measurements. We showed participants a video we had taken of a person's hand performing in a Libet experiment. In these videos the hand was seen with the button we used in the majority of our experiments. Behind the hand the Libet clock was clearly visible. Participants were asked, in separate blocks, to report M and W for the person engaged in a Libet task. In another separate block we also asked for estimates of F, which is the time at which the feedback beep sounded.

Our motivation for running the sham experiments was to determine whether observation of the other's action led to the same estimates of W and M that were obtained from participants reporting W and M for their own action. If they were the same, the hypothesis that they were observing an action and reporting on it in both cases would be supported. Certainly in observing another person press the button, there would be no way of knowing W, and it would need to be estimated postresponse. However, if in the real experiment they did report a W based on preresponse events, then the estimate in the sham experiment could not be generated on the same basis as in the real experiment. It would then be a coincidence if W were the same.

Another interpretation of the results of a sham experiment is that the viewer has an empathetic response to the actions being viewed and bases judgments of these actions on the empathetic response (Frith, 2002; Wohlschläger, Haggard, Gesierich, & Prinz, 2003; Wohlschläger, Engbert & Haggard, 2003). However, the empathetic action argument could not apply to simulation of a conscious decision because evidence for it would come only after the act. It would be too late to simulate it. The participant could not be judging on the basis of an internally generated W.

Judgment of M is a slightly different matter. The execution of the response is a visible action and is seen in both real and sham cases. In the sham case, however, the actions leading up to the response could not be seen. If M is estimated in the range normally found of 50 to 100 ms before the action, then the same finding in the sham experiment cannot be attributed to efference copies or other processes that come before the action.

The participants were shown a few trials so that they could see the task being enacted. They were read the instructions that were given to our participants in Banks and Isham (2009) and asked to report M, W, and F. Only two participants objected to reporting W. They pointed out rightly that they saw only the hand pressing the button but had no access to the person's decision as to when to press the button. They were told in response that they would see "subtle cues" that tipped off the moment of decision. Having been told this they turned to the screen and began the task.

The results are shown in Figure 5.3. The slopes for W, M, and F, respectively, were −.48, −.27, and −.52. The slope for W is shallower than the slope we found with active participation. The slope for M is close to the −.35 we got with the same response button used in the experiment whose results are plotted in Figure 5.2. If judgments had been uninfluenced by any illusion, M would have had a slope of zero and an intercept of zero. Allowing for the usual misestimation of M, the intercept would have been somewhere in the range of 50 to 100 ms, but the slope should still have been zero. Accurate judgments of F, the beep, would have produced an intercept of zero and a slope of −1.0. There is no way of knowing what an "accurate" judgment of W would be, if accuracy even applies to this measure.

We had not taken judgments of F previously and were surprised at the error obtained for an auditory signal that is not itself a product of the

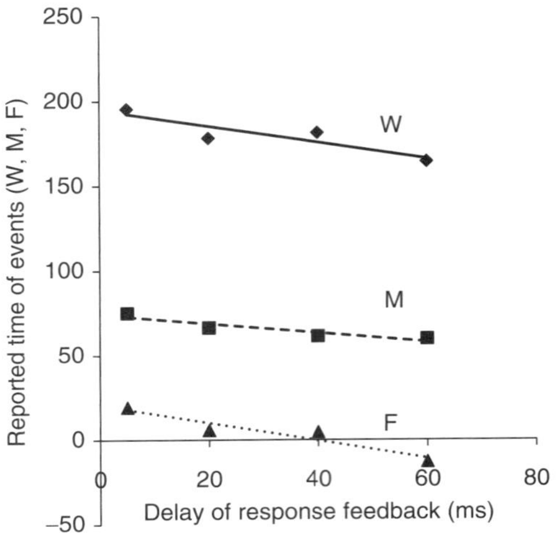


**Figure 5.3** Judgments of W, M, and F based on passively viewing a hand performing the Libet et al. (1983) judgment task.

participant's response. However, if F is perceived as the time of response such an error is to be expected. This error in location of F is confirmation that the beep alters the apparent time of response, as we have been assuming. The slope and intercept of the M participants estimated from viewing the sham experiment is close to what we obtained when participants were actively responding. This finding gives support for the position that participants are doing something similar in observing the action of others and their own. The slope of W could be less for observing than acting for several reasons. The parallel W, M, and F functions suggest that some common process underlies the functions. It could be that W and M are both determined by perception of the beep, and thus both are roughly parallel to F.

In another measurement of the sham W, we did not use a beep but simply had participants estimate the W for the person depicted in the video. Their estimates averaged 220 ms, which is close to the 195 ms intercept in this experiment, the intercept being the best estimate of what W would have been with no beep.

We had thought this sham experiment would give a measure of what people thought W was on the basis of folk theories of volition. They would base their judgment on how they think action is related to the decision and apply it to the judgment of another's action as they would to their own. We think this alternative hypothesis could be tested by giving the observer a competing motor task to perform during the observation. Such a competing task should suppress the empathetic response and produce a very different response or become extremely variable (c.f., Häberle, Schütz-Bosbach, Laboissière, & Prinz, 2008). If it turns out that the competing task causes the estimates to change greatly, that would be evidence that an empathetic response was involved in the estimate. If it turns out that attributions of intention to the person whose hand is visible in the video are not affected by the competing task, our premise that the judgment of W is based on intuitive theories of action would be supported.

## THE ISSUE OF THE CLOCK

One line of questioning about the late entry of conscious decision in the process of acting concerns the accuracy of measuring W with the moving dot method, otherwise known as the Libet clock. Could there be consistent errors in the reading of the clock? These errors might shift the reported W to a point that might either complicate or simplify and rationalize the interpretation of W.

Banks and Pockett (2007) surveyed a range of possible systematic errors in reading the clock. For example, there is the attentional problem in switching attention from the action to the position of the spot on the clock and back. They concluded that most possible errors in using the spot to note the time would be too small to make a meaningful difference in W and that others required assumptions difficult or impossible to test. Some of these possible errors would bias the report in one direction and some in the other. Some of these errors could even cancel each other out. Pockett and Miller (2007) experimentally tested and rejected seven possible factors that would significantly challenge the accuracy of the Libet clock method. In a review of the literature, Haggard (2005) concluded that Libet's clock "appears to offer one of the few viable methods for experimental studies of awareness of action."

Despite the confidence researchers seem to have in the Libet clock, there are persistent doubts. We decided that the best way to test these was to use an entirely different clock. We compared the Libet clock with a digital clock. The digital clock does not have the physical motion that is a major complaint about the Libet clock. We programmed the digital clock in MATLAB and showed the numbers on the same screen we used for the Libet clock. This digital clock presented two-digit numbers in sequence at 90 ms each. We also had the same clock but with the numbers presented in a random order. A random sequence of numbers does not allow the participant to make systematic errors based on guesses about the sequence.

The results are seen in Figures 5.4 and 5.5. Figure 5.4 shows the values of M found with the different clocks. As is seen, they vary considerably with the method of measurement. Figure 5.4 shows M as reported by use of each of the three clocks. The Libet clock gives the typical result, an M that is earlier than the button press. Surprisingly, the digital clock with the numbers in proper order gives an M that follows the button press by 60 ms. The randomized numerical clock gave an M that followed the button press by only 20 ms.

The report of M does not fall in the −50 to −100 ms range with the digital clock. Instead, the report of M changed reliably with the types of clock used, $F(2,20) = 4.919$, $p = .018$. The most interesting aspect of the data is the obvious fact that the judgment of M moves from a region prior to the actual response to one after it when the measurement is switched from the Libet clock to the digital clock. Post-hoc comparisons between each of these three clocks and time of keypress response show that reports of M for the Libet clock ($p = .036$) and the numeric clock ($p = .029$) are reliably different from the time of keypress, whereas the report of M in the randomized clock is not significantly different from the time of actual press, $p = .729$. This shift suggests that the error in M normally observed cannot be confidently attributed to the operation of the motor system. For example, neither feedback nor a feed-forward efferent copy need be assumed as an explanation of the usual error of estimating that M comes before the response (Obhi, 2007; Obhi et al., 2009). It seems unlikely that the differences between the clocks would

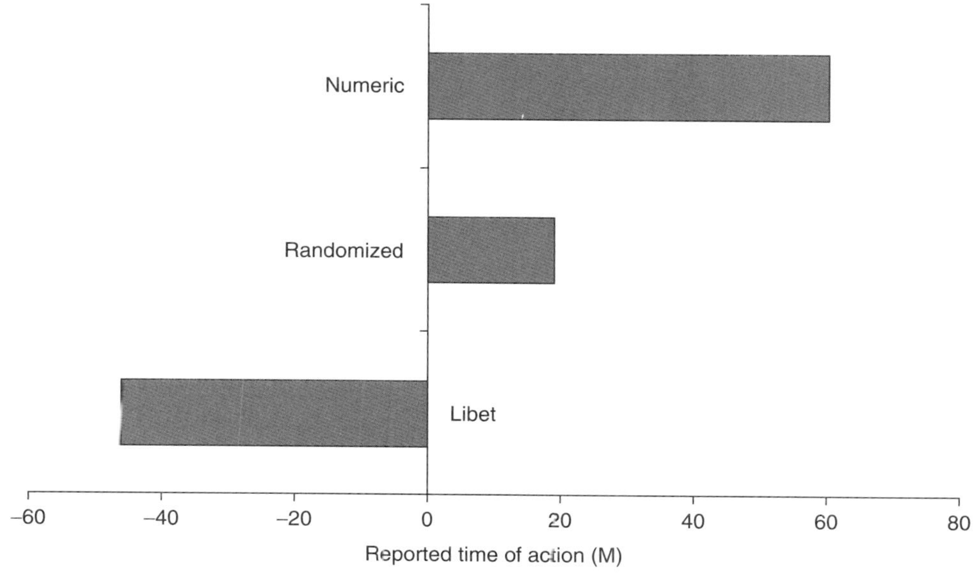


**Figure 5.4** Reports of M (time of pressing the button) based on the analog clock of Libet, a digital clock in which the numbers are presented in numerical order, and a digital clock identical to the other one except that the numbers are presented in random order.

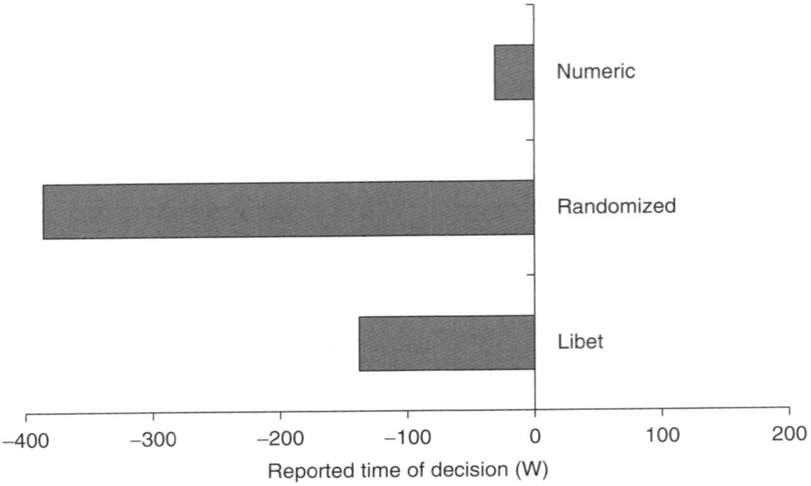


**Figure 5.5** Reports of W based on reading the three clocks reported in Figure 5.4.

come from differences in the motor systems. It is much more likely that the analog Libet clock and the digital clocks have different perceptual properties. The differences in results for the two kinds of clock are problematic for any theory of motor response based on M.

Figure 5.5 shows the result when W is estimated with the three clocks. Here we have a very different result. All three clocks yield a W that is prior to the response. The result with the Libet clock is in the normal range at −138 ms. The two digital clocks produced very different reports of W. The randomized digital clock gave a W of −385 ms and the digital clock in numerical order gave a W of −30 ms. The three clocks are reliably different from one another $F(2,8)=10.631$, $p=.006$. The three clocks all produced Ws prior to the response. The Soon et al. (2008) experiment also had a very large W, and they used a clock somewhat like our randomized clock. Their clock was alphabetic and unordered. It was presented at a 500 ms rate rather than our 90 ms rate, and reporting was by multiple choice among letters that could have been in view when W was reported. Their W was 625 ms (estimated from Soon et al., supplemental materials, Figure 1). The differences in reporting technique make this similarity to our finding all the more credible. However, as in the case of M, we have no way of knowing which, if any, of these Ws is "correct." If our theory of the generation of W is correct the concept of "correct" is not meaningful.

## GENERAL DISCUSSION

The findings of Libet et al. led to much concern and speculation about the meaning of W. It was intended to be a measure of the conscious moment of decision to act. The face validity of this measure is good. Participants know what is meant. Not one participant in our experiments has ever questioned the instruction to note the time when they made the decision. People in general accept that a decision to act must come at some time and that we know that time. When we learn that the brain had been preparing for the decision 300 ms to several seconds before the time that seems right as the moment of decision, our clear and distinct self-perceptions are brought uncomfortably into question.

The research we conducted adds to the discomfort. A delayed auditory signal that deceptively indicated the moment of response was able to move W later in time. Thus, W is not even fixed as an event somehow related to the mental or physiological activity that is involved in the response. While W moves forward with the beep, the EMG, which measures the beginning of the muscular response, does not. At the longer delays W comes *after* the EMG. The intuitively clear moment of decision then seems more like an afterthought, having no relation to the real action. It's enough to drive one to embrace epiphenomenalism!

The experiment reported in Figure 5.2 began as an attempt to see what aspect of the response is used as a landmark for W. It turned out, first, that the perception of response time (M) can also be moved by a deceptive auditory cue and, second, that the degree of force needed to close the response button was ineffective in influencing the perceived time of response or in modifying the effect of the auditory cue. Because the seemingly concrete act of pressing a button (M) is also shifted in time when a deceptive cue is present, it seems to be a reconstruction after the act rather than a report of what came before it. Obhi (2007) also mentioned that his effects on M were consistent with a post-response construction of the event.

In the sham experiment participants estimated W and M for the video of another person's hand pressing the button. Our intention was to use this as a test of the hypothesis that the report of W is based on an intuitive model of volition people apply to others as well as themselves. If they use the same model for others that they use for themselves, then they should give approximately the same reports of W and M in both cases. This is predicted because, if reports of their own actions come from observations of what their body is doing, they should be the same when observing others. The alternative hypothesis is that the reports of their own actions really are reports of internal events and would not translate to observations of others.

This is a hypothesis whose test is asymmetrical. If the sham and real estimates agree, there are several hypotheses besides our own that would explain the agreement. If the sham resulted in very different values for M and W, or if the sham estimates were extremely variable and inconsistent across participants, then our hypothesis that we apply an intuitive model to our own behavior as well as that of others would be rejected. Such an outcome would be consistent with Libet's assumption that participants' reports of W are reports of an internal event, and certainly not observations of their own behavior.

The sham results were close to results obtained from self-report and thus did not discriminate among several different theories of observational judgments. One alternative theory in particular is that people have an empathetic response when observing the actions of others (Frith, 2002), and the participants report on the basis of this simulation. We note, however, that the time W supposedly took place is before anything is observed and must be inferred from the action. It would seem that retrospective construction may happen in empathetic simulation as well as in self-reports.

The sham experiment also had participants estimate F, the time of the auditory signal. It appears that there is reciprocal influence here. Just as the signal affects the report of W and M, the actions affect the report of F. The result may be a blended multisensory perception. That is, the signal and the response become a single perceptual event. The parallelism of the functions in Figure 5.3 suggests that participants are reporting numbers based on a single event at each delay. We have found similar effects in judgments of real responses rather than the observational ("sham") actions reported here. The effects in Figure 5.3 are not specific to judgments of the actions of others.

Considerable research may be needed to outline the process involved in creating the parallel functions. There are a number of mysteries here. One is why M and W are parallel, when M is a report of an observable action, and W is not, and may be only a folk-concept.

Figures 5.4 and 5.5 show a set of findings we are currently extending. While many researchers have discussed artifacts that may be created by the type of clock Libet used, no one to our knowledge has used a completely different sort of clock in order to check the readings derived from the Libet clock. The results we report here show surprising differences between a digital clock and the Libet analog clock. If these results prove general across different sorts of digital clocks many conclusions will need to be revisited.

The Libet measurements have led to much discussion about their implications for philosophical theories of volition. One of these is the Causal Theory of Action (CTA; see Davidson, 1963;

Pacherie, 2008). The CTA defines an action on the basis of the intention that motivated it. Thus waving away a flying insect and calling to a friend may involve exactly the same action, but they are different acts because of their volitional history. Our concern with the CTA is that it depends on our having a formed intention that is prior to the act. If in the case of W we infer our intention from the act, the basis for the CTA is lost. While the Libet measurement is of a momentary and tightly constrained action, there are other sources of evidence (see Wegner, 2002, 2003, for example) that actions involving more complex putative intentions also subject to the same suspicion: Did the intention inform the action, or was the intention inferred from the action? At the very least these considerations would cause us to ask for more than a subjective report of intention on which to ground the CTA. It relies on an accurate epistemology of personal volition. Given the unreliability and malleability of introspective report, we think the CTA would require some analysis from psychological experiments on self-report such as ours.

Pacherie (2006, 2008) has an analysis of the phenomenology of volition that may help us sort out the ways in which the Libet measurements, our own findings, and research of the type performed by Wegner (2002, 2003) bear on such questions as freedom of will and intention. Philosophers have divided intentional acts into two components. Searle (2001), for example, distinguishes between prior intentions and intentions-in-action. Bratman (1987), Brand (1984), and Mele (1992; 2009) also make distinctions between two levels of intention, these being more general intentions and concrete ones that are expressed in the action itself. The more general ones precede action and may contain components beyond the action in question.

Pacherie divides volition into three categories. What she calls D-intentions, or distal intentions, are plans that extend into the next few minutes or the next few years. The specific actions may be only sketches, or may be planned only when the time comes to execute them. Proximal intentions, or P-intentions, are concerned with putting a plan derived from D-intentions into effect in a given situation. These are more concrete than D-intentions, but they do not specify every muscular component of the act. M-intentions are motor intentions, which are expressed in the action itself, and which are not accessible to consciousness except perhaps in their effects. A reasonable account of the Libet experimental procedure in these terms is that the D-intention is enacted at the beginning of the session. This is the overriding intentional framework for performance. In this sense, an intention to act exists throughout the experiment, not just at the time the motion is made. This intention includes the specification that at some moment the act will be executed. We know of no account of how this moment is chosen. However it is generated, all evidence points to the moment termed W as being much later than the inception of the process that leads to the action. Finally, the M-intentions are the motor programs that carry out the action. We can be conscious of the guidance and corrections in performing the action, but the lower-level muscular actions are not accessible. We don't know the delicate mechanisms that allow us to hold a teacup level so as not to spill, but we monitor the action and have some degree of control over it. Our knowledge of activity at the M-intention level has definite limits. Just consider how hard it is to remember which specific motions will cause pain in a sprained muscle.

Where is W in this scheme? The results reported in Banks and Isham suggest that W may be based on some aspect of monitoring. The shift in reported W can come both from hearing a deceptive auditory response signal and from viewing a delayed visual image of the hand pressing the response button. Such generality implies that the monitoring is done in a perceptual representation of the overall action, not muscular activity or brain activity that precedes the action. The fact that W can be *after* the EMG associated with executing the action renders dubious the idea that it is involved in the cause of the action.

Monitoring the execution of the action is consistent with the time W is reported. If it were involved with the early preparation of the action, it should be a second or more before the act. Another possibility is that W's time is influenced by an intuitive sense of when it ought to be, given the task and the situation. The intuitive model would be that W must come before the action, but not so long before that we would initiate the action and then absurdly have time to wait for it to happen. Such considerations would require W to be close to the range, or just beyond the range, of the perceptual moment of the action. If events within an approximately 100 ms window are integrated into a single perceptual event (see Eagleman, 2004, and Eagleman & Sejnowski, 2000), then a W of about 200 ms before the apparent moment of action would be reasonable. The longer Ws found with different measuring procedures could come from implicit changes in the assumptions in the task. Differences could also come from strictly perceptual effects, as in the results found with the digital clock in the measurements we report here.

The psychological, philosophical, and phenomenological discussions of intention and action, including our own, glibly bypass the central question of how a conscious intention can result in a real action, one that involves muscular activity and an expenditure of energy. We assume conscious efficacy but have no idea of how it works. Is this yet another elephant in the living room that no one is talking about?

In place of a theory that might explain conscious efficacy we seem to have intuitive models based on folk concepts of physical causality. Just as hitting a ball causes it to move, the idea of acting causes a muscle to move. Of course, the analogy is inaccurate. In the physical case we have transfer of kinetic energy from one object to another. In the case of mental causation we have mental processes setting something into action. We know that much of the process is not conscious, so introspection may be no help at all. There is no transfer of energy. A control process might be a better analogy, but we still don't know how it works.

Once we have a neurophysiological model of conscious causation, we may see our theories of volition go the way of theories of memory when brain mechanisms of memory began to be understood. The discovery of the role of the hippocampus and related structures caused a sea change in memory, a tsunami that swept interference theory away and changed even the questions we ask.

## REFERENCES


Banks, W. P. (Ed.). (2002). On timing relations between brain and world. *Consciousness and Cognition, 11*(2).

Banks, W. P., & Isham, E. A. (2009). We infer rather than perceive the moment we decided to act. *Psychological Science, 20,* 17–21.

Banks, W. P., & Pockett, S. (2007). Benjamin Libet's work on the neuroscience of free will. In M. Velmans & S. Schinder (Eds.), *Blackwell companion to consciousness* (pp. 657–670). Malden, MA: Blackwell.

Brand, M. (1984). *Intending and acting: Toward a naturalized action theory*. Cambridge, MA: MIT Press.

Bratman, M. E. (1987). *Intention, plans, and practical reason*. Cambridge, MA: Cambridge University Press.

Davidson, D. (1963). Actions, reasons, and causes. *Journal of Philosophy, 60,* 685–700.

Eagleman, D. M. (2004). The where and when of intention. *Science, 303,* 1144–1146.

Eagleman, D. M., & Sejnowski, T. J. (2000). Motion integration and postdiction in visual awareness. *Science, 287,* 2036–2038.

Frith, C. (2002). Attention to action and awareness of other minds. *Consciousness and Cognition, 11,* 481–487.

Häberle, A., Schutz-Bosbach, S., Laboissière, R., & Prinz, W. (2008). Ideomotor action in cooperative and competitive settings. *Social Neuroscience, 3,* 26–36.

Haggard, P. (2005). Conscious intention and motor cognition. *Consciousness and Cognition, 9,* 290–295.

Haggard, P., & Clark, S. (2003). Intentional action: Conscious experience and neural prediction. *Consciousness and Cognition, 12,* 695–707.

Hallett, M. (2007). Volitional control of movement: The physiology of free will. *Clinical Neurophysiology, 118,* 1179–1192.

Kornhuber, H. H., & Deecke, L. (1965). Hirnpotentialanderungen bei Willkurbewegungen und passiven Bewegungen des Menschen: Bereitschaftspotential und reafferente Potentiale. *Pflugers Archiv fur die Gesamte Physiologie des Menschen und der Tiere, 284,* 1–17.

Lashley, K. (1951). The problem of serial order in behavior. In L. A. Jeffress (Ed.), *Cerebral mechanisms in behavior* (pp. 112–146). Oxford, UK: Wiley.

Lau, H. C., Rogers, R. D., Haggard, P., & Passingham, R. E. (2004). Attention to intention. *Science, 303,* 1208–1210.

Lau, H. C., Rogers, R. D., & Passingham, R.E. (2007). Manipulating the experienced onset of intention after action execution. *Journal of Cognitive Neuroscience, 19,* 81–90.

Libet, B. (1985) Unconscious cerebral initiative and the role of conscious will in voluntary action. *Behavioral and Brain Sciences, 8*(4), 529–566.

Libet, B., Freeman, A., & Sutherland, K. (Eds.). (2000). *The volitional brain: Towards a neuroscience of free will.* Exeter, UK: Imprint Academic.

Libet, B., Gleason, C. A., Wright, E. W., & Pearl, D. K. (1983). Time of conscious intention to act in relation to onset of cerebral activity (readiness–potential): The unconscious initiation of a freely voluntary act. *Brain, 106,* 623–642.

Matsuhashi, M., & Hallet, M. (2008). The timing of the conscious intention to move. *European Journal of Neuroscience, 28,* 2344–2351.

Mele, A. R. (1992). *Springs of action: Understanding intentional behavior.* Oxford: Oxford University Press.

Mele, A. R. (2009). Effective Intentions: The power of conscious will. New York: Oxford.

Nachev, P., Wydell, H., O'Neill, K., Husain, M., & Kennard C. (2007). The role of the pre-supplementary motor area in the control of action. *Neuroimage, 36,* 155–163.

Obhi, S. S. (2007). Evidence for feedback dependent conscious awareness of action. *Brain Research, 1161,* 88–94.

Obhi, S. S., Planetta, P. J., & Scantlebury, J. (2009). On the signals underlying conscious awareness of action. *Cognition, 110,* 65–73.

Pacherie, E. (2006). Toward a dynamic theory of intention. In S. Pockett, W. Banks, & S. Gallagher (Eds.), *Does consciousness cause behavior? An investigation of the nature of volition* (pp. 145–167). Cambridge, MA: MIT Press.

Pacherie, E. (2008). The phenomenology of action: A conceptual framework. *Cognition, 107,* 179–217.

Passingham, R. E., & Lau, H. C. (2006). Free choice and the human brain. In S. Pockett, W. Banks, & S. Gallagher (Eds.), *Does consciousness cause behavior? An investigation of the nature of volition* (pp. 53–72). Cambridge, MA: MIT Press.

Pockett, S., & Miller, A. (2007). The rotating spot method of timing subjective events. *Consciousness and Cognition, 16,* 241–254.

Searle, J. (2001). *Rationality in action.* Cambridge, MA: MIT Press.

Soon, C. S., Brass, M., Heinze, H., & Haynes, J. (2008). Unconscious determinants of free decisions in the human brain. *Nature Neuroscience, 11,* 543–545.

Stetson, C., Cui, X., Montague, P. R., & Eagleman, D. M. (2006). Motor-sensory recalibration leads to an illusory reversal of action and sensation. *Neuron, 51,* 651–659.

Trevena, J. A., & Miller, J. (2002). Cortical movement preparation before and after a conscious decision to move. *Consciousness and Cognition, 11,* 162–190.

Wegner D. M. (2002). *The illusion of conscious will.* Cambridge, MA: MIT Press.

Wegner D. M. (2003). The mind's best trick: How we experience conscious will. *Trends in Cognitive Science, 7,* 65–69.

Wohlschläger, A., Engbert, K., & Haggard, P. (2003). Intentionality as a constituting condition for the own self and other selves. *Consciousness and Cognition, 12,* 708–716.

Wohlschläger, A., Haggard, P., Gesierich, B., & Prinz, W. (2003). The perceived onset time of self- and other-generated actions. *Psychological Science, 14,* 586–591.

# CHAPTER 6

# Volition: How Physiology Speaks to the Issue of Responsibility

*Mark Hallett*

## STARTING POINT

For a topic as complex and controversial as volition, it is critical to begin with definitions. Making definitions, at least in my mind, also brings a bit of clarity to the problem. Volition is the idea that people can freely choose to make (freely will) some of their movements. This regards "some" of their movements, not all. No one would claim that they are voluntarily extending their knee after the doctor taps their patellar tendon; that's a reflex. Some movement appears to be produced by aberrant activity in the brain, such as a seizure, and there is no issue about this either. Additionally, most people are not thinking about willing all the time they are making movements. Much of the time, one's everyday movements are done rather automatically. However, if asked or if someone focuses on these movements, most people would say that the movements are voluntary.

Thus the notion of volition can be put more simply, "I choose to move." The definition of "move" is not a problem: it is to generate force and/or the displacement of a body part in space-time. "I" (or you, or he/she) is not really a problem either if you are a monist. I am my brain, you are your brain, she is her brain. I am not separate from my brain. It is easy to fall into dualistic thinking in this regard, but if we are talking "I," we are talking "my brain." "Moveo, ergo sum" should not imply that there is a prime mover in addition to the brain, just as "cogito, ergo sum" should not imply (in a broader sense) a mind separate from the body.

So how about "choose"? This is more difficult. To "choose" may mean to decide, expressing or exerting free will. "Free will" can be interpreted in two ways. The first is more common: a force that initiates movement and/or decides which movement to make. This is certainly the folk psychology point of view, but so far this force has not been found. In fact, it is not even clear how to identify it. What would its anatomical and physiological characteristics be? What experiment could show its operation? Later, I will discuss movement genesis, which can be understood without reference to any "free will force."

The second interpretation of "free will" is as a perception of consciousness. The elements of consciousness are qualia, and free will is a quale. Indeed, this must be true. Even if free will is also a force, it must also be a quale for persons to recognize it. The folk psychology view is that this quale arises from, and occurs contemporaneously with, the action of the "free will force." But, of course, this is not necessarily the case. Qualia can be misleading. There could certainly be a quale of freely choosing, even if there is no such force. However, this perceptual view of free will means that people have it if they perceive it. Most normal people perceive that they have free will much of the time (at least when they think about it), but this is not the case in some neurological or psychiatric disorders (Hallett, 2007). Patients with schizophrenia can feel that their movements are externally controlled. Patients with psychogenic movement disorders feel that their movements are involuntary, even if physiological investigations show great similarity between their involuntary movements and their voluntary ones.

This sets the stage for current physiological investigations. We are able to study perceptions even if we do not understand consciousness. Hence, we are able to study what generates the quale or the perception of free will. If we do understand the quale, that might tell us something about whether free will is also a driving force.

One more definition: "agency" is a term that sometimes gets mixed up with "free will." Agency is the perception that I (or you or he/she) caused the movement that just occurred. Willing is the intention to move, whether or not it occurs. Agency requires a matching of will and an event. It is another quale. A report of agency, like volition, can also be misleading. It is not at all uncommon for people to have the perception that they caused something that they did not cause. This was demonstrated experimentally by Wegner and Wheatley (1999), who showed that subjects might report agency when externally produced movement was temporally coupled with a thought also externally induced. On the other hand, subjects may fail to report agency for a movement actually made if the feedback of the movement is temporally delayed (Farrer et al., 2008).

## PHYSIOLOGICAL INVESTIGATIONS

There are a number of questions that can be investigated. How does the brain make movement? What process is responsible for the quale of free will? What process is responsible for the quale of agency? A fundamental question in the understanding of the quale of free will is when it occurs in the course of making a movement. This is what I will consider first.

### The Timing of Free Will

The pioneering experiment that first identified the time of awareness of volition was reported by Libet et al. (Libet, Gleason, Wright, & Pearl, 1983). In this book honoring Libet, it is not necessary to recount the details of this classic experiment. The subjective time of intending to act is called W and the subjective time of actually moving is called M. Simultaneous EEG measured what Libet called the readiness potential, RP, which more commonly goes by the original German name, the *Bereitschaftspotential*, or BP. W occurred about 200 ms prior to EMG onset, and M occurred about 90 ms prior to EMG onset. The onset of the type I RP (for a preplanned movement) occurred about 850 ms prior to W, and the onset of the type II RP (a spontaneous movement) occurred about 375 ms prior to W. Libet and colleagues concluded "that cerebral initiation of a spontaneous, freely voluntary act can begin unconsciously, that is, before there is any (at least recallable) subjective awareness that a 'decision' to act has already been initiated cerebrally" (Libet et al., 1983).

These results have been reproduced by many others plus or minus a few milliseconds, so the basic data are really not in question. Haggard and Eimer looked carefully at the timing of W compared with BP onset and the onset of another measure, the lateralized readiness potential (LRP, the difference in the voltage of right and left central regions) in tasks where subjects moved either their right or their left hand (Haggard & Eimer, 1999). The onset of the LRP preceded W, indicating that movement selection also precedes awareness.

Let's consider other types of experiments that deal with the question of when. A modified version of the Libet clock experiment has been done with fMRI (Soon, Brass, Heinze, & Haynes, 2008). Subjects made movements of right or left finger at freely chosen times while watching a series of letters. They indicated the time of choice by indicating the letter they were seeing. Using a sophisticated analysis method, the researchers were able to predict with up to 60% probability the subject's right or left choice as long as 10 seconds prior to the movement. Does this mean that a movement is started on its inevitable course that long in advance of the actual movement? Likely not. The critical point is that the probability is not high, but might be what is expected 10 seconds prior to a movement. The brain likely starts thinking and planning early, and the probabilities oscillate. It would likely not be uncommon for the movement planning to be aborted. The probabilities will become higher closer to movement onset for those movements that actually occur.

The timing of perception of W and M can be influenced by transcranial magnetic stimulation (TMS) over the preSMA (presupplementary motor area) delivered "immediately after the action" or 200 ms later (Lau, Rogers, & Passingham, 2007). TMS had the effect of moving the W judgment earlier in time and the M judgment later in time. This effect was time-specific and did not occur with stimulation over the primary motor cortex. There are a number of interesting conclusions. One relevant here is that subjective timing of events that are felt to occur prior to the movement may be influenced after the movement. This suggests that the sense of W actually occurs after the movement.

Is it possible that the brain event of W might actually occur after the movement but be referred back in time to before the movement? This question leads us back to another of Libet's contributions, the issue of the latency between a real world sensory event and its perception. A person's subjective present is actually slightly in the real past (Eagleman, Tse, Buonomano, Janssen, Nobre, & Holcombe, 2005). This point, while at first surprising, is actually obvious. For example, it takes time for sensory information to reach the brain from peripheral receptors. Moreover, these times are different for different sensory modalities, and there has to be time to allow this information to be aligned for a unitary percept.

Libet studied this by determining the time of sensory awareness after trains of electrical stimuli applied directly to sensory cortex during neurosurgical procedures. It took 300–500 ms for awareness, and Libet called this the utilization time (Libet, Wright Jr., Feinstein, & Pearl, 1979). His idea was that the sensory stimulus was processed for this period of time and then subjectively referred back to the time that the sensory stimulus began (Ortinski & Meador, 2004). Given this approximate time estimate, and that W is about 200 ms prior to movement, it is not at all unlikely that the brain event of W does indeed occur after movement onset or, if initiated prior to movement, is still being processed after movement onset.

All the protocols discussed so far depend on subjective timing reported by the subject after the event. Recently, we have approached the problem in a different way (Matsuhashi & Hallett, 2008). We asked subjects to make movements at freely chosen times while listening to tones occurring at random times. The EEG was monitored. If a tone came after the thought to make a movement, but before the movement, the subject was to veto the movement. No introspective data are needed to interpret the data, and nothing is reconstructed retrospectively. The timing of all tones is plotted with respect to the onset of movements made. Some tones will be present prior to the thought of making a movement, which we called T (for thought). Other tones will be just before movement, indicating those tones present after the "point of no return," that time when movement can no longer be vetoed. Between the early tones and the late tones, there will be a gap indicating the time when the movements are vetoed. On average T occurred about 1.42 seconds prior to movement onset. As this is earlier than RPI of Libet, this fact by itself might indicate that thinking about the movement does occur prior to observable brain activity. However, in our experiments, we also recorded EEG, and the BP onset was 2.17 seconds before movement. (I will refer to this here as BP to differentiate it from type I RP and type II RP of Libet.) BP onset does differ in different experimental settings, but our methodology these days is more sensitive than that of Libet, and our BP timing is similar to many other contemporary experiments. So while T is still later than observable brain activity, it is much longer before movement than W. The interpretation of this is below, but one more result of these experiments is relevant: the point of no return was 0.13 seconds prior to movement onset.

Putting this together on a timeline is illustrated in Figure 6.1. Although there might be intimations of movement earlier, the brain starts the more definitive process of movement initiation, say 2 seconds, prior to movement. At T, 1.4 s prior to movement, persons can know that the movement is being readied if they are probed or asked about it even if they are not subjectively

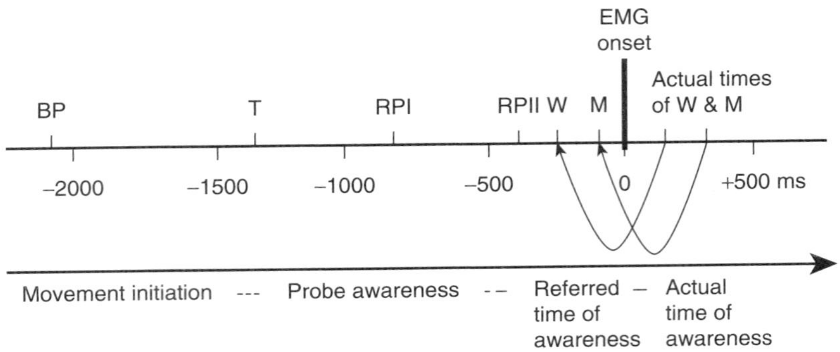


**Figure 6.1** Timeline of events in movement generation and perception of W and M, the qualia of willing and movement. BP = Bereitschaftspotential, T = time of thinking about movement, RP = readiness potential.

aware spontaneously. This type of situation is called probe awareness and has been demonstrated in other circumstances as well. This suggests that there is a brain state, where a process is occurring just below conscious level, but that it is available to consciousness if asked about it. Awareness of the brain event increases, either as a matter of time or a matter of increasing probability of going forward. Then the brain event of subjective spontaneous awareness, W, may begin several hundred ms prior to movement. However, apparently, it is still being processed after movement. When W is fully processed, it is referred back in time, perhaps to when the brain was beginning to generate the quale.

Thus, it is possible to do experiments on the quale of willing and get some sense of its timing. From the original Libet et al. experiment, W appeared to occur too late to be responsible for movement initiation, but the concept of W has been subject to much criticism, and it appears to still be in process after the movement occurs. Our measure of T is not subject to the same criticisms and appears to be more objective. Even though we appear to be probing thought at a stage when the "idea" of movement is still ordinarily subconscious, T still occurs later than observable brain events. This means that if there is a free-will force for movement generation, then it operates at an earlier time from the quale of willing. This is certainly different from the folk psychology view, which would say that "I freely choose to make a movement at the time that I perceive myself to be doing so."

Interestingly, Libet did not want to interpret his experiment to say that there was no force of free will prior to movement. He put it a different way: the movement may well originate unconsciously, but there still might be a force that could veto it before it is accomplished (Libet, 1999; Libet, 2006). Vetoing is free will, and there is time after W to veto. Vetoing should be possible up to the time of the point of no return, which in the Matsuhashi and Hallett experiment was 130 ms prior to movement. However, if W occurs at 200 ms prior to movement, the time to veto would be only 70 ms. Voluntary reaction time is more than 70 ms, so there actually is not sufficient time for there to be a "voluntary" decision to veto in reaction to the conscious event of W. Putting it this way means that there is actually not sufficient time to veto.

The notion of vetoing a movement has been designated "free won't" (Obhi & Haggard, 2004). Of course, "free won't" could also be initiated subconsciously and could be a process similar to that which generates movement. For example, there is a cortical potential prior to relaxation of a tonic movement that is similar to the Bereitschaftspotential (Terada, Ikeda, Nagamine, & Shibasaki, 1995). It should be possible to veto a developing movement before W. All of this would be taking place, however, subconsciously. The physiology of vetoing a planned movement has been studied (Brass & Haggard, 2007; Kuhn, Haggard, & Brass, 2008), and its physiology is different from movement genesis. In this circumstance a region in the dorsal fronto-median cortex is particularly active.

Is this all a tempest in a teapot? Who cares about twiddling thumbs in the laboratory? What really designates the intention to move? It could be argued that the decision to move is made when agreeing to do the experiment in the first place (Deecke & Kornhuber, 2003; Mele, 2006, 2007). The movements themselves are then a simple (perhaps, even nonvoluntary) consequence of that earlier choice. Moreover, there are data that indicate that the more specific the decision about future behavior, the more likely that behavior will actually occur. Experiments show that having an "implementation intention," a plan to implement a goal, is more effective than a general "goal intention" (Gollwitzer & Sheeran, 2006). What is the nature of these decisions? These are "thinking" and thinking is another element of consciousness that we do not fully understand. However, thinking, like movement, is a manifestation of brain function, and imagining movement activates many of the same structures that are activated by movement itself (Hanakawa, Dimyan, & Hallett, 2008). A decision like agreeing to do the experiment very likely biases the probabilities of movement selection. In any event, in order to do science, it is necessary to create reduced preparations with control of all the variables, like simple movements. As we learn more, we will be able to make the experiments more complex.

### How Decisions Are Made and Movement Is Generated

The physiology of movement generation is reasonably well known. Muscles make movements. They are controlled by the alpha-motoneurons in the spinal cord, which themselves are controlled by a large number of segmental and suprasegmental influences. The corticospinal tract delivers the most important suprasegmental control signals from the brain, and much of this derives from the primary motor cortex. Recordings from the primary motor cortex show a fairly direct relationship to muscle activity during movement. The old debate as to whether the motor cortex primarily codes for movement or muscles has largely been settled in terms of movement.

The first question that one might ask is, What is the physiology underlying the motor cortex producing a specific output? At any one time, the motor cortex could potentially produce a whole range of movements. Any particular neuron, and any particular collection of neurons, is under the influence of its synaptic input, a mixture of excitatory and inhibitory postsynaptic potentials (EPSPs and IPSPs). When the resultant membrane potential of the neuron at its axon hillock reaches a threshold level, it fires. (And, of course, this same process will be fundamentally responsible for other brain regions as well.)

So, the question then becomes, What controls the motor cortex? Input comes from the entire brain. The most influential proximal input comes from premotor cortex including the supplementary motor area. Input to premotor cortex comes from three general directions, subcortical influences from basal ganglia and cerebellum, parietal cortex, and frontal cortex. Parietal cortex is largely responsible for collecting information from all the senses, informing the brain about the current state of the environment, including the most recent stimuli that might require responses. The frontal cortex is largely responsible for collecting information from the brain itself, including limbic and homeostatic information. Subcortical, parietal, and frontal information converge onto premotor cortex neurons in specific patterns that have been associated with different types of movements, such as reaching or grasping (Rizzolatti & Luppino, 2001; Rizzolatti, Luppino, & Matelli, 1998).

There have been some demonstrations that movements occur when cellular activity in specific regions of the brain achieve a certain level of firing. One such nice example is saccadic initiation in monkeys in a reaction time experiment with ambiguous visual stimuli. Saccades are initiated when single cell activity in the frontal eye field (Stuphorn & Schall, 2002) or the lateral interparietal (LIP) area of the parietal lobe (Gold & Shadlen, 2007) reaches a certain level; more rapid reaction times occur when the cellular activity reaches the threshold level more rapidly. This has been modeled quantitatively (Gold & Shadlen, 2007) and extended to multiple choices (Churchland, Kiani, & Shadlen, 2008).

Research also has extended the quantitative analysis of decision making from sensory processing alone to the addition of value or reward. Reward can be defined as "anything that an animal will work to acquire" (Sugrue, Corrado, & Newsome, 2005). Reward is a benefit, but any choice might also have a cost measured as time, effort, and resource use. A parameter of value representation, depending on such a cost-benefit analysis, can be determined that can predict the relative probabilities of response. That is, in a multiple choice situation, the responses will be chosen according to reward probabilities (Sugrue et al., 2005). Reward determination is modulated strongly by dopamine. Dopamine can signal that a known stimulus is likely to produce a reward, can signal bidirectionally a prediction error if the reward does not match expectation, and can signal uncertainty of a predicted reward (Schultz, 2007a, 2007b).

The more that we know about a person's brain, its past history, and the current situation, the more possible it is to predict what a person will do. Even though the probability of the prediction can be very good, it will likely never be 100% in all circumstances. Why should that be? There are several reasons at least. Each of multiple choices may have some value and differing types of value, and these may be difficult to choose among. There will always be a trade-off between reward expectation and exploratory behavior (Haggard, 2008). Exploration is a good thing, perhaps even greater rewards can be obtained from a risky or uncertain choice. The brain is also noisy. There are many nodal points in the circuits leading to behavior, and any of them might well fire off randomly at a random time.

Thus, there is a great deal known about how the brain decides to do something at any particular time. However, as noted, it is unlikely that even if we have an enormous amount of information about a brain and the circumstances that behavior can be certainly predicted. Potentially, this leaves room for another factor, a free will factor. It is not necessary to postulate it, but, if present, it would have to work via these mechanisms. As noted earlier, at present, it is not clear how to identify it or even construct an experiment to demonstrate it.

### Anatomy of the Qualia of Willing and Agency

Many good experiments identify the anatomy and physiology of both willing and agency. The awareness of W (as well as M) could well derive from feedforward signals (corollary discharges) (Poulet & Hedwig, 2007) from the movement planning and the command for movement execution, since all of this certainly occurs prior to movement feedback. Indeed, it has been demonstrated that movement feedback is not necessary for W (Frith, 2002; Frith, Blakemore, & Wolpert, 2000). Using fMRI, when attention is directed to intention, there is greater activation in the preSMA, right dorsal prefrontal cortex, and left interparietal sulcus (Lau, Rogers, Haggard, & Passingham, 2004). Further evidence that the parietal lobe is relevant to the sense of voluntariness comes from experiments with the Libet clock in patients with parietal lobe lesions, who show a shorter interval between W and movement onset (Sirigu et al., 2004).

Agency has been investigated with fMRI modulating the relationship between voluntary movement and visual feedback. There appears to be an inverse relationship between activity in the inferior parietal lobe, more on the right side, and agency (Farrer, Franck, Georgieff, Frith, Decety, & Jeannerod, 2003). We have similar results in unpublished experiments. Clearly, more work is needed to firm up conclusions about the anatomy of the perceptions of volition and agency, but the types of experiments to demonstrate these are already yielding reasonable results.

## RESPONSIBILITY

The physiology says that our brains make our movements, and from what we know already, we have a good sense about the processes of how movement can be predicted in any circumstance. In more complex circumstances, we will need to know more information about a person, including past experiences. It is possible that this physiology will be a complete explanation, that an unknown factor of "free will" is not a necessary explanatory element. On the other hand, we have a subjective sense of freely choosing these movements. This quale occurs very late in the process, and it appears that it might be a perception of the brain as a consequence of feedforward signals as the movement is generated. It is clear that if there is a factor of free will helping to determine movement, it must precede our introspection of when it occurs.

Proceeding from the introductory theme, if a person is his/her brain, and the brain generates all behavior, then a person is always responsible for all behavior. There is no separate "he" that might not bear responsibility for what his brain does. There are some exceptions that might be considered minor. In a seizure, for example, the brain itself loses control, but it would be vanishingly rare for a seizure to cause organized behavior.

That the brain is always responsible is a somewhat simple conclusion, but should be followed (in appropriate circumstances) by the question, Why? Why did his brain generate that behavior? This may well be an analogous question to what is often asked now, Is the person responsible for the behavior? The essence of the question really is why that behavior was chosen. So the physiology clarifies the nature of the question, but may not actually simplify the inquiry. Behavior, like all other elements of a person, is a product of that person's genetics, experience, and current environment and internal state. Is a person hungry or angry? Is there an opportunity for rewarded behavior? What has a person's experience been in similar circumstances before? A person's behavior should be subject to influence by specific environmental interventions, such as reward and punishment, education, and social pressures.

In the end, if society is not happy with a person's behavior, it is a societal decision as to whether intervention is appropriate and, if so, what to do about it: punishment, medical remediation, or something else. The physiology does suggest that appropriate interventions may well be able, in many circumstances, to change behavior in the future. Focusing the question on "Why was the behavior done?" rather than just simply "Is the person responsible?" may be a better approach, first, in understanding the behavior, and, second, in finding the best remediation.

Let's consider the case of Jean Valjean, the character in Victor Hugo's novel *Les misérables*, who steals a loaf of bread because he cannot afford it and his sister and her family are starving. The question for the judicial system might be whether he is responsible or not for stealing that loaf. If he did do it, he is responsible, and he goes to jail automatically, because that what is done with thieves. On the other hand, if the system assumes he is responsible and asks why, then his situation can be readily understood, and the system might come up with a different suggested course of action, like finding him a job.

On the other hand, let's consider a person who underpaid his income tax. If the question is that of responsibility, then the answer is relatively easy, and a punishment might be defined by the book—perhaps a fine. However, if the consideration is why, and if it is determined that the person is wealthy and the motivation is greed, society might want to give a harsh penalty to deter such behavior by him and others. If the person was well motivated and tried to do the right thing, but got confused, it might be best to change the instructions on the tax form.

It is possible to get along without having to postulate that "free will" is driving behavior. The brain is complex, and many factors influence what it does, but we are often able to get a good idea of why specific behaviors occurred.

## ACKNOWLEDGMENTS

This work is supported by the NINDS Intramural Program. This essay is in part revised and updated from prior publications (Hallett, 2007, 2009). As a work of the U.S. government, it has no copyright.

## REFERENCES

Brass, M., & Haggard, P. (2007). To do or not to do: The neural signature of self-control. *Journal of Neuroscience, 27,* 9141–9145.

Churchland, A. K., Kiani, R., & Shadlen, M. N. (2008). Decision-making with multiple alternatives. *Nature Neuroscience, 11,* 693–702.

Deecke, L., & Kornhuber, H. H. (2003). Human freedom, reasoned will, and the brain: The Bereitschaftspotential story. In M. Jahanshahi & M. Hallett (Eds.), *The Bereitschaftspotential: Movement-related cortical potentials* (pp. 283–320). New York: Kluwer Academic/Plenum Publishers.

Eagleman, D. M., Tse, P. U., Buonomano, D., Janssen, P., Nobre, A. C., & Holcombe, A. O. (2005). Time and the brain: How subjective time relates to neural time. *Journal of Neuroscience, 25,* 10369–10371.

Farrer, C., Franck, N., Georgieff, N., Frith, C. D., Decety, J., & Jeannerod, M. (2003). Modulating the experience of agency: A positron emission tomography study. *Neuroimage, 18,* 324–333.

Farrer, C., Frey, S. H., Van Horn, J. D., Tunik, E., Turk, D., Inati, S., et al. (2008). The angular gyrus computes action awareness representations. *Cerebral Cortex, 18,* 254–261.

Frith, C. D. (2002). Attention to action and awareness of other minds. *Consciousness and Cognition, 11,* 481–487.

Frith, C. D., Blakemore, S., & Wolpert, D. M. (2000). Explaining the symptoms of schizophrenia: Abnormalities in the awareness of action. *Brain Research, Brain Research Reviews, 31,* 357–363.

Gold, J. I., & Shadlen, M. N. (2007). The neural basis of decision making. *Annual Review of Neuroscience, 30,* 535–574.

Gollwitzer, P. M., & Sheeran, P. (2006). Implementation intentions and goal achievement: A meta-analysis of effects and processes. *Advances in Experimental Social Psychology, 38,* 69–119.

Haggard, P. (2008). Human volition: Towards a neuroscience of will. *Nature Reviews, Neuroscience, 9,* 934–946.

Haggard, P., & Eimer, M. (1999). On the relation between brain potentials and the awareness of voluntary movements. *Experimental Brain Research, 126,* 128–133.

Hallett, M. (2007). Volitional control of movement: The physiology of free will. *Clinical Neurophysiology, 118,* 1179–1192.

Hallett, M. (2009). Physiology of volition. In G. F. R. Ellis, N. Murphy, & T. O'Connor (Eds.), *Downward causation and the neurobiology of free will.* Berlin: Springer.

Hanakawa, T., Dimyan, M. A., & Hallett, M. (2008). Motor planning, imagery, and execution in the distributed motor network: A time-course study with functional MRI. *Cerebral Cortex, 18,* 2775–2788.

Kuhn, S., Haggard, P., & Brass, M. (2008). Intentional inhibition: How the "veto-area" exerts control. *Human Brain Mapping, 30*(9), 2834–2843.

Lau, H. C., Rogers, R. D., Haggard, P., & Passingham, R. E. (2004). Attention to intention. *Science, 303,* 1208–1210.

Lau, H. C., Rogers, R. D., & Passingham, R. E. (2007). Manipulating the experienced onset of intention after action execution. *Journal of Cognitive Neuroscience, 19,* 81–90.

Libet, B. (1999). Do we have free will? *Journal of Consciousness Studies, 9,* 47–57.

Libet, B. (2006). The timing of brain events: Reply to the "Special Section" in this journal of September 2004, edited by Susan Pockett. *Consciousness and Cognition, 15,* 540–547.

Libet, B., Gleason, C. A., Wright, E. W., & Pearl, D. K. (1983). Time of conscious intention to act in relation to onset of cerebral activity (readiness-potential): The unconscious initiation of a freely voluntary act. *Brain, 106,* 623–642.

Libet, B., Wright, E. W., Jr., Feinstein, B., & Pearl, D. K. (1979). Subjective referral of the timing for a conscious sensory experience: A functional role for the somatosensory specific projection system in man. *Brain, 102,* 193–224.

Matsuhashi, M., & Hallett, M. (2008). The timing of the conscious intention to move. *European Journal of Neuroscience, 28,* 2344–2351.

Mele, A. R. (2006). *Free will and luck.* Oxford: Oxford University Press.

Mele, A. R. (2007). Decision, intentions, urges, and free will: Why Libet has not shown what he says he has. In J. Campbell, M. O'Rourke, & D. Shier (Eds.), *Explanation and caustion: Topics in comtemporary philosophy.* Boston: MIT Press.

Obhi, S. S., & Haggard, P. (2004). Free will and free won't. *American Scientist, 92,* 358–365.

Ortinski, P., & Meador, K. J. (2004). Neuronal mechanisms of conscious awareness. *Archives of Neurology, 61,* 1017–1020.

Poulet, J. F., & Hedwig, B. (2007). New insights into corollary discharges mediated by identified neural pathways. *Trends in Neurosciences, 30,* 14–21.

Rizzolatti, G., & Luppino, G. (2001). The cortical motor system. *Neuron, 31,* 889–901.

Rizzolatti, G., Luppino, G., & Matelli, M. (1998). The organization of the cortical motor system: New concepts. *Electroencephalography and Clinical Neurophysiology, 106,* 283–296.

Schultz, W. (2007a). Behavioral dopamine signals. *Trends in Neurosciences, 30,* 203–210.

Schultz, W. (2007b). Multiple dopamine functions at different time courses. *Annual Review of Neuroscience, 30,* 259–288.

Sirigu, A., Daprati, E., Ciancia, S., Giraux, P., Nighoghossian, N., Posada, A., et al. (2004). Altered awareness of voluntary action after damage to the parietal cortex. *Nature Neuroscience, 7,* 80–84.

Soon, C. S., Brass, M., Heinze, H. J., & Haynes, J. D. (2008). Unconscious determinants of free decisions in the human brain. *Nature Neuroscience, 11,* 543–545.

Stuphorn, V., & Schall, J. D. (2002). Neuronal control and monitoring of initiation of movements. *Muscle and Nerve, 26,* 326–339.

Sugrue, L. P., Corrado, G. S., & Newsome, W. T. (2005). Choosing the greater of two goods: Neural currencies for valuation and decision making. *Nature Reviews, Neuroscience, 6,* 363–375.

Terada, K., Ikeda, A., Nagamine, T., & Shibasaki, H. (1995). Movement-related cortical potentials associated with voluntary muscle relaxation. *Electromyography and Clinical Neurophysiology, 95,* 335–345.

Wegner, D. M., & Wheatley, T. (1999). Apparent mental causation: Sources of the experience of will. *The American Psychologist, 54,* 480–492.

# CHAPTER 7

## What Are Intentions?

*Elisabeth Pacherie and Patrick Haggard*

### INTRODUCTION

Neuroscientific work on intentions and voluntary actions has tended to focus on very short time scales, immediately before movement onset. As a prime example, the intentions investigated by Benjamin Libet are states that are first consciously experienced on average 200 ms before action onset. Libet's experiments showed that these conscious intentions were reliably preceded by a few hundred milliseconds by a negative brain potential, the so-called readiness potential. The existence of this antecedent unconscious brain activity indicated that the action was initiated unconsciously rather than by the conscious intention. This led Libet to the conclusion that we do not have full-blown "free will." However, he attempted to salvage a limited form of free will by suggesting that although we cannot consciously initiate actions, we can still consciously veto them in the 200 ms interval between conscious intention and action onset. Libet's conception of free will and his interpretation of his results have been widely discussed and criticized.

Here, we take as our starting point one of these lines of criticism, voiced notably by Shaun Gallagher (2006). Gallagher argues that it is misguided to attempt to frame the question of free will at the time scale and in terms of the very short-term motor intentions and control processes Libet considers. Rather, free will involves temporally extended deliberative processes and applies to intentional actions considered at levels of description typically higher and more abstract than descriptions in terms of motor processes and bodily movements. In earlier work, one of us (Pacherie, 2008) proposed a three-tiered hierarchical model of intentions, the DPM model, distinguishing distal or prospective intentions, proximal or immediate intentions, and motor intentions; the other (Haggard, 2008) offered a naturalized model of human volition involving a set of decision-making processes concerned with whether to act, what to do (and how), and when to act. If Gallagher is right about the temporal and intentional framework relevant for the exercise of free will, a discussion of free will must at least include not only the contribution of intentions to the final process of action initiation itself, but also the anterior decision processes that take place at the level of prospective intentions.

### 1. IMMEDIATE INTENTION AND ACTION INITIATION

Providing a satisfactory definition of intention is notoriously difficult. In this chapter, we assume that intention is a mental state, which may be associated with particular brain states. But what *kind* of mental state is an intention? We suggest that intentions have two distinguishing features. First, they are accessible to consciousness. Second, they bear some relation to subsequent action. This relation could be distinctive for two reasons: a causal reason or a content reason. Let us take a physical movement of the body (I raise my arm) as a paradigm of action. The causal reason suggests that the intention (I intend to raise my arm) is simply the mental state that causes the action of lifting my arm (Wittgenstein, 1953). Intentions thus explain why actions occur, and serve as the guarantors of volition. This view is clearly vulnerable to skeptical attack: folk psychology may find it convenient to have some appropriate explanation of a person's actions, and the concept of intention could be designed to fulfill this purpose. The fact that intentions do a good job of explaining actions does not therefore constitute evidence that they are a bona fide mental state.

The content argument suggests the content of the intention ("I will raise my arm") is somehow linked to the specific details of the arm-raising action. This view makes clearer predictions about what might constitute an intention. For example, if I perform two different actions, raising my left arm on one occasion and my right arm on another, the intentions for each action should have different contents, capable of explaining which arm is used for the action in each case. The content of intention should be discriminative, in the sense that it should predict specific details of action. The content argument emphasizes the continuity between decision and intention: when someone decides to do A rather than B, they may develop an intention whose specific content will relate to A rather than to B. A number of neuroscientific studies have attempted to decode the brain processes predicting the specific content of a subsequent action (Soon, Brass, Heinze, & Haynes, 2008; Haggard & Eimer, 1999). This level of motor content would typically be generated once the specific situation and context of action are established, and only immediately before action initiation. Because intention, viewed in this way, is very close to the details of motor execution, we use the term "immediate intention" to refer to it.

Interestingly, although Libet's work (Libet, Gleason, Wright, & Pearl, 1983) occupies a central role in modern scientific work on intention, he himself appeared to avoid the word. On the one hand, he speaks of the "unconscious initiation" of action. This refers to the set of brain processes that ultimately give rise to muscular movement. The readiness potential generated by the frontal motor areas of the brain is a convenient marker that these processes have begun, but Libet avoids making the simplistic claim that the onset of the readiness potential simply constitutes initiation. On the other hand, the conscious experience of immediate intention (W judgment) occurs several hundred milliseconds after the readiness potential onset, and only slightly before movement itself. If the W judgment is taken as the marker of conscious intention, then, our conscious intentions cannot be the cause or explanation of our actions, because intention follows neural initiation of action, rather than precedes it.

But is the W judgment really a marker of immediate conscious intention? Libet himself speaks of an "urge to act." Participants are supposed to report the moment when this urge begins. This is clearly one of the weaker points of the experimental method. How do participants know what they are supposed to report? Could the instruction to report urges somehow suggest to the subject that they should have a specific experience of immediate intention that would otherwise remain unconscious? Could the instruction suggest to subjects the need to report a moment slightly before action, even if they have no distinctive conscious experience at that moment? Participants might interpret the instructions in such experiments as "Behave as if you had free will, and make your reports of intention consistent with this concept of free will." If this were the case, then such experiments could not separate the influence of folk psychology from any genuine mental state of intention, making them vulnerable to skeptical attack, or even scientifically worthless.

## EVIDENCE FROM DIRECT CORTICAL STIMULATION

Clearly, experimental manipulations of intention that do not depend on instructions, and therefore avoid the worst problems of suggestion, are highly desirable. Perhaps the most informative data come from reports of direct cortical stimulation prior to neurosurgery for epilepsy. Methodologically, these data clearly differ from psychological experiments relying on participants' understanding of instructions. In fact, no instruction is given at all: the patient's behavior during stimulation is observed, and they are invited to report anything that they feel. Little detail is generally given about *how* the reporting is done. Few neurosurgical studies seem to address the problems of experimenter-led suggestion and response bias, for example, by including catch trials without stimulation. Nevertheless, these data have particular significance for the psychology of intention, and are therefore worth examining in some detail.

Direct stimulation data broadly support a distinction between initiation of action and conscious immediate intention. In particular, we shall argue that direct stimulation of the presupplementary motor area (preSMA) is accompanied by an anticipatory conscious experience of immediate intention. In contrast, direct stimulation of the deeper cingulate motor area (CMA) produces a strong *motivation* to perform a specific action, and can trigger action initiation, but without any particular *specific* conscious experience prior to action. In the neurosurgical literature, and in Libet's work also, the word "urge" is widely used. We argue that the same word is used with two quite different meanings, which have been unnecessarily confounded. On the one hand, an urge involves a conscious experience of being about to act. On the other hand, an urge involves a feeling of compulsion, or having to. We suggest these two components are localized to the preSMA and the CMA respectively. Rather than the general term "urge" we suggest that the terms immediate intention and motivation to act might be more appropriate.

### Pre-SMA Stimulation Can Evoke a State Resembling Immediate Intention

The awake patient reports a subjective experience or "urge to move" during stimulation of characteristic cortical regions, notably the supplementary motor area. The study closest to our interest is that by Fried et al. (1991). The paper reports responses to stimulation through intracranial grids over the mesial frontal cortex. In one patient, several reports of "urge" were obtained following low-amplitude stimulation over the supplementary motor area. The responses typically referred to a specific contralateral body part, as in "urge to move the right elbow." In some trials, different verbal formulas appear: "need to move," "feeling as if movement were about to occur." At higher stimulation intensities, actual movements were often evoked. The authors comment that the actual movement evoked was not necessarily commensurate with the urge. However, urge and movement at least referred to the same limb in the majority of trials reported for this patient.

The ability to evoke by external intervention a mental state that appears close to conscious intention is intriguing. However, several important methodological questions remain. How general are these sensations: they receive prominent attention in the report of one case, but it is unclear whether they were investigated and found to be absent, or merely not investigated, in the remaining cases? What phenomenal experience does the stimulation cause? Beyond the frequent use of the word "urge" there is little information on phenomenology. One particular concern would be whether the experience reported as "urge" is truly an anticipatory experience of central origin, and occurring in advance of movement. Could "urge" actually reflect subtle muscle contractions caused by low-intensity stimulation, which lacked the strength required to produce observable movement? Alternatively, could "urge" reflect a sensory experience, like the "tingling" sensation frequently reported following stimulation at sites close to those provoking "urge" (Fried et al, 1991)? The preSMA is known to receive sensory afferent input, probably after initial processing in somatosensory cortical areas (Mima et al, 1999). In conditions such as Tourette's syndrome and restless legs syndrome, the urge to move is strongly associated with, or is simply described as, a *sensory* quality localized in specific body parts, and relieved by movement of those body parts. If urges were essentially sensory in nature, they clearly would not be a good model for conscious intention. Interestingly, however, a recent review of a series of 52 patients who underwent electrical stimulation suggests sensory experiences are not a normal feature of preSMA stimulation, being recorded in only a single instance (Chassagnon, Minotti, Kremer, Hoffmann, & Kahane, 2008). In fact, they were much more common following stimulation of the posterior portion of the CMA. It seems likely that preSMA stimulation produces a specific conscious experience, distinct from both stimulation-evoked sensation and from peripheral sensation. This experience, like immediate intention, is motorically specific, and linked to an impending action.

### CMA Stimulation Produces Motivated but Automatized Actions

In fact, the stimulation of the CMA, and particularly of the region of the cingulate sulcus immediately below the preSMA, seems to correspond more closely to Libet's "unconscious initiation of a . . . voluntary act." Chassagnon et al. (2008) report four instances where CMA stimulation elicited reaching and grasping behaviors, "as if the patients were groping around and handling a small object in the dark." There is no specific report or evidence of urge *prior* to actual movement. An extended report of one patient in this series (Kremer, Chassagnon, Hoffmann, Benabid, & Kahane, 2001) shows that these behaviors had a compulsive, irresistible quality. This patient had a strong drive to perform the movement once stimulation began, making scanning eye movements and exploratory arm movements to identify a potential target for grasping. The patient is described as having an "urge to grasp something." However, it remains hard to locate this feeling of urge within the chain of events linked to the action. In particular, no quantitative data is given on two details that are of primary importance for the psychology of intention: the delay between stimulation onset and movement onset, and the delay between stimulation onset and any sense of "urge." We suggest that this patient showed "urge" in the motivational sense during CMA stimulation, but they did not experience the kind of anticipatory conscious awareness characteristic of immediate intentions.

A more extensive study of actions evoked by CMA stimulation in 83 epileptic patients was reported by Bancaud, Talairach, Geier, Bonis, Trottier, and Manrique (1976). Stimulation generally produced an increased state of arousal and attentiveness, often at low stimulation intensities. This was interpreted as a nonspecific form of attention to action. At higher stimulation intensities, a range of coordinated manual, buccal, and oculomotor actions were produced. Interestingly, if an object were given to the participant during stimulation, it would evoke complex series of object-appropriate movements. For example, when one patient was given a cigarette, they lit and smoked it in a compulsive manner, stopping smoking when stimulation ceased, and restarting when stimulation restarted. In other cases, patients compulsively ate food they were offered, or brought objects to the mouth and sucked them. Again, ceasing stimulation caused the action to end. When the experimenters physically restrained the patient's arms, the patient often strove to continue the action, especially at greater stimulation intensities. This sustained drive to achieve the action is not merely a matter of maintaining motor output in the face of perturbation, since in one case the patient transferred an object repeatedly between the hands to overcome the experimenter's interference.

What did the patients experience? While Bancaud et al. do not address this point systematically, the general attitude of the patients toward their own evoked actions appeared indifferent. Patients acknowledged the action they had performed immediately afterward, but did not generally give specific reasons why they performed it, nor did they appear surprised by actions that might prima facie seem strange. On questioning the next day, the patients did not find their actions under stimulation in any way surprising or unusual. One way of interpreting this unusual phenomenology of action would suggest that the CMA drives actions, without any reference to conscious intentions, desires, or reasons for action. For example, a patient presented with a fruit in the absence of stimulation would merely hold it. But once stimulated, the patient would grasp and eat the fruit for as long as the stimulation lasted. This compulsive eating was not part of a normal desire for food, since it ceased with the end of stimulation.

In summary, CMA stimulation transiently induced a syndrome similar to utilization behavior (Lhermitte, 1983). The overall impression is of a

CMA role in motivating and driving behavior, but not in anticipating, or monitoring or adjusting it to circumstances, nor in providing a conscious experience of an impending action. The state evoked by CMA stimulation therefore appears to be closer to a motivational drive than to an intentional decision. The evoked actions appear to happen **to** the patient, but are quite decoupled from their conscious mental life, and play no role in it. This explains why the patient does not produce convincing or detailed reasons to explain why they occurred.

### A Model of Frontal Contributions to Intentional Action

One simple model, which could encompass Libet et al.'s (1983) concept of conscious intention, is shown in Figure 7.1. Selection between competing alternative actions that are currently available might occur in dorsolateral prefrontal cortex (DLPFC) (Rowe, Toni, Josephs, Frackowiak, & Passingham, 2000). This process may involve conscious thought about the range of action alternatives, but only at the level of abstract action possibilities. The DLPFC selects the appropriate action, and forwards the decision to two separate cortical motor areas to implement it. On the one hand the decision is sent to the CMA, which provides a motivational drive to initiate the action. On the other hand the decision is sent to the preSMA, which provides a stage of flexible, contextual modulation of internally generated action, weaving the selected action into the ongoing flow of behavior and experience. This flexibility is required since a behavior may be appropriate in one context but not in another: even a strongly motivated action can and should sometimes be stopped or delayed. PreSMA therefore provides contextual arbitration, according to which a drive may be developed into an impending action plan, or alternatively inhibited. This contextualizing role of preSMA can explain three specific findings from the neurophysiological literature that may otherwise be hard to explain (see Haggard, 2008, for a detailed review). First, cells in the preSMA appear to play a key role in integrating single actions into coordinated superordinate sequences of behavior. Second, lesions in this area produce compulsive action tendencies, reminiscent of the automatized reaching and grasping evoked by CMA stimulation. Third, the preSMA plays a key role in arbitrating involving conflict between the various alternative actions that could be consistent with a given situation. The preSMA is therefore involved not in the raw drive to action, but in reconciling action drives with current contexts.

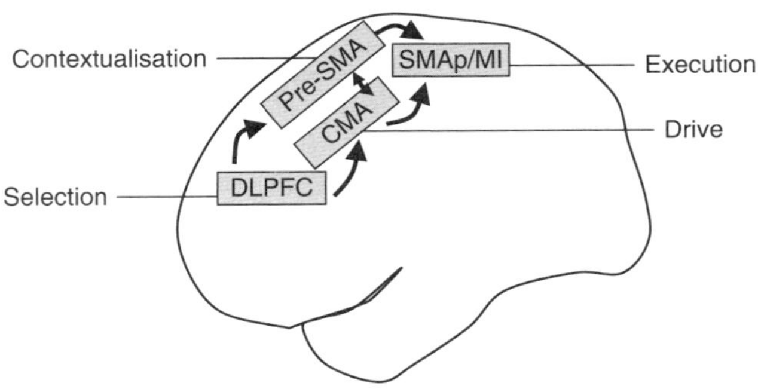


**Figure 7.1** A simple model of the division of labor between frontal cortical areas in the initiation of intentional action. Selection between alternative action plans occurs in the dorsolateral prefrontal cortex (DLPFC). The signal corresponding to the selected action is forwarded along two major neural pathways: to the cingulate motor area (CMA) to provide a motivated drive to perform the action, and to the presupplementary motor area (preSMA) to modulate the action according to current context, competing action representations, etc. Hypothesized interactions provide an arbitration between the push from drive and the constraints provided by context. Both areas have access to the main motor execution pathway via supplementary motor area proper (SMAp) and the primary motor cortex (M1).

Interestingly, the conscious experience of immediate intention seems to involve the same circuits that contextually constrain action drives. The conscious "urge" evoked by preSMA stimulation, which perhaps underlies W-judgments of intention in Libet-type experiments, would correspond to the moment of opening the gate between drive and motor action. The preSMA would then pass the contextualized action plan to the SMA-proper (SMAp), M1, and possibly CMA for execution. On this model, Libet is absolutely right that our actions are initiated unconsciously, by the normal functioning of the sensory and motor network of the cortex. The conscious experience of immediate intention occurs when the prefrontal executive opens the gates between this network and motor executive areas, such as M1, so that the drive built up within this network can now proceed to appropriate action execution.

### What Are Immediate Intentions?

The discussion above allows us to revisit our question, "what are immediate intentions?" From a neural point of view, immediate intentions are conscious experiences of impending action, generated by the motor systems of the medial frontal cortex. From a psychological point of view, two important aspects of immediate intention are worth emphasizing. First, immediate intentions are predictive, in the sense that they precede actions. Second, immediate intentions have an episodic, time-locked quality, rather than being abstract and semantic. Thus, the content of an immediate intention prefigures at least some of the specific motor details of the action itself. Immediate intentions are not linked to actions in a vague and general way, but in a motor-specific way (Haggard & Eimer, 1999), even in artificial cases such as preSMA stimulation (Fried et al, 1991). Put another way, immediate intentions incorporate the specific contextual detail, corresponding at least to the P-level and often to the M-level in the DPM hierarchy. An interesting conscious correlate of this episodic quality is the very integrated experience we have of our own voluntary action. Intention, action, and goal are not experienced as separate disconnected events, but as a tight and integrated flow. In particular, intentional actions, but not involuntary movements, display an effect called "intentional binding," whereby the experiences of action and effect are perceived as temporally compressed and bound together (Haggard et al, 2002; Haggard & Cole, 2007), as if part of a single episode.

## 2. PROSPECTIVE INTENTIONS

We share with other animals the capacity to act purposefully, but we also regularly make more or less complex plans for the future, and our later conduct is guided by these plans. We are, in Michael Bratman's words, planning agents, and this planning ability appears to be distinctively human. People can, and frequently do, form intentions focused on actions that may occur years or even decades later. Intentions to choose particular careers, to become prime minister, or to choose a destination for next year's holiday all offer examples. The length of time-scale associated with prospective intentions is virtually unlimited. These long-range intentions appear to be effectively connected with short-range intentions, and therefore with action itself. General intentions formed at one time-point cascade into much more detailed intentions prior to action execution.

However, almost nothing is known about how these long-range, prospective intentions connect to immediate, short-term intentions. Indeed, experimental studies of voluntary action deal hardly at all with the concept of prospective intention. On one view, the prospective intention in such studies consists in the participant's decision to participate in the experiment in the first place, and thus lies beyond what can be measured in the experimental setting itself.

We start this section with a brief review of Bratman's influential account of prospective intentions (or as he calls them future-directed intentions), what their main characteristics are, and what makes it useful to have them. We then turn to the issue what kind of cognitive processes are involved in the formation of prospective intentions and how these relate to the processes involved in immediate intentions.

### Bratman on Intentions

Bratman's account of future-directed intentions (Bratman, 1987) stresses the commitment to action that is a distinctive characteristic of intentions. When I intend today to go Christmas shopping tomorrow, I do not simply want or desire today that I go Christmas shopping tomorrow. Rather I am committed now to going shopping tomorrow. What exactly does this commitment involve? Bratman distinguishes two dimensions of a commitment to action: a volitional dimension and a reasoning-centered dimension. The volitional dimension concerns the relation of intention to action and can be characterized by saying that, "intentions are, whereas ordinary desires are not, conduct-*controlling* pro-attitudes. Ordinary desires, in contrast, are merely *potential influencers* of action" (1987, p. 16). In other words, unless something unexpected arrives that forces me to revise my intention, my intention today to go shopping tomorrow will control my conduct tomorrow. The reasoning-centered dimension of commitment is most directly linked to planning. At stake here are the roles played by intentions in the period between their initial formation and their eventual execution. First, intentions have what Bratman calls a characteristic *stability* or inertia: once we have formed an intention to *A*, we will not normally continue to deliberate whether to *A* or not. In the absence of relevant new information, the intention will resist reconsideration, we will see the matter as settled and continue to so intend until the time of action. Intentions are thus *terminators of practical reasoning* about ends or goals. Second, during this period between the formation of an intention and action, we will frequently reason from such an intention to further intentions, reasoning for instance from intended ends to intended means or preliminary steps. When we first form an intention, our plans are typically only partial, but if they are to eventuate into action, they will need to be filled in. Thus, intentions are also *prompters of practical reasoning* about means. Finally, the volitional and reasoning-centered dimensions of intentions together account for another important function of prospective intentions, namely their role in supporting both *intrapersonal and interpersonal coordination*. Because intentions have stability, are conduct-controlling, and prompt reasoning about means, they support the expectation that I will do tomorrow what I intend today to do tomorrow. Such expectations facilitate coordination. My intention to go Christmas shopping tomorrow supports my sister's expectation that I will, and she can go ahead and plan to join me in this shopping expedition. Similarly, I can go ahead and plan my activities for the day after tomorrow, on the assumption that by tomorrow evening I will be done with Christmas shopping.

As noted by Bratman himself, future-directed intentions have an air of paradox. They are typically stable but they are not irrevocable. Such irrevocability would be irrational, since things can change and our anticipation of the future is not infallible. This suggests that, having formed today an intention to do something tomorrow, I should persist in that intention tomorrow only if it would then be rational for me to form such an intention from scratch. But then, asks Bratman, why should I bother deciding today what to do tomorrow? Isn't that just a waste of time?

Bratman offers several complementary answers to that challenge. They stem from the fact that we are epistemically limited creatures, with limited cognitive and time resources for use in attending to problems, gathering information, deliberating about options, determining likely consequences, and so on. There are several reasons our epistemic limitations make it useful for us to form prospective intentions. First, if our actions were influenced by deliberation only at the time of action, this influence would be minimal, as time pressure isn't conducive to careful deliberation. Advance planning frees us from that time pressure and allows us to deploy the cognitive resources needed for successful deliberation. Second, intentions once formed have characteristic stability. They resist reconsideration. This doesn't mean we never reconsider. Intentions may be revoked. But as Bratman points out, revocability does not entail actual reconsideration. Unless new facts come to light, we will normally simply retain our intentions. Furthermore, in settling on a course of action, we have already rehearsed and weighted the considerations for and against that course of action. This prior rehearsal puts us in a better position to assess whether a new piece of information is actually relevant or not to our plans. If nonreconsideration is the default option, once an intention is formed the precious cognitive resources that were engaged in deliberation about ends are free be used for other tasks, including planning about means and ensuring both intra- and interpersonal coordination. To achieve complex goals, I must coordinate my present and future activities and coordinate with activities of other agents. If I now intend to go to the concert tomorrow night, I first need to procure a ticket and make sure I have a babysitter for the evening. If I were to leave it to the last minute to decide whether I go to the concert tonight or not, I may well be frustrated to find out that tickets are sold out or that the babysitter is not available. Thus, the success of many of our actions depends on our ability to coordinate our own activities over time and to coordinate them with the activities of other agents. This coordination is best achieved if we plan ahead of time.

So-called Buridan cases provide a third reason for forming intentions. We may be forced to choose between options that we find equally desirable. I may have an equal desire to go to a concert or to go see a play tomorrow evening. But if I am to do either, I had better decide now among these options. For one thing, it may not be worth my while looking for further information in the hope of finding new reasons to decide between them, as the effort and time needed to gather further information may well exceed the potential benefits of, say, enjoying the concert slightly more than I would have the play. Moreover, once again, intrapersonal and interpersonal coordination require that I reach a decision. I need to know whether to buy a ticket for the play or for the concert, and if I wish friends to join me, I need to let them know whether I intend to go to the concert or to go see the play.

## Future-Oriented Cognition and Mental Time Travel

Prima facie, it would seem that the reasons that make it useful for us to form prospective intentions also apply to other species. Limited cognitive resources and a need for coordination are not unique to humans. So why is it that we alone appear to exhibit such distinctive planning abilities? One obvious answer is that other species are even more limited then we are in their cognitive resources; a complementary answer is that how much need and use we have for planning also depends on the kind of environment we live in. There wouldn't be much use for planning in an environment that was completely unpredictable, for planning exploits regularities and in such an environment there would be none to exploit. On the other hand, in an environment both simple and reasonably predictable, there may be cheaper ways of coping than those involving advance planning. Suddendorf and Corballis, (2007) describe several ways in which behavior may be future-oriented without involving a capacity to think about the future as such. First, future-directed behavior may be instinctual, as when, through natural selection, a species has evolved behavioral predispositions to exploit significant long-term regularities. For instance, an animal can gather food for hibernation, although it has yet to experience a winter. Second, future-directed behavior may be driven by procedural learning, allowing an individual to track short-term regularities. For instance, through association, a conditioned stimulus can predict the future arrival of an unconditioned response and trigger a future-directed response. Third, future-directed behavior may exploit semantic memory about regularities, which provides the basis for inferential and analogical reasoning and allows learning in one context to be voluntarily transferred to another. Procedural learning allows for greater flexibility than instinctual patterns of behavior, allowing behavior to be modulated by individual experience; semantic memories provide even greater behavioral flexibility as they can be triggered endogenously rather than being stimulus bound. Yet, the environment in which humans live is unique in both its ecological and its social complexity. Humans also have an extraordinary range of desires and motivations, going far beyond the basic drives and simpler desires present in other species. Dealing with this spectacular environmental, social, and motivational complexity may require in turn forms of future-oriented cognition that exhibit unique flexibility and versatility.

A prime candidate for this more flexible form of future-oriented cognition is *mental time travel*, the faculty that allows a person to mentally project herself backward in time to relive past events or forward to pre-live events (Suddendorf & Corballis, 1997, 2007; Suddendorf & Busby, 2003, 2005; Wheeler, Stuss, & Tulving, 1997). Mental travel in the past, known as episodic memory, has been intensively studied (e.g., Tulving, 1983, 2005). Mental travel into the future, in contrast, has only recently begun to draw attention. Recent work indicates that mental travel into the past and into the future are closely related, involving similar cognitive processes—a combination of episodic memory and imagination under executive control—and recruiting strongly overlapping neural systems (D'Argembeau & Van der Linden, 2006; Hassabis, Vann, & Magurie, 2007; Klein, 2002; Gerrans, 2007). Several researchers have argued that mental time travel into the future is a crucial cognitive adaptation, enhancing planning and deliberation by allowing a subject to mentally simulate and evaluate contingencies, and thus enhancing fitness, and that mental time travel into the past is subsidiary to our ability to imagine future scenarios (Dudai & Carruthers, 2005; Suddendorf & Corballis, 2007).

Mental time travel, whether into the past or into the future, involves episodic memory and inherits its two main characteristics. First, it is not about regularities but about constructing or reconstructing the *particularities of specific events*. Second, mental time travel involves *autonoesis*, i.e., awareness of a self as the subject of actual, recalled, or imagined experience. But what are exactly the benefits that accrue from using mental time travel rather than simply reasoning from general knowledge stored in semantic memory in planning future actions? As we have seen, prospective intentions involve making a number of decisions. The intention is first formed when one reaches a decision about what to do. Once the intention is formed, one must still typically make a number of decisions about how to implement the chosen goal. Another important decision, not explicitly considered by Bratman, concerns when to act. What can mental time travel contribute to these what-decisions, how-decisions, and when-decisions?

### What-decisions

Not all what-decisions involve explicit conscious deliberation. Some decisions are pretty straightforward. If my closest friend invites me to her wedding, of course I'll accept the invitation and form the intention to attend the wedding. If, however, being on the job market, I am offered academic positions in two different universities, I might spend quite a while weighing the pros and cons of each option before reaching a decision. Yet, it may be that performing a logical cost-benefit analysis of the two options does not suffice to motivate me to choose one over the other, even if this analysis yields a clear advantage for one of the options. Rather, I might have to imaginatively rehearse future experiences occupying one or the other position as part of the process of deliberation.

Patients with damage to the ventromedial prefrontal cortex (VMPFC) are often described as having impaired ability for planning and decision-making despite retaining intact capacities for explicit reasoning. Philip Gerrans, (2007) argues that this impairment is best explained by a deficit in mental time travel. In his view, Damasio's somatic marker hypothesis (Damasio, Tranel, & Damasio, 1991; Bechara, Damasio, Damasio, & Lee, 1999), according to which the deficits of VMPFC patients result from a failure to link an implicit emotional response—a somatic marker—with an explicit representation of a situation, is deficient in two ways. First, it uses an account of emotions that explains salience and motivation in terms of valence and within this framework interprets somatic markers as valencing systems whose activation is required to produce suitable motivation. However, recent research shows that the mechanisms that make objects salient and motivate behavior are independent neurally and cognitively from those that determine valence. The mesolimbic dopamine system plays a central role in salience/motivation by predicting reward (rather than valence), while valencing appears to be realized by a number of other systems, including the opioid and benzodiazepine systems (Berridge & Robinson, 2003;

Berridge, 2007; Robinson & Berridge, 2003). Second, the somatic marker hypothesis underspecifies the nature of the explicit representations involved in decision-making. These representations can either be declarative, as when one performs cost-benefit analysis by manipulating probabilities, or episodic, as when one uses past experiences to imagine future ones. According to Gerrans then, the planning and decision-making deficits of VMPFC patients result not so much from their inability to associate semantic markers to their explicit declarative representations as from their inability to perform mental time travel, that is to imagine themselves living out future scenarios and thus activating the motivationally relevant contingencies salient in these imagined experiences.

If this conception of the link between mental time travel and motivation is on the right track, mental time travel could also help explain one unique characteristic of human planning. According to the Bischof-Köhler hypothesis (Bischof-Köhler, 1985; Suddendorf & Busby, 2005), nonhuman animals cannot anticipate future needs or drive states. Humans, in contrast, can plan for the future not just on the basis of their current motivational states but also on the basis of what they anticipate their future motivational states to be. The ability to project oneself forward in time and imagine future scenarios may be an important key to motivation regulation.

### How-decisions

The construction of plans for future actions depends in part on semantic memory, since it is crucial to their success that the plans we come up with be consistent with our general knowledge about the world. Yet, filling in the details of a plan may depend on our ability to imagine future episodes, since they provide the particularities that will help us fine-tune the plan to the particular occasion. However, trade-offs need to be considered, since mental time travel is effortful and cognitively costly. When I form the prospective intention to go to my office tomorrow rather than to work from home, there is no need for me to mentally rehearse the route to my office. The route is familiar enough that I can trust myself to do the right thing when the time comes. Suppose, however, that I have an appointment tomorrow in some other part of the city I am less familiar with. In that case, it may be worthwhile rehearsing possible ways of getting there and using memories of past episodes to decide between options. For instance, I may remember that changing lines at this station takes forever and involves walking along endless, badly lit, corridors, or I may remember getting stuck in heavy traffic on a given bus line. Or imagine again, I am about to visit Beijing for the first time and have no clue what the public transportation is like there. In such a case it may be a waste of time and energy imagining potential future scenarios for how to get around in Beijing. The scenarios I come up with may be far off the mark and completely useless in the end; better just wait and see.

More generally, whether we make how-decisions early or late and the extent to which we use mental time travel to make those decisions depends on a number of factors, among them: how predictable we think the future situation is; how knowledgeable we are; whether our knowledge is mostly declarative or based on prior personal experience; how motivated we are (as rehearsing a future scenario may help reinforce motivation); how novel or difficult the prospective action is; how neurotic our personality is. In addition, there appear to be important individual differences in the ability to project oneself into possible future events. A recent study (D'Argembeau & Van der Linden, 2006) provides evidence that the individual differences in dimensions known to affect memory for past events similarly influence the experience of projecting oneself into the future. People less adept at recalling in vivid detail past episodes of their life, are also less able to simulate specific future events. Note that these results also provide support for the view that mental time travel into the past and mental time travel into the future rely on similar mechanisms.

### When-decisions

A prospective intention is an intention to perform an action at some future time. But if the intention is to eventuate into action, it is important that the time of action be specified. An initial when-decision can take at least two forms. The time of action can be specified in explicit temporal fashion, say as "next Tuesday" or "on the first of November" or it can be specified in relation to some specific future event, say "when I next meet Charles" or "as soon as the bell rings." Work in the field of prospective memory sheds light on interesting differences between the time-based and the event-based strategies.

Prospective memory is a field of cognitive psychology dealing with remembering to perform an action in the future (e.g., I must remember to stop to buy fruit on my way home from work). The starting point for prospective memory is clearly an intention to perform an action at a future time. Most experimental studies deal with event-based prospective memory, in which a specific event that will occur in the future is used as a cue for an action. Translating a long-range intention into action then becomes a matter of identifying that the cue has occurred, and retrieving the appropriate action in response to it. Several studies of "implementation intentions" in applied psychology (Gollwitzer, 1999) suggest this strategy is effective: intended actions such as taking medication are more likely to occur if people link their implementation to a specific external event. According to Gollwitzer, (1999), what explains the efficacy of implementation intentions is the fact that their formation triggers two sets of processes. First, when an implementation intention is formed, mental representations of the relevant situational cues become highly activated, leading to heightened accessibility, and thus a better detection, of these cues when they are encountered (Aarts, Dijksterhuis, & Midden, 1999; Gollwitzer, 1999; Webb & Sheeran, 2007). Second, implementation intention formation not only enhances the accessibility of the specified situational cue, but also forges an association between that cue and a response that is instrumental for obtaining one's goal, thus making action initiation more immediate and efficient.

Such "implementation intentions" may take advantage of the fact that externally cued intentions are normally more strongly held, in the sense of being harder to overturn, than internally generated intentions (Fleming, Mars, Gladwin, & Haggard, 2009).

Prospective memory can also be time-based, rather than event-based. In time-based prospective memory, an intended action is performed at a designated future time, without any particular cue event occurring at that time. Thus, time-based prospective memory seems to be purely endogenous, while event-based prospective memory effectively reduces endogenous actions to cue-triggered reactions. The distinction between the two forms is supported by the dissociation between different rostral prefrontal activations in time-based and event-based prospective memory tasks (Okuda et al., 2007).

Recent studies of time-based prospective memory suggest an interesting role for unconsciously initiated processes, similar to Libet's action initiation, in linking long-range intentions to eventual action. Kvavilashvili and Fisher (2007) asked participants to call an experimenter at a self-chosen time one week after an initial briefing session. In the intervening week, they noted the circumstances in which they remembered this intention, using a diary. Although the authors refer to these memory events as "rehearsals" they were primarily automatic and uncued events, in which the intention to make the phone call simply "popped into" the participant's mind, without obvious cue or antecedent. The frequency of these recall events increased dramatically in the day before the phone call was due, but this increase was less dramatic in those participants who in fact failed to return the phone call on time.

## 3. LINKING PROSPECTIVE INTENTIONS TO IMMEDIATE INTENTIONS

Actions are not always the product of prospective intentions, they may often simply be the outcome of immediate intentions, formed on the spot, so to speak. But let us focus on cases where actions are preceded and brought about by prospective intentions. What is the additional contribution, if any, of immediate intentions to such actions?

Recall that in the section 1 we characterized the content of immediate intentions as involving episodic representations. Forming an immediate intention involves fitting one's endogenous goal to the current situation, using contextual information to generate a representation of a specific episode of acting. When one has a prospective intention to perform an action, how much work there is left for an immediate intention to do at the moment of action itself will depend on how episodic the content of the prospective intention already is. This will in turn depend on the extent to which the agent made use of mental time travel in forming and shaping his prospective intentions. For example, a person forming a prospective intention may become fully involved in mental time travel and may simulate the full details of how and when the action will occur. Conversely, one can have a genuine prospective intention while knowingly leaving it for later to decide on the means. At one extreme of a continuum is the "neurotic planner," at the other end is the "optimistic improviser."

The neurotic planner makes extensive use of mental time travel, imaginatively combining and recombining elements from prior stored episodes to generate, early on, precise scenarios concerning the action to be performed and the situation in which it is to be performed. His strategy is to generate as much episodic information as he can as early as he can. When mental time travel serves well, this front-loading strategy leaves little left for immediate intentions to do.

Using Gollwitzer's terminology, we can say that neurotic planners tend to make early detailed how- and when-decisions, thus forming implementation intentions. A key feature of this strategy of early planning is that it allows for later automatization. As Gollwitzer points out, implementation intentions automatize action initiation: "The goal-directed behavior specified in an implementation intention is triggered without conscious intent once the critical situational context is encountered" (Gollwitzer, 1999, p. 498). Thus, the use of external cues to trigger action seems partly to shift the action from an endogenous or voluntary one to a stimulus-driven or reactive one.

In contrast, the optimistic improviser generates little episodic information early on. She makes a what-decision, possibly a time-based when-decision, but keeps her options open as to how and in what specific situation the action is to be performed. She is committed to generating relevant episodic information in real time, at the moment of the action itself. The prospective intentions of agents following this strategy contain as yet too little episodic information to yield action. To fill this informational gap between her prospective intention and action initiation, the agent will have to form an immediate intention specifying the missing information. This means that the agent must retain some endogenous control over action initiation and cannot delegate it to automatic responses to environmental triggers.

Episodic information must be generated in order to produce a specific action. It can be generated either early (neurotic planner) or later (optimistic improviser). These are in some sense alternative reciprocal responses to the common challenge of deciding exactly what one will do. Despite the personality-based labels we used, early versus late planning isn't just a matter of temperament. Each strategy may be better suited to some situations than to others. Early planning has its dangers. If the agent's anticipations were not correct, the external cues on which action initiation depends may fail to materialize. Or, worse perhaps, the cues may be present and automatically trigger the action when other unanticipated and unattended aspects of the situation make it unadvisable to pursue as planned. The late planner may be more flexible, but she risks unpreparedness when the time of acting comes. Having left it to the last moment to deliberate about means, when she finally does so she also risks reopening the Pandora's box of deliberation about ends. What-decisions and how-decisions aren't strictly compartmentalized. The costs and efforts involved in deliberating about how to *A* under time pressure, may lead one to reconsider whether to *A* in the first place, when giving up *A*-ing may well tempt us as the less costly option.

Often, and perhaps most of the time, our planning strategies will be mixed strategies, taking into account various factors beyond mere temperament; among them, the expected predictability of relevant future situations, one's store of relevant semantic and episodic information, one's degree of motivation, the degree of novelty or difficulty of the planned action, and how strong one thinks time constraints will be at the time of acting. The generation of episodic information about future actions will thus be distributed over time in various ways according to our assessment of these factors. One example of these differing distributions comes from the contrast between an event-based and time-based prospective memory. In event-based prospective memory, specific details of the action episode are already present in the prospective intention itself. In contrast, time-based prospective memory lacks any concrete details about the specific context in which the action will occur. Most people can and do use both forms of planning. This flexibility in the temporal distribution of episodic information is a fundamental dimension of the psychology of intention. The skilled planner is the one who knows how best to take advantage of this flexibility.

## 4. CONCLUSION

The concept of intention can do useful work in psychological theory. We have made a distinction between prospective and immediate intentions. Many authors have insisted on a qualitative difference between these two regarding the type of content, with prospective intentions generally being more abstract than immediate intentions (e.g., Searle, 1983; Pacherie, 2008). However, we suggest that the main basis of this distinction is temporal: prospective intentions necessarily occur before immediate intention and before action itself, and often long before them. In contrast, immediate intentions occur in the specific context of the action itself. Yet both types of intention share a common purpose, namely that of generating the specific information required to transform an abstract representation of a goal-state into a concrete episode of instrumental action directed toward that goal. To this extent, the content of a prospective and of an immediate intention can actually be quite similar. The main distinction between prospective and immediate intentions becomes one of when, i.e., how early on, the episodic details of an action are planned.

In our view, the conscious experience associated with intentional action comes from this process of fleshing out intentions with episodic details. In the field of episodic memory, representations of episodes are thought to include an autonoetic type of consciousness (Tulving, 1983). We suggest that intentional actions reach conscious awareness at the point where they become specific action episodes. However, the time when this occurs can vary. We have argued that episodic detail can be generated either as part of advance planning, in the form of prospective intentions, or as part of an immediate intention in real time. In the former case, one might have a conscious mental image of what one will do, but the doing itself may be automatized and only marginally conscious. In the latter case, one may have a specific conscious experience linked to the initiation of action, along the lines studied by Libet.

## ACKNOWLEDGMENTS

Elisabeth Pacherie was supported by a project grant from Agence Nationale de la Recherche (ANR-07-NEURO-039-03).

Patrick Haggard was supported by a Royal Society Research Fellowship, a Leverhulme Trust Research Fellowship, and a project grant from ESRC.

## REFERENCES

Aarts, H., Dijksterhuis, A., & Midden, C. (1999). To plan or not to plan? Goal achievement or interrupting the performance of mundane behaviours. *European Journal of Social Psychology, 29,* 971–979.

Bancaud, J., Talairach, J., Geier, S., Bonis, A., Trottier, S., & Manrique, M. (1976). Behavioral manifestations induced by electric stimulation of the anterior cingulate gyrus in man. *Revue Neurologique (Paris), 132,* 705–724.

Bechara, A., Damasio, H., Damasio, A., & Lee, G. P. (1999). Differential contributions of the human amygdala and ventromedial prefrontal cortex to human decision-making. *Journal of Neuroscience, 19,* 5473–5481.

Berridge, K. C. (2007). The debate over dopamine's role in reward: The case for incentive salience. *Psychopharmacology, 191,* 391–431.

Berridge, K. C., & Robinson, T. E. (2003). Parsing reward. *Trends in Neurosciences, 26*(9), 507–513.

Bischof-Köhler, D. (1985) Zur Phylogenese menschlicher Motivation [On the phylogeny of human motivation]. In L. H. Eckensberger & E. D. Lantermann (Eds.), Emotion und Reflexivität (pp. 3–47). Vienna: Urban & Schwarzenberg.

Bratman, M. E. (1987). *Intention, plans, and practical reason*. Cambridge, MA: Harvard University Press.

Chassagnon, S., Minotti, L., Kremer, S., Hoffmann, D., & Kahane, P. (2008). Somatosensory, motor, and reaching/grasping responses to direct electrical stimulation of the human cingulate motor areas. *Journal of Neurosurgery, 109,* 593–604.

Damasio, A. R., Tranel, D., & Damasio, H. (1991). Somatic markers and the guidance of behaviour: Theory and preliminary testing. In H. S. Levin, H. M. Eisenberg, A. L. Benton (Eds.), *Frontal lobe function and dysfunction* (pp. 217–229). New York: Oxford University Press.

D'Argembeau, A. & Van der Linden, M. (2006) Individual differences in the phenomenology of mental time travel: The effect of vivid visual imagery and emotion regulation strategies. *Consciousness and Cognition, 15,* 342–350.

Dudai, Y., & Carruthers, M. (2005). The Janus face of Mnemosyne. *Nature, 434,* 567.

Fleming, S. M., Mars, R. J., Gladwin, T. E., & Haggard, P. (2009). When the brain changes its mind: Flexibility of action selection in instructed and free choices. *Cerebral Cortex, 19*(10), 2352–2360.

Fried, I., Katz, A., McCarthy, G., Sass, K. J., Williamson, P., Spencer, S. S., et al. (1991). Functional organisation of human supplementary motor cortex studies by electrical stimulation. *Journal of Neuroscience, 11,* 3656–3666.

Gallagher, S. 2006. Where's the action? Epiphenomenalism and the problem of free will. In W. Banks, S. Pockett, & S. Gallagher (Eds.), *Does Consciousness Cause Behavior? An Investigation of the Nature of Volition* (pp. 109–124). Cambridge, MA: MIT Press.

Gerrans, P. (2007). Mental time travel, somatic markers and "myopia for the future." *Synthese, 159*(3), 459–474.

Gollwitzer, P. M. (1999). Implementation intentions: Strong effects of simple plans. *American Psychologist, 54,* 493–503.

Haggard, P., Clark S., & Kalogeras, J. (2002). Voluntary action and conscious awareness. *Nature Neuroscience, 5*(4), 382–5.

Haggard, P. (2005). Conscious intention and motor cognition. *Trends in Cognitive Science, 9*(6), 290–295.

Haggard, P. (2008). Human volition: Towards a neuroscience of will. *Nature Reviews: Neuroscience, 9,* 934–946.

Haggard, P., & Cole, J. (2007). Intention, attention, and the temporal experience of action. *Consciousness and Cognition, 16*(2), 211–220.

Haggard, P., & Eimer, M. (1999). On the relation between brain potentials and the awareness of voluntary movements. *Experimental Brain Research, 126,* 128–133.

Hassabis, D. K. D., Vann, S. D., & Maguire, E. A. (2007). Patients with hippocampal amnesia cannot imagine new experiences. *Proceedings of the National Academy of Sciences, 104,* 1726–1731.

Klein, S. B. (2002). Memory and temporal experience: The effects of episodic memory loss on an amnesic patient's ability to remember the past and imagine the future. *Social Cognition, 20,* 353–379.

Kremer, S., Chassagnon, S., Hoffmann, D., Benabid, A. L., & Kahane, P. (2001). The cingulate hidden hand. *Journal of Neurology, Neurosurgery, and Psychiatry, 70,* 264–265.

Kvavilashvili, L., & Fisher, L. (2007). Is time-based prospective remembering mediated by self-initiated rehearsals? Role of incidental cues, ongoing activity, age, and motivation. *Journal of Experimental Psychology: General, 136,* 112–132.

Lhermitte, F. (1983). "Utilization behaviour" and its relation to lesions of the frontal lobes. *Brain, 106,* 237–255.

Libet, B., Gleason, C. A., Wright, E. W., & Pearl, D. K. (1983). Time of conscious intention to act in relation to onset of cerebral activity (readiness-potential). *Brain, 106*(3), 623–642.

Mima, T., Ikeda, A., Yazawa, S., Kunieda, T., Nagamine, T., Taki, W., et al. (1999). Somesthetic function of supplementary motor area during voluntary movements. *Neuroreport, 10,* 1859–1862.

Okuda, J., Fujii, T., Ohtake, H., Tsukiura, T., Yamadori, A., Frith, C. D., et al. (2007). Differential involvement of regions of rostral prefrontal cortex (Brodmann area 10) in time- and event-based prospective memory. *International Journal of Psychophysiology, 64,* 233–246.

Pacherie, E. (2008). The phenomenology of action: A conceptual framework. *Cognition, 107*(1), 179–217.

Robinson, T., & Berridge, K. C. (2003). Addiction. *Annual Review of Psychology, 54,* 25–53.

Rowe, J. B., Toni, I., Josephs, O., Frackowiak, R. S., & Passingham, R. E. (2000). The prefrontal cortex: Response selection or maintenance within working memory? *Science, 288,* 1656–1660.

Searle, J. (1983). *Intentionality.* Cambridge, UK: Cambridge University Press.

Soon, C., Brass, M., Heinze, H. J., & Haynes, J. D. (2008). Unconscious determinants of free decisions in the human brain. *Nature Neuroscience, 11,* 543–545.

Suddendorf, T., & Busby, J. (2003). Mental time travel in animals? *Trends in Cognitive Sciences, 7,* 391–396.

Suddendorf, T., & Busby, J. (2005). Making decisions with the future in mind: Developmental and comparative identification of mental time travel. *Learning and Motivation, 36,* 110–125.

Suddendorf, T., & Corballis, M. C. (1997). Mental time travel and the evolution of the human mind. *Genetic, Social, and General Psychology Monographs, 123,* 133–167.

Suddendorf, T., & Corballis, M. C. (2007). The evolution of foresight: What is mental time travel, and is it unique to human? *Behavioral and Brain Sciences, 30,* 299–351.

Tulving, E. (1983) *Elements of episodic memory.* Oxford: Clarendon Press.

Tulving, E. (2005). Episodic memory and autonoesis: Uniquely human? In H. S. Terrace & J. Metcalfe (Eds.), *The missing link in cognition: Origins of self-reflective consciousness* (pp. 3–56). Oxford: Oxford University Press.

Webb, T. L., & Sheeran, P. (2007). How do implementation intentions promote goal attainment? A test of component processes. *Journal of Experimental Social Psychology, 43,* 295–302.

Wheeler, M. A., Stuss, D. T., & Tulving, E. (1997). Toward a theory of episodic memory: The frontal lobes and autonoetic consciousness. *Psychological Bulletin, 121,* 331–354.

Wittgenstein, L. (1953). *Philosophical investigations.* Oxford: Blackwell.

# CHAPTER 8

## Beyond Libet: Long-term Prediction of Free Choices from Neuroimaging Signals

*John-Dylan Haynes*

### INTRODUCTION

It is a common folk-psychological intuition that we can freely choose between different behavioral options. Even a simple, restricted movement task with only a single degree of freedom can be sufficient to yield this intuition, say in an experiment where a subject is asked to "move a finger at some point of their own choice." Although such a simple decision might not be perceived as important as say a decision to study at one university or another, most subjects feel it is a useful example of a specific type of freedom that is often experienced when making decisions: They have the impression that the outcome of many decisions is not predetermined at the time they are felt to be made, and instead they are still "free" to choose one or the other way.

This belief in the freedom of decisions is fundamental to our human self-concept. It is so strong that it is generally maintained even though it contradicts several other core beliefs. For example, freedom appears to be incompatible with the nature of our universe. The deterministic, causally closed physical world seems to stand in the way of "additional" and "unconstrained" influences on our behavior from mental faculties that exist beyond the laws of physics. Interestingly, in most people's (and even in some philosophers'[1]) minds, the incompatible beliefs in free will and in determinism coexist happily without any apparent conflict. One reason why most people don't perceive this as a conflict might be that our belief in freedom is so deeply embedded in our everyday thoughts and behavior that the rather abstract belief in physical determinism is simply not strong enough to compete. The picture changes, however, with direct scientific demonstrations that our choices are determined by the brain. People are immensely fascinated by scientific experiments that directly expose how our seemingly free decisions are systematically related to prior brain activity.

In a seminal experiment, Benjamin Libet and colleagues investigated the temporal relationship between brain activity and a conscious intention to perform a simple voluntary movement (Libet, Gleason, Wright, & Pearl, 1983). Subjects viewed a "clock" that consisted of a light point moving on a circular path rotating once every 2.56 seconds. Subjects were asked to flex a finger at a freely chosen point in time and to remember and report the position of the moving light point when they first felt the urge to move. The reported position of the light could then be used to determine the time when the person consciously formed their intention, a time subsequently called "W," as a shorthand for the conscious experience of "wanting" or "will." Libet recorded EEG signals from movement-related brain regions while subjects were performing this task. It had previously been known that negative deflections of the EEG signal can be observed immediately preceding voluntary movements (Kornhuber & Deecke, 1965). These so-called readiness-potentials (RP) originate from a region of cortex known as the supplementary motor cortex (SMA), which is involved in motor preparation. Libet and colleagues were interested in whether the readiness-potential might begin to arise even before the person had made up their mind to move. Indeed they found that the readiness-potential already began to arise a few hundred milliseconds before the "feeling of wanting" entered awareness. This systematic temporal precedence of brain activity before a freely timed decision was subsequently taken as evidence that the brain had made the decision to move *before* this decision entered awareness. It was proposed that the readiness potential reflects the primary cortical site where the decision to move is made (Eccles, 1982).

Due to their far-reaching implications that unconscious brain processes might cause what appears to be a free choice, Libet's groundbreaking experiments immediately met severe criticism. Following the analysis of Hume (1777) two empirical criteria are required to argue for a causal relationship between two events, say event B (brain) causing event W (will). First, there has to be a *temporal precedence* of B before W, and second there has to be a *constant connection* between events B and W. It has been debated whether Libet's experiments fulfill either of these criteria. Several authors have questioned whether there is indeed a temporal precedence between readiness potential and intention, in particular by arguing that the timing judgments are unreliable (Breitmeyer, 1985; Van de Grind, 2002). It has long been known that there are substantial inaccuracies in determining the timing and position of moving objects (Moutoussis & Zeki, 1997; Rollman, 1985; Van de Grind, 2002; Wundt, 1904). Thus, the choice of a moving light point to report the timing is far from optimal.

A different line of arguments addresses the constant connection between B and W. Libet reports data averaged across a number of trials. Although this shows that on average there is a readiness potential before the urge to move, it doesn't show whether this holds for every single trial, which would be necessary to provide evidence for a constant connection. For example, the early onset of the RP might be an artifact of temporal smearing and might reflect only the onset of the earliest urges to move (Trevena & Miller, 2002). This could only be assessed by measuring the onset time of individual RPs, which is a particularly challenging signal processing problem that requires advanced decoding algorithms (Blankertz et al., 2003).

A further important shortcoming of Libet's experiment is that it only investigates RPs, which means it is restricted to signals originating from movement-related brain regions. This leaves unclear how other areas might contribute to the build-up of decisions. This is particularly important because several other regions of prefrontal cortex have frequently been shown to be involved in free choice situations (e.g., Deiber, Passingham, Colebatch, Friston, Nixon, & Frackowiak, 1991), although it remains unclear to which degree they are involved in preparing a decision. Another shortcoming of RPs is that they only emerge in a narrow time window immediately preceding a movement, leaving unclear whether they indeed reflect the earliest stage where a decision is cortically prepared. In fact it has been argued that the close temporal proximity of RP and conscious awareness of the urge to move means that these two processes are scientifically indistinguishable (Merikle & Cheeseman, 1985).

Taken together, some of the problems with the original Libet experiment could be overcome by investigating whether other brain regions might begin to prepare a decision across longer time spans. Interestingly, it had been shown even before the original Libet experiments that prefrontal cortex prepares voluntary movements across longer periods than is visible from the readiness potential alone (Groll-Knapp, Ganglberge, & Haider, 1977). Thus, activity in prefrontal brain regions might be a much better predictor of the outcome of decisions than readiness potentials. However to date, studies on voluntary movement preparation in prefrontal cortex have not simultaneously measured the timing of the self-paced urge to move along with the corresponding brain activity.

## THE MODIFIED LIBET EXPERIMENT

To overcome these and other shortcomings of the Libet experiments, we performed a novel variant of the original task (Soon, Brass, Heinze, & Haynes, 2008). We used functional magnetic resonance imaging (fMRI), a technique that measures changes in the oxygenation level of blood, which are in turn caused by neural activity. Functional magnetic resonance imaging has a much higher spatial resolution than EEG. It uses a measurement grid with a resolution of around 3 mm to independently measure the brain activity at each position in the brain. Because the fMRI signal has a low *temporal* resolution (typically around 0.5 Hz) and lags several seconds behind neural activity, it does not allow one to resolve the fine-grained cascade of neural processes in the few hundred milliseconds just before the will enters awareness. However it is highly suitable for looking back from the W event at each position in the brain and across longer time spans. Our focus on longer time spans and the low sampling rate of the fMRI signal enabled us to relax our requirement on temporal precision of the timing judgment, thus overcoming a severe limitation of Libet's original experiments. We replaced the rotating clock with a randomized stream of letters that updated every 500 ms. Subjects had to report the letter that was visible on the screen when they made their conscious decision. This mode of report has the additional advantage of being unpredictable, which minimizes systematic preferences for specific clock positions.

Subjects were asked to freely decide between two response buttons while lying in an MRI scanner (Fig. 8.1A). They fixated on the center of the screen where the stream of letters was presented. While viewing the letter stream they were asked to relax and freely decide at some point in time to press either the left or right button. In parallel they should remember the letter presented when their decision to move reached awareness. After subjects made up their mind and pressed their freely chosen response button, a "response mapping" screen appeared, where subjects used a second button press to indicate at which time they had made their decision. This response mapping screen showed three letters plus a hash symbol ("#") arranged randomly on the four corners of an imaginary square centered on fixation. Each of these positions corresponded to one of four buttons operated by the left and right index and middle fingers. Subjects were to press the button corresponding to the letter that was visible on the screen when they consciously made their decision. When the letter was not among those presented on the screen they were asked to press the button corresponding to the hash symbol. Then, after a delay the letter stream started again and a new trial began. Note that due to the randomization of the position of letters in the response mapping screen, the second response is uncorrelated with the first, freely chosen response. Importantly, in order to facilitate spontaneous behavior, we did not ask subjects to balance the left and right button selections. This would require keeping track of the distribution of button selections in memory and would also encourage preplanning of choices. Instead, we selected subjects that spontaneously chose a balanced number of left and right button presses without prior instruction based on a behavioral selection test before scanning.

## DECODING CHOICES FROM BRAIN ACTIVITY PATTERNS

An important innovation was that we used a "decoder" to predict how a subject was going to decide from their brain activity (see Fig. 8.1B). We examined for each time point preceding the intention whether a given brain region carried information related to the specific outcome of a decision, that is the urge to press *either* a left *or* a right button, rather than reflecting unselective motor preparation. To understand the advantage of "decoding" it can help to review the standard analysis techniques in fMRI studies. Most conventional neuroimaging analyses perform statistical analyses on one position in the brain at a time, and then proceed to the next position (Friston et al., 1995). This yields a map of statistical parameters that plots how strong a certain effect is expressed at each *individual* position in the brain. But this neglects any information that is present in the distributed spatial patterns of fMRI signals. Typically, the raw data are also spatially smoothed, so any fine-grained spatial patterning is lost. It has recently emerged,

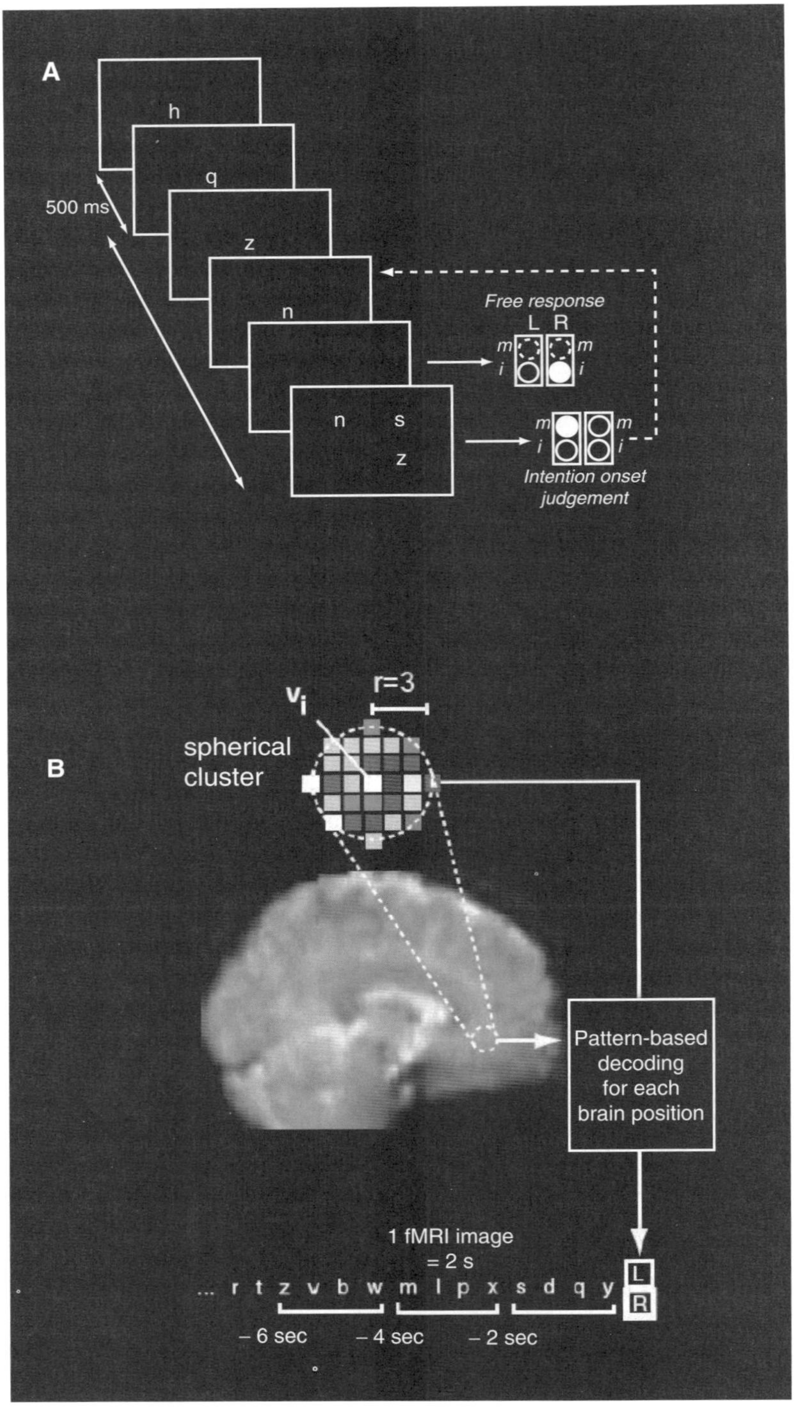


**Figure 8.1** (A) The revised Libet task. Subjects are given two response buttons, one for the left and one for the right hand. In parallel there is a stream of letters on the screen that changes every 500 ms. They are asked to relax and to decide at some spontaneous point of their own choice to press either the left or the right button.

**Figure 8.1** (*Cont.*) Once the button is pressed they are asked to report which letter was on the screen when they made up their mind. (**B**) Pattern-based decoding and prediction of decisions ahead of time. Using a searchlight technique (Kriegeskorte et al., 2006; Haynes et al., 2007; Soon et al., 2008) we assessed for each brain region and each time point preceding the decision whether it is possible to decode the choice ahead of time. Decoding is based on small local spherical clusters of voxels that form three-dimensional spatial patterns. This allowed us to systematically investigate which brain regions had predictive information at each time point preceding the decision.

however, that these fine-grained fMRI patterns contain information that is highly predictive of the detailed contents of a person's thoughts (Kamitani & Tong, 2005; Haynes & Rees, 2005, 2006). This is in accord with a common view that each region of the brain encodes information in a distributed spatial pattern of activity (Tanaka, 1997). This information is lost for conventional analyses. The full information present in brain signals can only be extracted by jointly analyzing multiple locations using pattern-based decoding algorithms. Conventional analyses can only reveal whether a brain area is more or less active during a task (say immediately preceding a decision). In contrast, we used the novel pattern-based decoding analyses not to investigate the overall level of activity but to extract a *maximal amount* of predictive information contained in the fine-grained spatial pattern of activity. This information allows one to predict the *specific* choice a subject is going to make on each trial.

In order to first validate our method we investigated from which brain regions the specific decision could be decoded *after* it had been made and the subject was already executing the motor response (**Fig. 8.2**, top). This served as a sanity check, because it is clear that one would expect to find the decision to be encoded in the motor cortex. We thus assessed for each brain area and each time point after the decision whether it was possible to decode from the spatial pattern of brain signals which motor response the subject was *currently* executing. As expected, two brain regions encoded the outcome of the subject's decision during the execution phase. These were primary motor cortex and SMA. Thus, the sanity check demonstrates the validity of the method. Please note that, as expected, the informative fMRI signals are delayed by several seconds relative to the decision due to the delay of the hemodynamic response.

Next we addressed the key question of this study, whether any brain region encoded the subject's decision *ahead* of time. We found that indeed, two brain regions predicted prior to the conscious decision whether the subject was about to choose the left or right response, even though the subject did not know yet which way they were about to decide (**Fig. 8.2**, bottom). The first region was in frontopolar cortex (FPC), BA10. The predictive information in the fMRI signals from this brain region was present already 7 seconds prior to the subject's decision. This period of 7 seconds is a conservative estimate that does not yet take into account the delay of the fMRI response with respect to neural activity. Because this delay is several seconds, the predictive neural information will have preceded the conscious decision by up to 10 seconds. There was a second predictive region located in parietal cortex (PC) stretching from the precuneus into posterior cingulate cortex. It is important to note that there is no *overall* signal increase in the frontopolar and precuneus/posterior cingulate during the preparation period. Rather, the predictive information is encoded in the spatial pattern of fMRI responses, which is presumably why it has only rarely been noticed before. Please note that due to the temporal delay of the hemodynamic response the small lead times in SMA/preSMA of up to several hundred milliseconds reported in previous studies (Libet et al., 1983; Haggard & Eimer, 1999) are below the temporal resolution of our method. Hence, we cannot exclude that other regions contain predictive information in the short period *immediately preceding* the intention.

## The Role of BA 10

The finding of unconscious, predictive brain activity patterns in Brodman area 10 (BA 10) is interesting because this area is not normally discussed in connection with free choices. This is

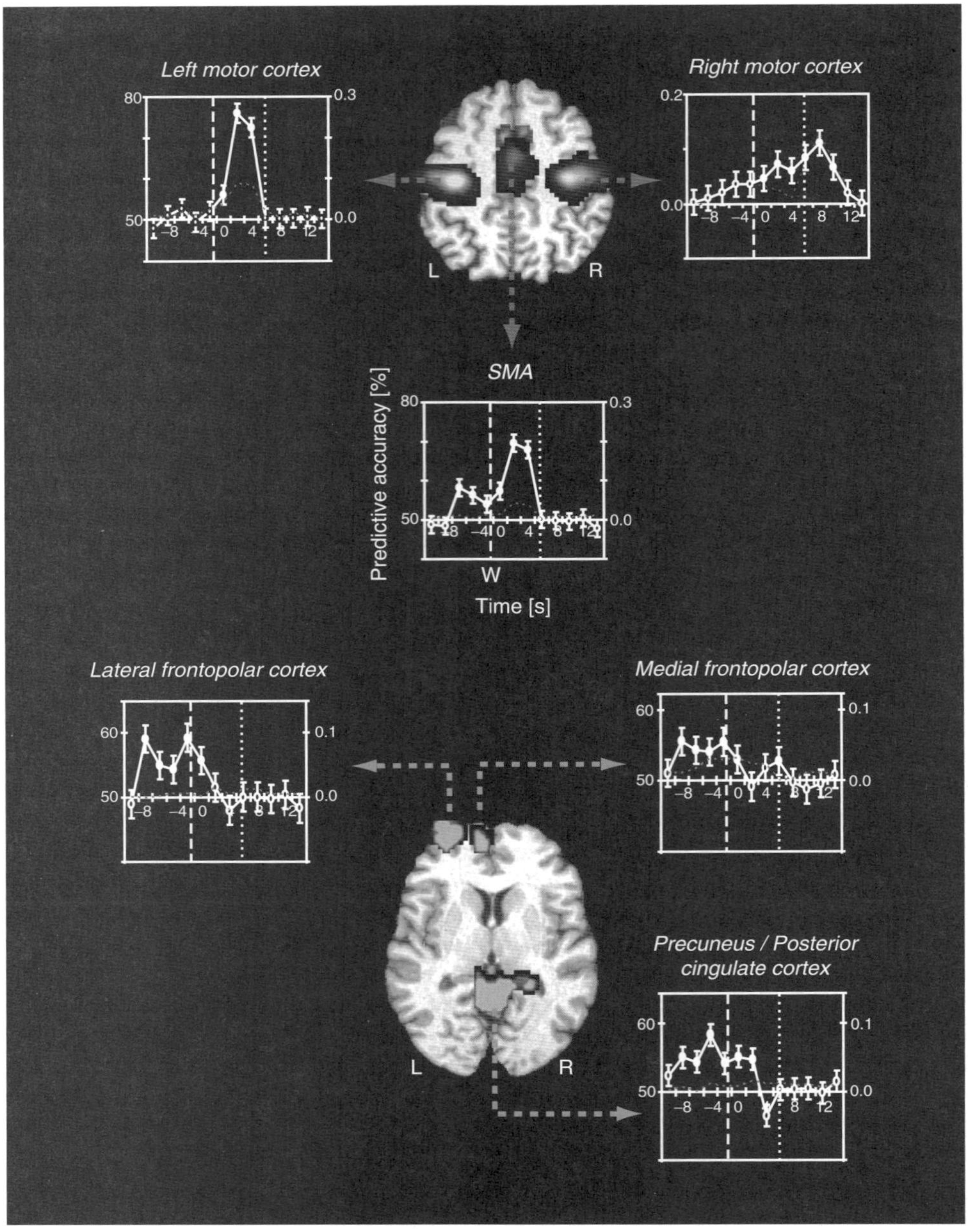


**Figure 8.2** **(Top)** First we assessed which brain regions had information about a subject's decision after it had been made and the subject was currently pressing the button corresponding to their choice. As expected, this yielded information in motor cortex and supplementary motor cortex. **(Bottom)** Second, we assessed which brain regions had predictive information about a subject's decision even before the subject knew how they were going to decide. This yielded regions of frontopolar cortex and precuneus/posterior cingulate cortex, which had predictive information already 7 seconds before the decision was made.

presumably due to the fact that conventional analyses will only pick up regions with *overall* changes in activity, but not regions where only the *patterning* of the signal changes in a choice-specific fashion. However, it has been repeatedly demonstrated using other tasks that BA 10 plays an important role in encoding and storage of intentions. It has long been known that lesions to BA 10 lead to a loss of prospective memory, thus disrupting the ability to hold action plans in memory for later execution (Burgess, Quayle, & Frith, 2001). In a previous study from our group we have shown that BA 10 also stores intentions across delay periods after they have reached consciousness, especially if there is a delay between decision and execution (Haynes, Sakai, Rees, Gilbert, Frith, & Passingham, 2007). Although BA 10 has only rarely been implicated in preparation of voluntary actions, a direct comparison across different brain regions has revealed that the earliest cortical region exhibiting preparatory signals before voluntary movements is frontopolar cortex (Groll-Knapp et al., 1977). BA 10 is also cytoarchitectonically very special. It has a very low cell density, but each cell forms a large number of synapses, meaning that it is a highly associative brain region (Ramnani & Owen, 2003). One could speculate that this would allow for locally recurrent processing that could support the storage of action plans in working memory. Furthermore, BA 10 is believed to be the area that has most disproportionately grown in size in humans compared to nonhuman primates (Ramnani & Owen, 2003).

### Two Preparatory Circuits: "What" versus "When"

When taking a closer look, it becomes apparent that multichoice versions of the Libet experiment involve not just one but two decisions to be made (Haggard & Eimer, 1999; Soon et al., 2008). On the one hand a decision needs to be made as to *when* to decide, on the other hand a decision has to be made as to *which button* to choose. Brass and Haggard (2008) have referred to this as "when" and "what" decisions. So far we have decoded the "what" decisions, so next we also conducted a further decoding analysis where we assessed to which degree the timing of the decision, (as opposed to its outcome) can be decoded. The time of conscious intention could be significantly predicted from preSMA and SMA. The earliest decodable information on timing was available 5 seconds before a decision. This might suggest that the brain begins to prepare self-paced decisions through two independent networks that only converge at later stages of processing. The classical Libet experiments, which were primarily concerned with "*when*" decisions, found short-term predictive information in the SMA. This is compatible with our prediction of the timing from preSMA and SMA. In contrast, as our results show, a "*what*" decision is prepared much earlier and by a much more extended network in the brain.

## SANITY CHECKS

Our findings point toward long-leading brain activity that is predictive of the outcome of a decision even before the decision reaches awareness. This is a striking finding, and thus it is important to critically discuss several possible sources of artifacts and alternative interpretations. Of particular interest is to make sure that the report of the timing is correct, and that the information does not reflect a carryover from previous trials.

### Early Decision—Late Action?

One question is whether the subjects are really performing the task correctly. For example, they might decide early, say at the beginning of the trial, which button to press, and then simply wait for a few seconds to execute their response. This could be the case if, say, the entire group of subjects had been grossly disregarding the instructions. A similar argument has already been made against the Libet experiment. It is conceivable that as the decision outcome *gradually* enters awareness, subjects adopt a very conservative criterion for their report and wait for the awareness to reach its "peak" intensity (Latto, 1985; Ringo, 1985). Fortunately, there are reasons that make it implausible that subjects simply waited to report that the decision that had already begun to reach awareness. In situations where subjects know which button they are going to press, the corresponding movement is already prepared all the way up to primary motor cortex. In contrast, in our study the motor cortex contains information only at a very late stage of processing, following the conscious decision which movement to make. This suggests that subjects did not decide early and then simply wait.

### Carryover from Previous Trial?

Importantly, it is also possible to rule out that the early prediction presumably reflects a carryover of information from the previous trial. First, the distribution of response sequences clearly resembles an exponential distribution without sequential order, as would be expected if subjects decide randomly from trial to trial which button to press. This is presumably because, in contrast to previous studies, we did not ask subjects to balance left and right button presses across trials, thus encouraging decisions that were independent of previous trials. Also, in our experiments subjects often took a long time until they made a decision, which might explain why subjects behaved more randomly than in traditional random choice experiments, where subjects systematically violate randomness when explicitly asked to rapidly generate random sequences (Nickerson, 2002). Second, our chosen statistical analysis method, fitting a so-called finite impulse response function, is designed to separate the effects of the current trial from the previous and the following trial. This approach is highly efficient as long as both types of responses are equally frequent, with variable intertrial intervals, as here. Third, the early onset of predictive information in prefrontal and parietal regions cannot be explained by any trailing blood-oxygenation-dependent (BOLD) signals from the previous trials. The onset of information occurs approximately 12 seconds after the previous trial, which is far beyond the relaxation time of the hemodynamic response. Also, the predictive information increases with temporal distance from the previous trial, which is not compatible with the information being an overlap from the previous trial. Fourth, time points that overlap into the next trial also revealed no carryover of information. Taken together, the high predictive accuracy preceding the decision reflects prospective information encoded in prefrontal and parietal cortex related to the decision in the current trial.

## IMPLICATIONS FOR THE FREE-WILL DEBATE?

Our study shows that the brain can begin to unconsciously prepare decisions several seconds before they reach awareness. Does our study thus have any novel implications for the debate on free will that has so far heavily relied on Libet's experiments? The potential implications of Libet's experiments for free will have been discussed at great length in the literature, which has helped sharpen what the contribution of such simple free choice paradigms might be. Obviously they do not address real-world decisions that have high motivational importance, they are not based on long-term reward expectations, and they do not involve complex reasoning. Our and Libet's decisions have only little motivational salience for the individual and are experienced as random rather than being based on in-depth trial to trial reasoning. However our and Libet's findings do address one specific intuition regarding free will, that is the naïve folk-psychological intuition that at the time when we make a decision the outcome of this decision is free and not fully determined by brain activity. As discussed above, this intuition is scientifically implausible anyway, simply because it stands in contradiction to our belief in a deterministic universe. However, the direct demonstration that brain activity predicts the outcomes of decisions before they reach awareness has additional persuasive power. Dissociations between awareness and brain processing are nothing unusual; they have been demonstrated in motor control before (Fourneret & Jeannerod, 1998). What our findings now show is that a whole cascade of unconscious brain processes unfolds across several seconds and helps prepare subjectively free, self-paced decisions.

## CAUSALITY?

An important point that needs to be discussed is to which degree our findings support any causal relationship between brain activity and the conscious will. For the criterion of *temporal precedence* there should be no doubt that our data finally demonstrate that brain activity can predict a decision long before it enters awareness. A different point is the criterion of *constant connection*. For a constant connection one would require that the decision can be predicted with 100% percent accuracy from prior brain activity. Libet's original experiments were based on averages, so no statistical assessment can be made about the accuracy with which decisions can be predicted. Our prediction of decisions from brain activity is statistically reliable, but far from perfect. The predictive accuracy of around 60% can be substantially improved if the decoding is custom-tailored for each subject. However even under optimal conditions this is far from 100%. This could have several reasons. One possibility is that the inaccuracy stems from imperfections in our ability to measure neural signals. Due to the limitations of fMRI in terms of spatial and temporal resolution it is clear that the information we can measure can only reflect a strongly impoverished version of the information available from a direct measurement of the activity in populations of neurons in the predictive areas. A further source of imperfection is that an optimal decoding approach needs a large (ideally infinite) number of training samples to learn exactly what the predictive patterns should be. In contrast, the slow sampling rate of fMRI imposes limitations on the training information available. So, even if the populations of neurons in these areas would in principle allow a perfect prediction, our ability to extract this information would be severely limited. However these limitations cannot be used to argue that one day with better methods the prediction will be perfect; this would constitute a mere "promissory" prediction. Importantly, a different interpretation could be that the inaccuracy simply reflects the fact that the early neural processes might *in principle* simply not be fully, but only partially predictive of the outcome of the decision. In this view, even full knowledge of the state of activity of populations of neurons in frontopolar cortex and in the precuneus would not permit to fully predict the decision. In that case the signals have the form of a biasing signal that influences the decision to a degree, but additional influences at later time points might still play a role in shaping the decision. Until a perfect predictive accuracy has been reached in an experiment, both interpretations—incomplete prediction and incomplete determination—remain possible.

## FUTURE PERSPECTIVES

An important question for future research is whether the signals we observed are indeed decision-related. This might sound strange given that they predict the choices. However, this early information could hypothetically also be the consequence of stochastic, fluctuating background activity in the decision network (Eccles, 1985), similar to the known fluctuations of signals in early visual cortex (Arieli, Sterkin, Grinvald, & Aertsen, 1996). In this view, the processes relevant for the decision would occur late, say in the last second before the decision. In the absence of any "reasons" for deciding for one or the other option the decision network might need to break the symmetry, for example by using stochastic background fluctuations in the network. If the fluctuations in the network are, say, in one subspace, the decision could be pushed toward 'left," and if the fluctuations are in a different subspace the decision could be pushed toward "right." But how could fluctuations at the time of the conscious decision be reflected already seven seconds before? One possibility is that the temporal autocorrelation of the fMRI signal smears the ongoing fluctuations across time. However, the fMRI signal itself is presumably not causally involved in decision-making, it is only an indirect way of measuring the *neural* processes leading up to the decision. Thus the relevant question is the temporal autocorrelation of neural signals, which seems incompatible with a time scale of 7–10 seconds. Nonetheless in future experiments we aim to investigate even further how tightly the early information is linked to the decision. One prediction of the slow background fluctuation model is that the outcome of the decision would be predictable even in cases where a subject does not know that they are going to have to make a decision or where a subject does not know what a decision is going to be about. This would point toward a predictive signal that does not directly computationally contribute to decision making.

A further interesting point for future research is the comparison of self-paced with rapid decisions that occur in response to sudden and unpredictable external events. At first sight it seems implausible that rapid, responsive decisions could be predicted ahead of time. How would we be able to drive a car on a busy road if it always took us a minimum of 7 seconds to make a decision? However, even unpredictable decisions are likely to be determined by "cognitive sets" or "policies" that are likely to have a much longer half-life in the brain than mere seven seconds.

Finally, it would be interesting to investigate whether decisions can be predicted in real-time before a person knows how they are going to decide. Such a real-time "decision prediction machine" (DP-machine) would allow us to turn certain thought experiments (Marks, 1985; Chiang, 2005) into reality, for example by testing whether people can guess above chance which future choices are predicted by their current brain signals even though a person might not have yet made up their mind. Such forced-choice judgments would be helpful in revealing whether there is evidence for subtle decision-related information that might enter a person's awareness at an earlier stage than would be apparent in the conventional Libet tasks (Marks, 1985). A different experiment could be to ask a person to press a button at a time point of their own choice, with the one catch that they are not allowed to press it when a lamp lights up (Chiang, 2005). Using real-time decoding techniques it might then be possible to predict the impending decision to press the button and to control the lamp to prevent the action. The phenomenal experience of performing such an experiment would be interesting. For example, if the prediction is early enough, the subject is not even aware that they are about to make up their mind and should have the impression that the light is flickering on and off randomly. It would be possible to use the DP-machine to inform the subject of their impending decision and get them to "veto" their action and not press a button. Currently such "veto" experiments rely on trusting a person to make up their mind to press a button and then to rapidly choose to terminate their movement (Brass & Haggard, 2007). A DP-machine would finally allow one to perform true "veto" experiments. If it were possible not only to predict *when* a person is going to decide, but also *which specific option* they are going to take, one could ask them to change their mind and take the *opposite* option. It seems plausible that a person should be able to change their mind across a period as long as seven seconds. However, there is a catch: How can one change one's mind if one doesn't even know what one has chosen in the first place? If it were one day realized, such a DP-machine would be a similarly useful device in helping us realize the determination of our free decisions as an autocerebroscope (Feigl, 1967) is in helping understand the relationship between our conscious thoughts and our brain activity.

## ACKNOWLEDGMENTS

This work was funded by the Max Planck Society, the German Research Foundation, and the Bernstein Computational Neuroscience Program of the German Federal Ministry of Education and Research. The author would like to thank Ida Momennejad for valuable comments on the manuscript.

## NOTE

1. The author is an incompatibilist.

## REFERENCES

Arieli, A., Sterkin, A., Grinvald, A, Aertsen, A. (1996). Dynamics of ongoing activity: Explanation of the large variability in evoked cortical responses. *Science, 273,* 1868–1871.

Blankertz, B., Dornhege, G., Schäfer, C., Krepki, R., Kohlmorgen, J., Müller, K. R., et al. (2003). Boosting bit rates and error detection for the classification of fast-paced motor commands based on single-trial EEG analysis. *IEEE Transactions on Neural and Rehabilitation Systems Engineering, 11,* 127–131.

Brass, M., Haggard, P. (2007). To do or not to do: The neural signature of self-control. *Journal of Neuroscience, 27,* 9141–9145.

Brass, M., & Haggard, P. (2008). The what, when, whether model of intentional action. *Neuroscientist, 14,* 319–325.

Breitmeyer, B. G. (1985). Problems with the psychophysics of intention. *Behavioral and Brain Sciences, 8,* 539–540.

Burgess, P. W., Quayle, A., & Frith, C. D. (2001). Brain regions involved in prospective memory as determined by positron emission tomography. *Neuropsychologia, 39,* 545–555.

Chiang, T. (2005) What's expected of us. *Nature, 436,* 150.

Deiber, M. P., Passingham, R. E., Colebatch, J. G., Friston, K. J., Nixon, P. D., & Frackowiak, R. S. (1991). Cortical areas and the selection of movement: A study with positron emission tomography. *Experimental Brain Research, 84,* 393–402.

Eccles, J. C. (1982). The initiation of voluntary movements by the supplementary motor area. *Archiv fur Psychiatrie und Nervenkrankheiten, 231,* 423–441.

Eccles, J. C. (1985). Mental summation: The timing of voluntary intentions by cortical activity. *Behavioral and Brain Sciences, 8,* 542–543.

Feigl, H. (1967). *The "mental" and the "physical": The essay and a postscript.* Minneapolis: University of Minnesota Press.

Fourneret, P., & Jeannerod, M. (1998). Limited conscious monitoring of motor performance in normal subjects. *Neuropsychologia, 36,* 1133–1140.

Friston, K. J., Holmes, A. P., Poline, J. B., Grasby, P. J., Williams, S. C., Frackowiak, R. S., et al. (1995). Analysis of fMRI time-series revisited. *Neuroimage, 2,* 45–53.

Groll-Knapp, E., Ganglberge, J. A., & Haider, M. (1977). Voluntary movement-related slow potentials in cortex and thalamus in man. *Progress in Clinical Neurophysiology, 1,* 164–173.

Haggard, P., & Eimer, M. (1999). On the relation between brain potentials and the awareness of voluntary movements. *Experimental Brain Research, 126,* 128–133.

Haynes, J. D., & Rees, G. (2005) Predicting the orientation of invisible stimuli from activity in human primary visual cortex. *Nature Neuroscience, 8,* 686–691.

Haynes J.D., & Rees, G. (2006). Decoding mental states from brain activity in humans. *Nature reviews Neuroscience, Jul;7(7),* 523–534.

Haynes, J. D., Sakai, K, Rees, G., Gilbert, S., Frith, C., & Passingham, R. E. (2007) Reading hidden intentions in the human brain. *Current Biology, 17,* 323–328.

Hume, D. (1977). An Enquiry concerning Human Understanding, edited by Tom L. Beauchamp, Oxford/New York: Oxford University Press, 1999.

Kamitani, Y., & Tong, F. (2005). Decoding the visual and subjective contents of the human brain. *Nature Neuroscience, 8,* 679–685.

Kornhuber, H. H. & Deecke, L. (1965) Hirnpotentialänderungen bei Willkürbewegungen und passiben Bewegungen des Menschen: Bereitschaftspotential und reafferente Potentiale. *Pflügers Archiv für die Gesamte Physiologie, 284,* 1–17.

Kriegeskorte, N., Goebel, R., & Bandettini, P. (2006). Information-based functional brain mapping. *Proceedings of the National Academy of Sciences, 103,* 3863–3868.

Latto, R. (1985). Consciousness as an experimental variable: Problems of definition, practice, and interpretation. *Behavioral and Brain Sciences, 8,* 545–546.

Libet, B., Gleason, C. A., Wright, E. W., & Pearl, D. K. (1983). Time of conscious intention to act in relation to onset of cerebral activities (readiness-potential): The unconscious initiation of a freely voluntary act. *Brain, 106,* 623–642.

Libet, B. (1985). Unconscious cerebral initiative and the role of conscious will in voluntary action. *Behavioral and Brain Sciences, 8,* 529–566.

Marks, L. E. (1985). Toward a psychophysics of intention. *Behavioral and Brain Sciences, 8,* 547–548.

Merikle, P. M., & Cheesman, J. (1985). Conscious and unconscious processes: Same or different? *Behavioral and Brain Sciences, 8,* 547–548.

Moutoussis, K., & Zeki, S. (1997) Functional segregation and temporal hierarchy of the visual perceptive systems. *Proceedings of the Royal Society B, 264,* 1407–1414.

Nickerson, R. S. (2002). The production and perception of randomness. *Psychological Review, 109,* 330–357.

Ramnani. N, & Owen, A. M. (2004). Anterior prefrontal cortex: insights into function from anatomy and neuroimaging. *Nature reviews. Neuroscience, Mar;5(3),* 184–94.

Ringo, J. L. (1985). Timing volition: Questions of what and when about W. *Behavioral and Brain Sciences, 8,* 550–551.

Rollman, G. B. (1985). Sensory events with variable central latencies provide inaccurate clocks. *Behavioral and Brain Sciences, 8*, 551–552.

Soon, C. S., Brass, M., Heinze, H. J., & Haynes, J. D. (2008). Unconscious determinants of free decisions in the human brain. *Nature Neuroscience, 11*, 543–545.

Tanaka, K. (1997). Mechanisms of visual object recognition: Monkey and human studies. *Current Opinion in Neurobiology, 7*, 523–529.

Trevena, J. A., & Miller, J. (2002). Cortical movement preparation before and after a conscious decision to move. *Consciousness and Cognition, 11*, 162–190.

Van de Grind, W. (2002). Physical, neural, and mental timing. *Consciousness and Cognition, 11*, 241–264.

Wundt, W. (1904). *Principles of physiological psychology* (Vol. 2). London: Sonnenschein; New York: Macmillan.

# CHAPTER 9

## Forward Modeling Mediates Motor Awareness

*Francesca Carota, Michel Desmurget, and Angela Sirigu*

According to the *Merriam-Webster's Collegiate Dictionary*, consciousness defines "the quality or state of being aware especially of something within oneself." Following Watson's behaviorist revolution (Watson, 1913), consciousness was deemed nonscientific and its investigation was considered to be the preserve of theologians and philosophers like Descartes (1641/1992), Spinoza (1677/1994), or Bergson (1888/2007). This view eroded recently in the face of neuropsychological evidence suggesting that consciousness is not a spiritual trait, but an emerging property of neural activities. When the brain is damaged our capacity to generate conscious intentions to act can be severely impaired (Haggard, 2005). At the same time, our ability to be aware of our motor responses can be dramatically altered (Frith, Blakemore, & Wolpert, 2000). For instance, some patients can become spectator of alien movements they produce without will (Scepkowski & Cronin-Golomb, 2003). Others can lose the subjective experience of wanting to move (Sirigu et al., 2004). Others can obstinately claim that they are moving a paralyzed arm (Orfei et al., 2007). Others can report movements in a limb that no longer exists (Ramachandran & Hirstein, 1998). Others can be tricked into identifying as their own, a movement performed by someone else (Sirigu, Daprati, Pradat-Diehl, Franck, & Jeannerod, 1999). Others can lose their ability to generate conscious motor images of their actions (Sirigu, Duhamel, Cohen, Pillon, Dubois, & Agid, 1996), etc.

Identification of awareness as a valid object for scientific exploration triggered a large number of studies in normal subjects. A first line of research investigated our ability to become aware of our intentions to move (Haggard, 2005, 2008). It was mainly found that the conscious experience of intending to move occurs after the onset of brain activity (Libet, Gleason, Wright, & Pearl, 1983; Haggard & Eimer, 1999; Sirigu et al., 2004). In another group of experiments, researchers focused on "action-effects" mismatches. In this type of paradigm, the effects of an action are manipulated in such a way that they no longer match the initial intention of the subject. It was shown that reafferent sensations associated with the ongoing movement were widely unavailable to consciousness (Goodale, Pelisson, & Prablanc, 1986; Wolpert, Ghahramani, & Jordan, 1995; Fourneret & Jeannerod, 1998). This result conflicts partially with other evidence showing that the way we consciously perceive our movements is not independent of action execution. In other words, although sensory-motor mismatches do not always reach consciousness, the sensory consequences of our actions can deeply influence the subjective experience attached to the realization of these actions (Haggard, Clark, & Kalogeras, 2002; Moore & Haggard, 2008).

The present chapter focuses on the issue of motor awareness. Our goal is to tackle some of the inconsistencies above by addressing three main questions: (1) What exactly are we aware of when making a movement? (2) What is the contribution of afferent and efferent signals to motor awareness? (3) What are the neural bases of motor awareness?

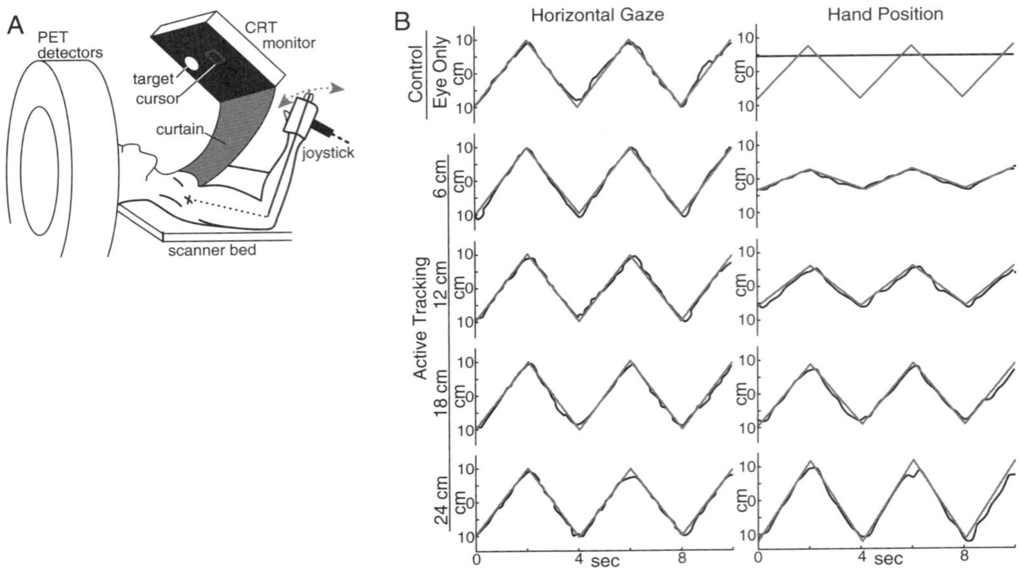


**Figure 9.1** **(A)** Experimental apparatus. The subjects were supine in the PET scanner with their right hand holding a joystick. A computer monitor was suspended over the eye of the subject. The task was to track a computer-driven target (circle) with a joystick-driven box (square). **(B)** Behavioral recording corresponding to 10 s of data for different gain values of the joystick. Changes in gain were not detected by the subjects. (Reprinted with permission from Turner et al. 2003).

## WHAT EXACTLY ARE WE AWARE OF WHEN MAKING A MOVEMENT?

Most of the functioning of the motor system occurs without awareness. Some examples of this fact can be found in postural regulations (Wing, Flanagan, & Richardson, 1997), nonverbal communication skills (Dijksterhuis & Bargh, 2001), eye movements during perception of complex scenes (Yarbus, 1967), and on-line control of goal-directed movements (Desmurget & Grafton, 2003). Other examples lie in several studies showing that the motor system can remain unaware of large sensory distortions occurring during the movement. For instance, Turner and colleagues required human subjects to perform a tracking task (Fig. 9.1) (Turner, Desmurget, Grethe, Crutcher, & Grafton, 2003). During task performance, a white circle moved horizontally across a monitor at constant speed (10 cm/s) between endpoints 20 cm apart. The circle reversed direction of movement with no delay on reaching left and right endpoints. Subjects were instructed to keep the circle within a red square controlled by a hand-held joystick. On different sessions, the gain of the relationship between joystick movement and cursor displacement was modified in such a way that joystick displacements of 6, 12, 18, and 24 cm produced cursor displacements of 20 cm. None of the 13 subjects involved in the study exhibited awareness that the joystick-to-cursor relation changed from session to session. A similar observation was reported by Wolpert and colleagues during a planar point-to-point reaching task (Wolpert et al., 1995). The subjects received a visual feedback of their movement through a mirror positioned above the pointing table. For the purpose of the study, the feedback was altered so as to increase the perceived curvature of the movement (Fig. 9.2).

The perturbation was zero at both ends of the movement and reached its maximum (4 cm) at the midpoint of the movement. This distortion was not consciously perceived by the subjects, who progressively restored straight paths in the visual space by generating curved hand movements in a direction opposite to the

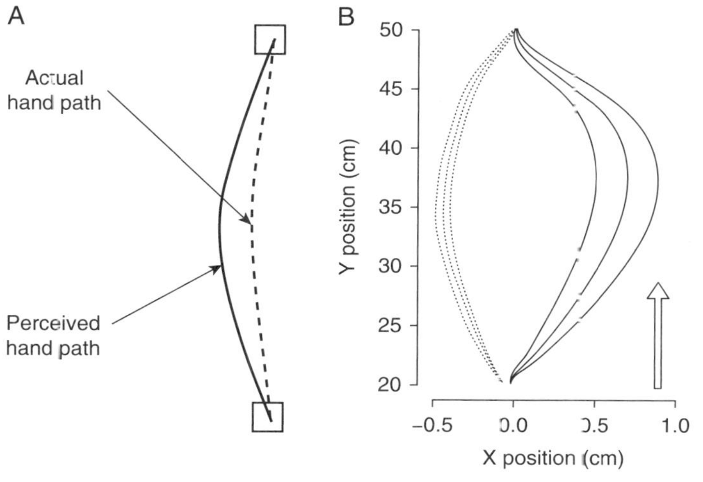


**Figure 9.2** (**A**) Illustration of the visual distortion. (**B**) Control trajectories (dotted lines) compared with postadaptation traces (solid lines). The arrow shows movement direction. (From Wolpert et al., 1995).

experimentally induced curvature. In a comparable study, Fourneret and Jeannerod required healthy humans to trace sagittal lines on a graphic tablet (Fourneret & Jeannerod, 1998). Visual feedback of the movement was provided to the subjects through a mirror positioned above the tablet. In some trials, this feedback was shifted so that the line traced by the subjects deviated to the right or the left by a substantial amount (up to 10 deg). To perform a straight movement, the subjects had thus to produce a lateral response. They were able to do so quite easily. However, they kept reporting that their movement was straight in the sagittal direction. They remained unaware of their motor adjustment, suggesting, in the terms of the authors, that "normal subjects are not aware of signals generated by their own movements" (Fourneret & Jeannerod, 1998, p. 1133). Further evidence supporting this conclusion is provided by the so-called subliminal double-step paradigm. In this paradigm, the subjects are required to "look and point" to visual targets displayed in the peripheral visual field. During saccadic gaze displacement the target location is modified. This procedure is interesting for at least three reasons. First, due to saccadic suppression, the target jump is not perceived consciously by the subjects (Matin, 1982). Second, because saccadic responses to stationary targets involve an initial saccade undershooting the target position and a secondary corrective saccade achieving accurate target acquisition (Harris, 1995), the target jump does not alter the intrinsic organization of the oculomotor system. Third, because pointing movements to stationary targets are corrected, after movement onset, when spatial information about target location is updated at the end of the saccadic shift (Desmurget, Turner, Prablanc, Russo, Alexander, & Grafton, 2005), the target jump does not alter the intrinsic organization of the manual response. In fact, one may summarize these observations by saying that pointing directed at stationary or unconsciously displaced targets are identical from a functional point of view. The intrasaccadic modification of target location simply causes the system to generate larger corrections. What is interesting is that these corrections are not detected by the subjects who remain completely unaware of even profound changes in path curvature and individual joint trajectories (Fig. 9.3) (Desmurget, Grea, Grethe, Prablanc, Alexander, & Grafton, 2001; Desmurget, Epstein, Turner, Prablanc, Alexander, & Grafton, 1999; Desmurget, Gaveau, Vindras, Turner, Broussolle, & Thobois, 2004; Prablanc & Martin, 1992).

However, it is now established that these corrections are "sensed" by the perceptual system. As shown by Johnson and Haggard (2005),

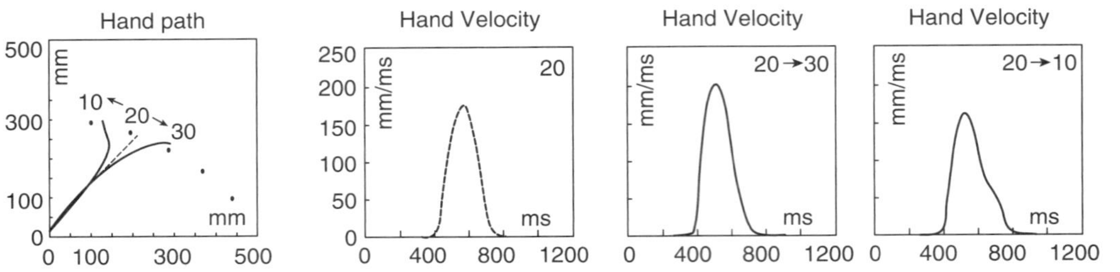


**Figure 9.3** Hand paths and corresponding velocity profiles for reaching movements directed at stationary (dotted lines) and subliminally displaced targets (solid lines). (Adapted from Martin and Prablanc, 1991).

when required to reproduce the trajectory of single and double-step responses, after movement completion, healthy subjects perform really well. They generate straight and curved paths respectively for the single and double-step trials. In other words, the motor system "knows" that hand paths have been altered in double-step trials, but this knowledge does not reach consciousness.

Based on data above, it is tempting to speculate that we are not aware of the kinematics and sensory details of the movement. As long as the desired state is achieved, the system does not care about the modus operandi, and no basic information about motor commands reaches consciousness. Even large discrepancies between the intended and actual sensory signals are disregarded if they can be corrected. Additional support for this view comes from adaptation studies that have compared abrupt and progressive sensory perturbations (Malfait & Ostry, 2004; Michel, Pisella, Prablanc, Rode, & Rossetti, 2007). In force field adaptation paradigms, for instance, when the perturbing force is introduced abruptly, the subjects cannot correct the experimentally induced error, they miss the goal and become aware of the perturbation. Now, if the same level of distortion is reached through a gradual process, on-line corrective loops can handle the error, the goal is always achieved, and the subjects remain unaware of the perturbation (Malfait & Ostry, 2004).

To summarize, these data show that the motor system is mainly aware of its intention, in other words, of what it wants to do. As long as the goal is achieved, nothing reaches awareness about the details of the ongoing movements, even when substantial corrections have to be implemented to attain the intended state.

## WHAT IS THE CONTRIBUTION OF AFFERENT AND EFFERENT SIGNALS TO MOTOR AWARENESS?

Addressing the relative contribution of afferent and efferent signals to motor awareness amounts to addressing a simple question: how do we know we are moving? This interrogation is not new, as shown by the famous "William Debate," which opposed Wilhelm Wundt and William James, more than a century ago (Petit, 1999). For James, knowledge about our movements was constructed a posteriori on the basis of sensory reafferent inputs. For Wundt, by contrast, this knowledge was available a priori, on the basis of the motor efferent output. Although years of research have not solved the controversy, substantial progress has been made. In light of this progress a reasonable conclusion might be that both Wundt and James were partially right.

### Motor Awareness and Efferent Signals

A first line of evidence suggesting that the efferent signal is important for motor awareness comes from studies on self-recognition. In one of these studies, Tsakiris and colleagues (Tsakiris, Haggard, Franck, Mainy, & Sirigu, 2005) investigated passive movements of the right index finger. This finger was moved through a lever operated by the left hand of the experimenter or the subject. Visual feedback about the movement was manipulated so that subjects observed their own or someone else's right hand. Self-recognition was significantly more accurate when the subjects were the authors of the action, i.e., when an efferent output was generated. This result strongly suggests that efferent information is important for constructing motor awareness in the context of self-generated actions.

At a second level, strong evidence for a role of efferent signals in motor awareness comes from studies in which the subjects report being aware of performing a movement, although no sensory signal is present. In a recent experiment, Kristeva and colleagues (Kristeva, Chakarov, Wagner, Schulte-Monting, & Hepp-Reymond, 2006) required a deafferented patient (GL) to perform self-paced flexions of the index finger. In control subjects, this task triggered contralateral movement-evoked potentials in the sensorimotor area. No such response was found in GL. However, this absence of sensory input did not prevent the patient from being aware of her movement. She knew that she was moving, which indicated, in the terms of the authors, that "she had a normal motor awareness" (Kristeva et al., 2006, p. 634). Of course, she had no "perceptual awareness" in the sense that she had no "feeling" about her movement. In fact, GL was "aware" that she was moving but she could not determine whether she was moving as expected. A similar observation was reported by Lafargue and colleagues, with the same patient (Lafargue, Paillard, Lamarre, & Sirigu, 2003). These authors required GL and seven healthy subjects to produce a target force with the right hand and then match this force with the left hand. Despite variations in the motor command that were larger than in controls, GL was able to perform the task with good accuracy. She was aware, not only that she was moving, but also of the level of force that she was applying.

Finally a third major evidence for the central origin of motor awareness comes from hemiplegic patients with anosognosia (Bisiach & Geniniani, 1991; Orfei et al., 2007). Some of these patients fail to recognize or appreciate the severity of their deficit. Others try to "explain it away" by arguing, for instance, that they are tired or not willing to move. Others finally, claim stubbornly that they are moving, despite their paralysis. In these patients, motor awareness arises from a normal efferent command, in the absence of sensory afference. A representative example is provided by Ramachandran in a well-known review (Ramachandran, 1996, p. 124): Doctor: "Can you clap." Patient: "Of course I can clap." Doctor: "Will you clap for me." At this point, the patient initiates clapping movements with the right hand, as if clapping with an imaginary hand near the sagittal plane. The discussion resumes. Doctor: "Are you clapping?" Patient: "Yes, I am clapping." To explain this result, it is often suggested that the brain mechanisms that normally compare the expected and actual peripheral reafferences are damaged, which prevent the subjects from knowing that they are not moving (Berti et al., 2005; Fotopoulou, Tsakiris, Haggard, Vagopoulou, Rudd, & Kopelman, 2008). In other words, the hemiplegic patients behave like deafferented subjects: they exhibit normal motor awareness but cannot determine whether their movement is unfolding as expected. Anosognosia has a different source in both groups of patients (absence of signal Vs destruction of the comparator), but it amounts to the same type of overt deficit.

In conclusion, the data above indicate, when considered together, that the efferent motor signal is critical and sufficient for the emergence of motor awareness. This efferent contribution is often thought to rely on forward modeling (Haggard, 2005; Sirigu et al., 2004; Frith, Blakemore, & Wolpert, 2000; Berti, Spinazzola, Pia, & Rabuffeti, 2007; Fotopoulou et al., 2008), a process that simulates the effect of the neural command and predicts the current and final states of the motor system (Miall, Christensen, Cain, & Stanley, 1993; Wolpert & Flanagan, 2001; Desmurget & Grafton, 2000, 2003). Schematically, the idea can be summarized as follows. When the subject initiates a movement, an efferent signal is issued, indicating first that the movement has started and second that the hand is at a given location, with a given velocity. Literally, this signal tells the brain that the movement is unfolding, thus leading to motor awareness. However, it does not tell the brain that the movement is unfolding as expected. This is the role of sensory reafferences.

### Perceptual (Veridical) Awareness and Afferent Inputs

There is clear evidence that sensory inputs can give rise to motor awareness. It is well known, for instance, that passive limb displacements are easily detected and reproduced by human subjects (Klockgether, Borutta, Rapp, Spieker, & Dichgans, 1995; Baud-Bovy & Viviani, 2004). In the same vein, it has been shown that vibratory stimulations of the muscle tendons can give rise to illusory movements. In a very elegant study, Albert and colleagues (Albert, Bergenheim, Ribot-Ciscar, & Roll, 2006) used a microneurographic technique to record Ia afferent messages from the six primary movers of the ankle joint, during imposed "writing like" movements. The Ia afferent pattern was then defined for each group of muscles and used as a template to pilot six small vibrators attached to the muscle tendons. Eleven different movements were considered. Following each trial, the subjects were instructed to draw with a hand-held stylus, and name, the shape of the evoked movement. The results indicated that the participants were able to achieve this task with a remarkable accuracy, thus showing that the Ia afferent feedback of a given movement evokes the illusion of the same movement (Fig. 9.4).

At first glance, this conclusion seems to contradict the evidence reported above that we are aware not of the kinematic details of the movement but of our conscious intentions (see first section). However, this apparent contradiction may be understood in reference to the process of forward modeling. Indeed, in the case of a peripheral stimulation, there is no expected input to which the actual input can be compared. As a consequence, when the sensory flow reaches the cortex, an error signal is generated. It is tempting to speculate that the inability of the motor system to deal with this signal gives rise to motor awareness. Another (nonexclusive) explanation might be related to the characteristic of passive-movement tasks. Indeed, in these tasks the subjects are generally required to pay close attention to the stimulus, which may facilitate motor awareness. As shown recently, muscle spindle sensitivity changes dramatically when attention is consciously directed to the recognition of a mechanically imposed two-dimensional movement (Hospod, Aimonetti, Roll, & Ribot-Ciscar, 2007).

Interestingly, a recent neuroimaging study suggested that a systematic mismatch between a preserved efferent command and an absent peripheral input could be the core factor explaining conscious phantom sensations in patients with amputations of the upper limb. As reported by the authors of the study (Giraux & Sirigu, 2003, p. S109):

> "Following peripheral injuries, motor commands can still be issued by the intact sensorimotor structures and are probably at the origin of the phantom sensations, directly or through internal "copies" of these motor commands fed back to other cortical areas such as the parietal and premotor cortices. However, since efferent motor signals produce no movement, and hence no proprioceptive input, a mismatch must occur between the normally correlated efferent and reafferent information, yielding an error signal."

In turns this error signal produces motor awareness.

Beyond the observations above, it may be worth noting that the comparison between peripheral and central signals is not straightforward from a computational point of view, even in "normal" conditions. Because of the existence of substantial delays in sensorimotor loops, this comparison has to be performed through predictive processes. Schematically, these processes are hypothesized to work as follows. Prior to movement, forward modeling is used to predict the sensory outcome of the action. This prediction is used to estimate the state of the moving limb for 70 ms or so (the time required to process sensory inputs; Desmurget & Grafton, 2003). After these 70 ms, the sensory signal becomes available. However, this signal is not related to the current hand position ($t_{current}$) but to the position that the hand had around movement onset ($t_{onset}$). Thus, to be useful, the peripheral input has to be compared with the predicted input for $t_{onset}$. This can be done if the system stores the characteristics of the expected input in a "delayed buffer" and if the delay is equivalent to the time necessary to process sensory information (Miall, Weir, Wolpert, & Stein, 1993). If the stored prediction ($t_{onset}$) matches the actual input, nothing happens. By contrast, if a discrepancy is detected, an error signal is issued and the estimation of the current motor state ($t_{current}$)

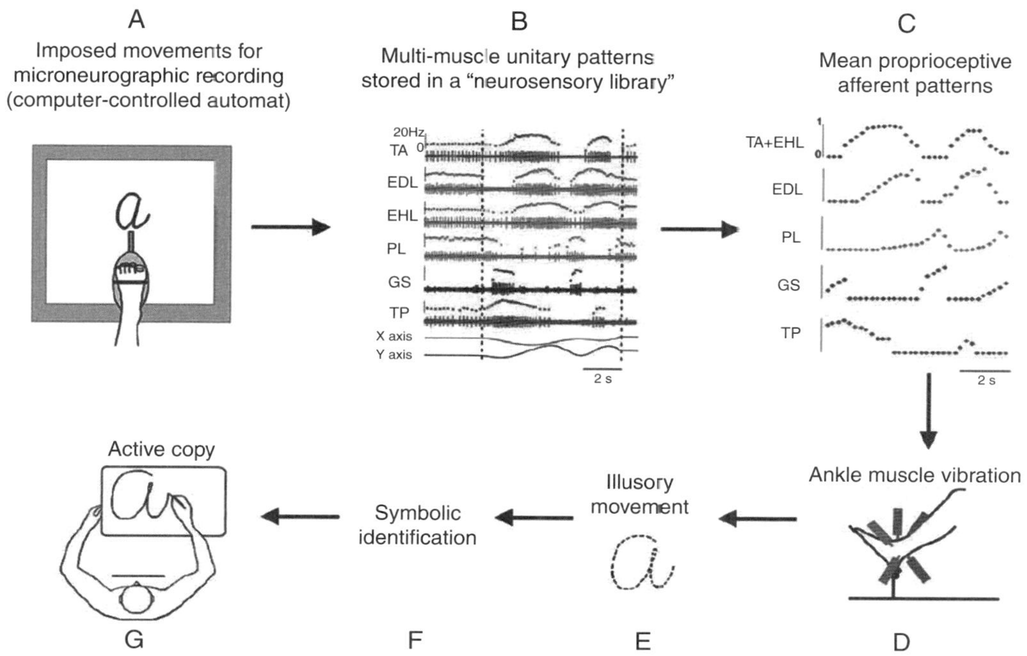


**Figure 9.4 Sensory signals trigger motor awareness.** **(A)** The subject traces a letter with his/her ankle joint. **(B)** Unitary Ia afferences are recorded for the six primary movers of the ankle joint. **(C)** Unitary responses are averaged. **(D)**) The averaged responses are used to pilot six vibrators placed over the six primary movers of the ankle joint. **(E)** The subject perceives a movement. **(F)** The subject identifies the shape of the movement. **(G)** The subject traces the perceived movement on a graphic tablet, with his/her hand. (From Albert et al., 2006).

is updated accordingly. As shown in the first section of this chapter, if the goal is reached, this "cooking" remains totally unconscious. Now, if the error is too big and cannot be corrected, a conscious warning is emitted. As an illustration of this point, imagine, for instance, that a subject initiates a motor response that is blocked at movement onset by an experimental device, unbeknownst to the subject. For at least 70 ms, this subject will be "aware" of the movement. However, after this delay, an error signal will be issued, indicating that the hand is not moving. This signal will reach consciousness, except, of course, if the process that compares the actual and predicted sensory reafferences is impaired because of a neural lesion. In this case, the subject will be aware of a movement that did not occur, as happens in hemiplegic patients with anosognosia (Berti et al., 2005).

## WHAT ARE THE NEURAL BASES OF MOTOR AWARENESS?

As emphasized in the previous sections, brain damages can give rise to major abnormalities in the awareness of action. A review of the clinical literature reveals that lesions within two specific regions are especially likely to produce such abnormalities: the posterior parietal cortex and the premotor cortex.

### The Posterior Parietal Cortex and Motor Awareness

In the sections above, we provided evidence that motor awareness results from predictive computations. During the last decade, numerous studies have linked these predictive computations to the functioning of the posterior parietal cortex (PPC) (Desmurget et al., 2001; Desmurget et al., 1999; Desmurget & Grafton, 2003; Blakemore &

Sirigu 2003; Pellijeff, Bonilha, Morgan, McKenzie, & Jackson, 2006; Ogawa, Inui, & Sugio, 2007). It was shown, for instance, that on-line movement corrections to subliminally displaced visual targets (see above) are inhibited when a transcranial stimulation pulse is delivered over the PPC at movement onset (Desmurget et al., 1999). In the same vein, it was found that the process of state estimation is severely disrupted when the parietal cortex is damaged (Wolpert, Goodbody, & Husain, 1998). A patient suffering from such damage on the left side became unable to maintain a representation of her right limbs over time. She reported feelings like "losing her right arm." Also, in the bus, she was sometimes surprised to "find" her right leg in the middle of the aisle, as other passengers tripped over her foot. A compatible observation was reported by Sirigu and colleagues in a group of patients with lesions restricted to the parietal cortex (Sirigu et al., 1996). In contrast to control subjects or an individual with a lesion to the primary motor cortex, these patients were dramatically impaired at predicting, through mental imagery, the time necessary to perform either hand gestures or visually directed pointing movements. In another study carried out by the same group (Sirigu et al., 1999), it was found that patients with parietal brain damages could sometimes present some level of anosognosia. In this study, the patients were required to perform hand movements. These movements were recorded with a video camera, and fed back to the patients through a mirror positioned above their hand (Fig. 9.5).

However, in some trials, the hand displayed in the mirror was not the real hand of the patients, but the hand of an experimenter executing a similar response. Results indicated that the patients were more impaired than healthy subjects at recognizing their own hand. Of particular interest were the trials in which the patients produced inaccurate clumsy gestures. In nearly 90% of these trials, the patients believed that they were observing their own hand when watching a smooth and accurate movement performed by the experimenter. This is not surprising, considering that the movements executed by the experimenter did closely match the conscious intention of the patients.

From a theoretical point of view, if forward modeling underlies motor awareness and if the PPC mediates forward modeling, then two predictions can be made: (1) lesions of the PPC should induce major abnormalities in the awareness of action; (2) the subjects should become aware of their movements a few tens of milliseconds after EMG onset, when sensory signals become available. This second prediction derives from the assumption that lesion of the PPC prevents the system from anticipating the characteristics of the reafferent sensory input. Without this input, an error message is issued in response to the attempt to compare the efferent and afferent signals. This error message triggers motor awareness (see above). A pattern of response compatible with these predictions was recently reported by Sirigu and colleagues in a group of parietal patients (Sirigu et al., 2004). The authors used a paradigm initially designed by Libet and colleagues (Libet et al., 1983). In this paradigm, subjects have to fixate a spot rotating on a screen. They initiate a voluntary press-button movement with the right index finger whenever they feel a desire to do so. At random time after this movement, the rotating spot is stopped, indicating to the subjects to report where the spot was when they first felt their desire to move ("Will to move," W-Judgment). Libet et al. found that the W-Judgment occurred 206 ms before EMG onset in normal subjects. A slightly longer delay (239 ms) was reported by Sirigu et al., based not on EMG onset but on the time at which the button was pressed by the subject. Interestingly, this delay was almost abolished in patients with parietal lesions. For these patients the W-Judgment occurred about 50 ms before movement onset. However, for a press-button task, the delay between EMG onset and the mechanical response can easily reach 110–120 ms (Hasbroucq, Tandonnet, Micallef-Roll, Blin, & Possamai, 2003). This indicates that motor awareness occurred probably around 60–70 ms after actual movement onset in the parietal patients studied by Sirigu and colleagues. Such a latency is compatible with the idea that motor awareness did emerge, in the patients, not from the efferent command, but from the processing of the peripheral input, potentially by the premotor cortex.

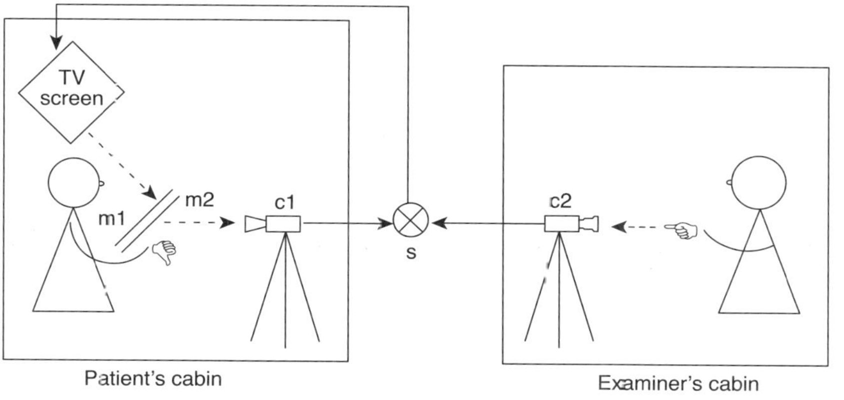


**Figure 9.5** Schematic representation of the experimental apparatus used to present veridical or false visual feedback about their ongoing hand movement to control subjects and parietal patients. (From Sirigu et al., 1999).

### The Premotor Cortex and Veridical Motor Awareness

The main evidence that the premotor cortex is involved in veridical motor awareness comes from a lesion mapping study (Berti et al., 2005). In this study, Berti and colleagues investigated the anatomical distribution of brain lesions in right-brain–damaged patients with anosognosia for hemiplegia. As previously stated, these patients stubbornly deny their motor impairment. They keep claiming that they can move their paralyzed limb with no deficit. Berti and colleagues identified the premotor cortex (area 6) as the most frequently damaged area in these patients. It was concluded that this region monitors the actual movement by comparing the actual and expected sensory reafferences. This hypothesis is consistent with the fact that the premotor cortex receives sensory reafferences about the ongoing movement (Hummelsheim, Bianchetti, Wiesendanger, & Wiesendanger, 1988; Scott, Sergio, & Kalaska, 1997; Fogassi, Raos, Franchi, Gallese, Luppino, & Matelli, 1999; Raos, Franchi, Gallese, & Fogassi, 2003). However, there is little evidence in the literature indicating that this region is involved in forward modeling. Most studies suggest that this process is more likely to rely on the functioning of the cerebellum and the parietal cortex (Wolpert et al., 1998; Desmurget et al., 2001; Desmurget et al., 1999; Blakemore & Sirigu, 2003; Miall et al., 2007; Miall & King, 2008). Further studies will be necessary to address the origin of this discrepancy.

## CONCLUSIONS

In this chapter, we have briefly reviewed evidence that the motor system is mainly aware of its intention. As long as the goal is achieved, nothing reaches awareness about the kinematic details of the ongoing movements, even when substantial corrections have to be implemented to attain the intended state. Also, we showed that motor awareness relies mainly on the central predictive computations carried out within the posterior parietal cortex. The outcome of these computations is contrasted with the peripheral reafferent input to build a veridical motor awareness. Some evidence exists that this process involves the premotor areas.

## REFERENCES

Albert, F., Bergenheim, M., Ribot-Ciscar, E., & Roll, J. P. (2006). The Ia afferent feedback of a given movement evokes the illusion of the same movement when returned to the subject via muscle tendon vibration. *Experimental Brain Research, 172,* 163–174.

Baud-Bovy, G., & Viviani, P. (2004). Amplitude and direction errors in kinesthetic pointing. *Experimental Brain Research, 157,* 197–214.

Bergson, H. (1888/2007). *Essai sur les données immédiates de la conscience*. Paris: Puf.

Berti, A., Bottini, G., Gandola, M., Pia, L., Smania, N., Stracciari, A., et al. (2005). Shared cortical anatomy for motor awareness and motor control. *Science, 309,* 488–491.

Berti, A., Spinazzola, L., Pia, L., & Rabuffeti, M. (2007). Motor awareness and motor intention in anosognosia for hemiplegia. In P. Haggard, Y. Rossetti, & M. Kawato (Eds.), *Sensorimotor foundations of higher cognition series: Attention and performance XXII*. New York: Oxford University Press.

Bisiach, E., & Geniniani, G. (1991). Anosognosia related to hemiplegia and heminopia. In G. P. Prigatano & D. L. Scahcter (Eds.), *Awareness of deficit after brain injury* (pp. 17–39). New York: Oxford University Press.

Blakemore, S. J., & Sirigu, A. (2003). Action prediction in the cerebellum and in the parietal lobe. *Experimental Brain Research, 153,* 239–245.

Descartes, R. (1641/1992). *Méditations métaphysiques*. Paris: Flammarion.

Desmurget, M., Epstein, C. M., Turner, R. S., Prablanc, C., Alexander, G. E., & Grafton, S. T. (1999). Role of the posterior parietal cortex in updating reaching movements to a visual target. *Nature Neuroscience, 2,* 563–567.

Desmurget, M., Gaveau, V., Vindras, P., Turner, R. S., Broussolle, E., & Thobois, S. (2004). On-line motor control in patients with Parkinson's disease. *Brain, 127,* 1755–1773.

Desmurget, M., & Grafton, S. (2000). Forward modeling allows feedback control for fast reaching movements. *Trends in Cognitive Sciences, 4,* 423–431.

Desmurget, M., & Grafton, S. (2003). Feedback or forward control: End of a dichotomie. In S. Johnson (Ed.), *Cognitive neuroscience perspectives on the problem of intentional action* (pp. 289–338). Boston: MIT Press.

Desmurget, M., Grea, H., Grethe, J. S., Prablanc, C., Alexander, G. E., & Grafton, S. T. (2001). Functional anatomy of nonvisual feedback loops during reaching: A positron emission tomography study. *Journal of Neuroscience, 21,* 2919–2928.

Desmurget, M., Turner, R. S., Prablanc, C., Russo, G. S., Alexander, G. E., & Grafton, S. T. (2005). Updating target location at the end of an orienting saccade affects the characteristics of simple point-to-point movements. *Journal of Experimental Psychology: Human Perception and Performance, 31,* 1510–1536.

Dijksterhuis, A., & Bargh, J. A. (2001). The perception-behavior expressway: Automatic effects of social perception on social behavior. *Advances in Experimental Social Psychology, 33,* 1–40.

Fogassi, L., Raos, V., Franchi, G., Gallese, V., Luppino, G., & Matelli, M. (1999). Visual responses in the dorsal premotor area F2 of the macaque monkey. *Experimental Brain Research, 128,* 194–199.

Fotopoulou, A., Tsakiris, M., Haggard, P., Vagopoulou, A., Rudd, A., & Kopelman, M. (2008). The role of motor intention in motor awareness: An experimental study on anosognosia for hemiplegia. *Brain, 131,* 3432–3442.

Fourneret, P., & Jeannerod, M. (1998). Limited conscious monitoring of motor performance in normal subjects. *Neuropsychologia, 36,* 1133–1140.

Frith, C. D., Blakemore, S. J., & Wolpert, D. M. (2000). Abnormalities in the awareness and control of action. *Philosophical Transactions of the Royal Society B: Biological Sciences, 355,* 1771–1788.

Giraux, P., & Sirigu, A. (2003). Illusory movements of the paralyzed limb restore motor cortex activity. *Neuroimage, 20*(Suppl. 1), S107–S111.

Goodale, M. A., Pelisson, D., & Prablanc, C. (1986). Large adjustments in visually guided reaching do not depend on vision of the hand or perception of target displacement. *Nature, 320,* 748–750.

Graziano, M. S., Taylor, C. S., & Moore, T. (2002). Complex movements evoked by microstimulation of precentral cortex. *Neuron, 34,* 841–851.

Haggard, P. (2005). Conscious intention and motor cognition. *Trends in Cognitive Sciences, 9,* 290–295.

Haggard, P. (2008). Human volition: Towards a neuroscience of will. *Nature Reviews Neuroscience, 9,* 934–946.

Haggard, P., Clark, S., & Kalogeras, J. (2002). Voluntary action and conscious awareness. *Nature Neuroscience, 5,* 382–385.

Haggard, P., & Eimer, M. (1999). On the relation between brain potentials and the awareness of voluntary movements. *Experimental Brain Research, 126,* 128–133.

Harris, C. M. (1995). Does saccadic undershoot minimize saccadic flight-time? A Monte-Carlo study. *Vision Research, 35,* 691–701.

Hasbroucq, T., Tandonnet, C., Micallef-Roll, J., Blin, O., & Possamai, C. A. (2003). An electromyographic analysis of the effect of levodopa on the response time of healthy subjects. *Psychopharmacology (Berlin), 165,* 313–316.

Hospod, V., Aimonetti, J. M., Roll, J. P., & Ribot-Ciscar, E. (2007). Changes in human muscle spindle sensitivity during a proprioceptive attention task. *Journal of Neuroscience, 27,* 5172–5178.

Hummelsheim, H., Bianchetti, M., Wiesendanger, M., & Wiesendanger, R. (1988). Sensory inputs to the agranular motor fields: A comparison between precentral, supplementary-motor and premotor areas in the monkey. *Experimental Brain Research, 69,* 289–298.

Johnson, H., & Haggard, P. (2005). Motor awareness without perceptual awareness. *Neuropsychologia, 43,* 227–237.

Klockgether, T., Borutta, M., Rapp, H., Spieker, S., & Dichgans, J. (1995). A defect of kinesthesia in Parkinson's disease. *Movement Disorders, 10,* 460–465.

Kristeva, R., Chakarov, V., Wagner, M., Schulte-Monting, J., & Hepp-Reymond, M. C. (2006). Is the movement-evoked potential mandatory for movement execution? A high-resolution EEG study in a deafferented patient. *Neuroimage, 31,* 677–685.

Lafargue, G., Paillard, J., Lamarre, Y., & Sirigu, A. (2003). Production and perception of grip force without proprioception: is there a sense of effort in deafferented subjects? *European Journal of Neuroscience, 17,* 2741–2749.

Libet, B., Gleason, C. A., Wright, E. W., & Pearl, D. K. (1983). Time of conscious intention to act in relation to onset of cerebral activity (readiness-potential): The unconscious initiation of a freely voluntary act. *Brain, 106*(3), 623–642.

Malfait, N., & Ostry, D. J. (2004). Is interlimb transfer of force-field adaptation a cognitive response to the sudden introduction of load? *Journal of Neuroscience, 24,* 8084–8089.

Matin, E. (1982). Saccadic suppression and the dual mechanism theory of direction constancy. *Vision Research, 22,* 335–336.

Miall, R. C., Christensen, L. O., Cain, O., & Stanley, J. (2007). Disruption of state estimation in the human lateral cerebellum. *PLoS Biology, 5,* e316.

Miall, R. C., & King, D. (2008). State estimation in the cerebellum. *Cerebellum, 7,* 572–576.

Miall, R. C., Weir, D. J., Wolpert, D. M., & Stein, J. F. (1993). Is the cerebellum a Smith predictor? *Journal of Motor Behavior, 25,* 203–216.

Michel, C., Pisella, L., Prablanc, C., Rode, G., & Rossetti, Y. (2007). Enhancing visuomotor adaptation by reducing error signals: Single-step (aware) versus multiple-step (unaware) exposure to wedge prisms. *Journal of Cognitive Neuroscience, 19,* 341–350.

Moore, J., & Haggard, P. (2008). Awareness of action: Inference and prediction. *Consciousness and Cognition, 17,* 136–144.

Ogawa, K., Inui, T., & Sugio, T. (2007). Neural correlates of state estimation in visually guided movements: An event-related fMRI study. *Cortex, 43,* 289–300.

Orfei, M. D., Robinson, R. G., Prigatano, G. P., Starkstein, S., Rüsch, N., Bria, P., et al. (2007). Anosognosia for hemiplegia after stroke is a multifaceted phenomenon: A systematic review of the literature. *Brain, 130,* 3075–3090.

Pellijeff, A., Bonilha, L., Morgan, P. S., McKenzie, K., & Jackson, S. R. (2006). Parietal updating of limb posture: An event-related fMRI study. *Neuropsychologia, 44,* 2685–2690.

Petit, J.-L. (1999). Constitution by movement: Husserl in light of recent neurobiological findings. In F. Petitot, F. J. Varela, B. Pachoud, & J.-M. Roy (Eds.), *Naturalizing phenomenology: Issues in contemporary phenomenology and cognitive science* (pp. 220–245). Stanford, CA: Stanford University Press.

Prablanc, C., & Martin, O. (1992). Automatic control during hand reaching at undetected two-dimensional target displacements. *Journal of Neurophysiology, 67,* 455–469.

Ramachandran, V. S. (1996). What neurological syndromes can tell us about human nature: Some lessons from phantom limbs, capgras syndrome, and anosognosia. *Cold Spring Harbor Symposia on Quantitative Biology, 61,* 115–134.

Ramachandran, V. S., & Hirstein, W. (1998). The perception of phantom limbs: The D. O. Hebb Lecture. *Brain, 121*(9), 1603–1630.

Raos, V., Franchi, G., Gallese, V., & Fogassi, L. (2003). Somatotopic organization of the lateral part of area F2 (dorsal premotor cortex) of the macaque monkey. *Journal of Neurophysiology, 89,* 1503–1518.

Scepkowski, L. A., & Cronin-Golomb, A. (2003). The alien hand: Cases, categorizations, and anatomical correlates. *Behavioral and Cognitive Neuroscience Reviews, 2,* 261–277.

Scott, S. H., Sergio, L. E., & Kalaska, J. F. (1997). Reaching movements with similar hand paths but different arm orientations: Vol. 2. Activity of individual cells in dorsal premotor cortex and parietal area 5. *Journal of Neurophysiology, 78,* 2413–2426.

Sirigu, A., Daprati, E., Ciancia, S., Giraux, P., Nighoghossian, N., Posada, A., et al. (2004). Altered awareness of voluntary action after damage to the parietal cortex. *Nature Neuroscience, 7,* 80–84.

Sirigu, A., Daprati, E., Pradat-Diehl, P., Franck, N., & Jeannerod, M. (1999). Perception of self-generated movement following left parietal lesion. *Brain, 122*(10), 1867–1874.

Sirigu, A., Duhamel, J. R., Cohen, L., Pillon, B., Dubois, B., & Agid, Y. (1996). The mental representation of hand movements after parietal cortex damage. *Science, 273,* 1564–1568.

Spinoza, B. (1677/1994). *L'éthique.* Paris: Gallimard.

Tsakiris, M., Haggard, P., Franck, N., Mainy, N., & Sirigu, A. (2005). A specific role for efferent information in self-recognition. *Cognition, 96,* 215–231.

Turner, R. S., Desmurget, M., Grethe, J., Crutcher, M. D., & Grafton, S. T. (2003). Motor subcircuits mediating the control of movement extent and speed. *Journal of Neurophysiology, 90,* 3958–3966.

Watson, J. B. (1913). Psychology as the behaviorist views it. *Psychological Review, 20,* 158–177.

Wing, A. M., Flanagan, J. R., & Richardson, J. (1997). Anticipatory postural adjustments in stance and grip. *Experimental Brain Research, 116,* 122–130.

Wolpert, D. M., & Flanagan, J. R. (2001). Motor prediction. *Current Biology, 11,* R729–R732.

Wolpert, D. M., Ghahramani, Z., & Jordan, M. I. (1995). Are arm trajectories planned in kinematic or dynamic coordinates? An adaptation study. *Experimental Brain Research, 103,* 460–470.

Wolpert, D. M., Goodbody, S. J., & Husain, M. (1998). Maintaining internal representations: The role of the human superior parietal lobe. *Nature Neuroscience, 1,* 529–533.

Yarbus, A. L. (1967). *Eye movements and vision.* New York: Plenum Press.

# CHAPTER 10

# Volition and the Function of Consciousness

*Tashina L. Graves, Brian Maniscalco, and Hakwan Lau*


## ABSTRACT

*What are the psychological functions that could only be performed consciously? People have intuitively assumed that many acts of volition are not influenced by unconscious information. These acts range from simple examples such as making a spontaneous motor movement, to higher cognitive control. However, the available evidence suggests that under suitable conditions, unconscious information can influence these behaviors and the underlying neural mechanisms. One possibility is that stimuli that are consciously perceived tend to yield strong signals in the brain, which makes us think that consciousness has the function of such strong signals. However, if we could create conditions where the stimuli could yield strong signals but not the conscious experience of perception, perhaps we would find that such stimuli are just as effective in influencing volitional behavior. Future studies that focus on clarifying this issue may tell us what the defining functions of consciousness are.*


## INTRODUCTION

Many acts of volition seem to require conscious effort. We consciously initiate spontaneous motor movements. We cancel planned actions at will. We deliberately avoid particular actions. We intentionally shift our action plans in order to pursue different goals. Sometimes, theorists say, these are the functions of consciousness, as if evolution has equipped us with the gift of consciousness just to perform these acts. Without consciousness, presumably, we would only be able to perform much simpler actions that are no more sophisticated than embellished reflexes.

In this chapter we review available evidence to see if these intuitive claims are empirically supported. Recent studies in cognitive neuroscience suggest that many of these complex processes can actually be performed without consciousness. Or at least, many of them can be directly influenced by unconscious information. This calls into question the true function of consciousness, if not to enable us to deliberate our actions. We end by discussing what is logically required for an experiment to demonstrate the true function of consciousness.

## SPONTANEOUS MOTOR INITIATION

Motor actions that are made not in immediate or direct response to external stimuli can be said to be spontaneously initiated. These are also sometimes called self-paced or self-generated actions. For instance, one may choose to casually flex one's wrist while sitting in a dark room, out of one's own free choice and timing, not to react to anything in particular. Some philosophers have argued that in cases like that, it should seem obvious that the action is caused by one's conscious intention (Searle, 1983). Whereas one may argue that fast reactions to external stimuli may be driven by unconscious reflexes (e.g., a runner leaping forward upon hearing the starting whistle), the immediate cause of spontaneous actions seems to be the conscious intention itself. Subjectively, it seems as though one forms the intention to act and then immediately performs the action.

However, it has been shown that preparatory activity in the brain starts as early as 1–2 seconds before spontaneous actions are executed—a much longer time than seems to take place between intention and execution. This piece of one of the most perplexing findings in cognitive neuroscience was originally reported by Kornhuber and Deecke in the 1960s (Kornhuber & Deecke, 1965). In this study, they placed electrodes on the scalp to measure electroencephalography (EEG) and asked subjects to perform a motor movement at a time of their own choosing. The EEG data were time-locked to the point of motor execution (as measured by muscle contraction indicated by electromyography (EMG) and averaged over many trials. This produced an event-related potential (ERP) known as the *Bereitschaftspotential* (BP) or readiness potential (RP).

The readiness potential peaks at around the point of action execution, but it begins slowly rising about 1–2 seconds before that (Fig. 10.1). It is most pronounced at electrodes near the vertex (Cz in the EEG coordinate system), which is directly above the medial premotor areas (including the supplementary motor area [SMA], presupplementary motor area [preSMA], and the cingulate motor areas below them). It is generally believed that one major source of the readiness potential lies in the medial premotor areas (Ball, Schreiber, Feige, Wagner, Lücking, & Kristeva-Feige, 1999; Erdler et al., 2000; Weilke et al., 2001; Cunnington, Windischberger, Deecke, & Moser, 2003). The demonstration of the readiness potential calls into question whether spontaneous movements are really caused by the preceding conscious intentions. Perhaps the brain starts to prepare for the actions long before we consciously initiate them.

Just how big is the gap between the start of the readiness potential and the feeling of conscious intention? Benjamin Libet and colleagues empirically studied the timing of the conscious intention in relation to the readiness potential and the action (Libet, Gleason, Wright, & Pearl, 1983) and reported that subjects on average report the onset of intention to be about 250 ms before motor execution. These studies used a clock paradigm in which subjects watched a dot revolving around a clock face at a speed of 2.56 seconds per cycle, while they flexed their wrist spontaneously (Fig. 10.2). After the action was finished, subjects were required to report the location of the dot when they "first felt the urge" to produce the action, i.e., the onset of intention. For instance, the subject might say it was at the 3 o'clock or 4 o'clock position when they first felt the intention. This way, the subjects could time and report the onset of their intention, and the experimenter could then work out actually when the action was produced, and hence the temporal distance between the two.

Many people feel uncomfortable with the fact that the onset of the readiness potential seems to be so much earlier than the onset of intention, and some have tried to explain away the gap. The Libet clock method has also received considerable criticism. It involves timing across modalities, and could be susceptible to various biases (Libet, 1985; Gomes, 1998; Joordens, van Duijn, & Spalek, 2002; Klein, 2002; Trevena & Miller, 2002). However, it is unlikely that all these biases are in the direction that would help to narrow the gap between the onsets of the readiness potential and intention. Some have actually suggested that the different biases may point to different directions and thus just cancel each other out (Klein, 2002). Also, in the original experiments by Libet and colleagues, there were control conditions that tested for the basic accuracy of the clock. They asked subjects to use the clock to time either the onset of movement execution, or in another condition to time the onset of tactile stimuli presented externally by the experimenter. Since the actual onsets of these events are objectively measurable, they could estimate the subjective error of onset reports produced by the clock method. They found the error to be in the order of about 50 ms, (e.g., people misestimate the time of action execution to be 50 ms earlier than it actually is). This size of error is considerably smaller than the gap between the onsets of the readiness potential and intention.

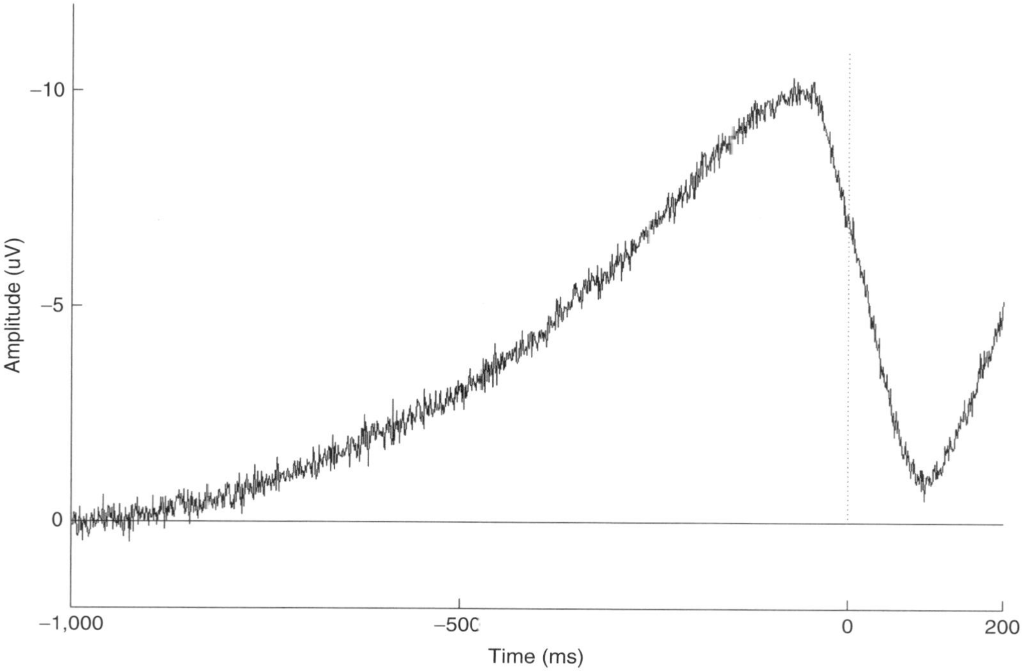


**Figure 10.1** A schematic depiction of the readiness potential (RP) preceding spontaneous movements. The RP is usually recorded at the top of the scalp, above medial frontal premotor areas. It gradually ramps up, beginning about 1-2 seconds before movement and peaking around the time of movement execution (marked as time = 0 above).

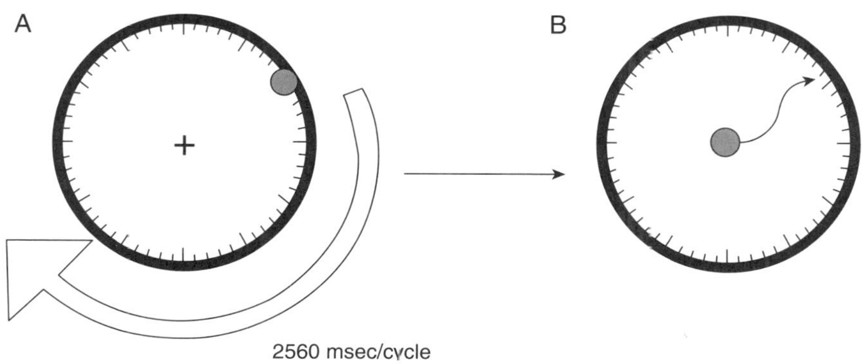


**Figure 10.2 The Libet clock paradigm.** **(A)** The subject views a dot rotating slowly (2.56 seconds per cycle) around a clock face and waits for an urge to move to arise spontaneously. When the urge arrives, the subject makes a movement (e.g. a key press). **(B)** After making the movement, the subject estimates the earliest time at which the intention to move was experienced. To carry out this time estimate, the subjects either verbally indicate the location of the dot where the intention was first felt, or move a cursor to that location (as in this example). In a common control condition, the subject uses the clock to estimate the time of movement rather than the onset of intention. Figure edited and adapted from Lau et al., 2007.

Libet and colleagues have tried to study the onset of the readiness potential more carefully, discarding trials that might have been "contaminated" by preplanning of action well before the action (for instance, by counting to 10 and then triggering the movement), as reported by the subjects. By only looking at the trials where the actions were supposed to be genuinely spontaneous, Libet and colleagues reported that the onset of the readiness potential is only about 500 ms before action execution (Libet, Wright, & Gleason, 1983). However, this is still clearly earlier than the reported onset of intention. And by discarding so many trials, it may be that the analysis simply lacked the power to detect an earlier onset.

Some have argued that the onset of readiness potential might be an artifact due to the averaging needed to produce the ERP (Miller & Trevena, 2002). However, Romo and Schultz (1987) have recorded from neurons in the medial premotor areas while monkeys made self-paced movements. It was found that some of neurons in this region in fact fired as early as 0.6–2.6 seconds before movement onset. From the reported results it was also clear that this pattern of early firing for these neurons was consistent across trials. One other recent study has reported that the spatial pattern of fMRI activity from this region, at up to 5 seconds before action, can statistically predict the timing of action above chance level (Soon, Brass, Heinze, & Haynes, 2008).

Others have argued that the readiness potential may not reflect the specific and causal aspects of motor initiation. However, as mentioned earlier, it is likely that the readiness potential partly originates from the medial premotor areas. Lesion to these areas can abolish the production of spontaneous actions (Thaler, Chen, Nixon, Stern, & Passingham, 1995). These areas also contain neurons that code specific action plans (Shima & Tanji, 1998; Tanji and Shima, 1996). Further, when people use the Libet clock paradigm to time their own intentions, there is attentional modulation of activity in the medial preSMA (Lau, Rogers, Haggard, & Passingham, 2004), as if people were reading information off the area that is likely to be a source of the readiness potential.

The basic results of Libet and colleagues have also been replicated in several different laboratories (e.g., Lau et al., 2004; Haggard & Eimer, 1998; Soon, Brass, Heinze, & Haynes, 2008). In general, the same pattern is found, that the onset of intention is either around or later than 250 ms before action execution, which seems to confirm our intuition that conscious intentions seem to be followed by motor actions almost immediately. In fact, given that the readiness potential starts as early as 1–2 seconds before action execution, it is hard to imagine how the onset of intention could coincide with or precede the readiness potential, unless one thinks of intention as a kind of prior intention (Searle, 1983), like the general plan that is formed at the beginning of the experimental session when the subject agrees to produce some actions in the next half an hour or so. We shall discuss this kind of higher-cognitive "intention" later in the chapter. However, the intention we are concerned with here is the immediate "urge" to produce the motor action (Libet, Wright, & Gleason, 1982).

Taken together, the evidence suggests that conscious intention, i.e., the immediate feeling of motor initiation, is unlikely to be the "first unmoved mover" in triggering spontaneous motor movements. It is likely to be preceded by unconscious brain activity that may contribute to action initiation. Perhaps the feeling of conscious intention to perform a motor movement is actually the detection of the response potential. Under this view, consciousness is nothing more than the detection of a signal that has passed a certain threshold. If so, why does this detection occur hundreds to thousands of milliseconds after the response potential, rather than as soon as the response potential occurs? The answer may lie in signal detection theory.

The response potential is a slowly increasing neural signal that must be detected against a background of noise. The signal is hard to detect at onset, because it starts out very weak. If the detection criterion is too low, there will be constant false alarms due to noise in the system. However, it is also important that the criterion not be too high, because then the signal might be detected very late, if at all. An optimal criterion would lead to responses with an average close to the actual onset of the signal and would also be consistent. That is, it would not produce responses that are extremely varied from one trial to the next. Probabilistic simulations done in the authors' lab (Nikolov et al., *in review*) have shown that when the criterion is at an optimal level for an increasing signal, the expected time of detection is on average later than the onset. This results from the trade-off between accuracy and bias. The detections are consistent, due to a lower number of false alarms, but there is a bias toward late detection, hence the lag between the beginning of the response potential and the "urge" to perform an action.

## CONSCIOUS VETO?

If the decision to perform an action is initiated unconsciously, perhaps our awareness of intention comes into play by allowing us to "veto," or cancel, that action. The fact that we have the ability to "veto" our actions has been demonstrated experimentally. Libet and colleagues (Libet et al., 1983) as well as other researchers (Brass & Haggard, 2007) have performed experiments where subjects prepare for an action and then cancel it in the last moment, just before it is executed. The question is whether the awareness of intention is critical to the ability to veto an action. It may not be if the choice to veto is preceded by unconscious activity, like the intention to act is preceded by the readiness potential, or actions are sometimes unconsciously vetoed without awareness.

Some recent evidence suggests that the conscious intention may not facilitate a veto. As mentioned earlier, when people were using the Libet clock to time the onset of their intentions, there was attentional modulation of activity in the preSMA (Lau et al., 2004). These data have subsequently been further analyzed (Lau, Rogers, & Passingham, 2006), and it has been shown that subjects who showed a large degree of attentional modulation tended to also report the onset of intention to be early. One interpretation could be that attention biases the judgment of onset to be earlier. It was found in another experiment that this was also true when people used the Libet clock to time the onset of the motor execution. The higher the level of fMRI activity modulated by attention, the earlier subjects reported the onset to be, even though on average subjects reported the onsets to be earlier than they actually were, as if experiencing a false alarm—incorrectly interpreting noise as the presence of a signal. This means a bias to the negative (i.e., early direction) produced more erroneous rather than more precise reports.

In general, the principle of attentional prior entry (Shore, Spence, & Klein, 2001) suggests that attention to an event speeds up its perception and negatively biases the reported onset. If this were true in the case of the Libet experiments, this could mean that attention might have exaggerated the 250ms onset, i.e., had subjects not been required to attend to their intentions in order to perform the timing tasks, the true onset of conscious intention may well be much later than 250 ms prior to action execution. This calls into question whether we have enough time to consider the veto.

Another study reported that some patients with lesion to the parietal cortex reported the onset of intention to be as late as 50 ms prior to action execution (Sirigu et al., 2004). If the awareness of intention allows one to veto actions, one might expect these patients to have much less time to consciously evaluate spontaneous intentions and cancel the inappropriate ones. This could be quite disastrous to daily life functioning. Yet there were no such reports about these patients.

Finally, in another study (Lau, Rogers, & Passingham, 2007), single pulses of transcranial magnetic stimulation (TMS) were sent to the medial premotor areas (targeting the preSMA). Again, subjects were instructed to produce spontaneous movements and to time the onset of intentions and movement execution using the Libet clock. Surprisingly, although TMS was applied *after* motor execution, it has an effect on the reported onsets. No matter whether TMS was applied immediately after action execution or with a 200 ms delay, the stimulation exaggerated the temporal distance between the reported onsets of intention and movement, as if people reported a prolonged period of conscious intending. One interpretation is that TMS injected noisy activity into the area, and the intention-monitoring mechanism did not distinguish this from endogenously generated activity that is supposed to represent intention, causing early false alarms. However, what is crucial is the fact that the reported onsets can be manipulated even after the action is finished. This seems to suggest that our awareness of intention may be constructed after the facts, or at least not completely determined before the action is finished. If conscious intentions are not formed before the action, they certainly cannot play any role in facilitating veto, let alone causing it.

This interpretation may seem wild, but it is consistent with other proposals. For instance, on the basis of many ingenious experiments manipulating subjects sense of agency, Wegner (2002) has suggested that the conscious will is an illusion. The sense of agency is often inferred post hoc, based on many contextual factors. Wegner cites experiments to support these claims. One example is a study on "facilitated communication" (Wegner, Fuller, & Sparrow, 2003). Subjects (playing the role of "facilitators") were asked to place their fingers on two keys of a keyboard, while a confederate (playing the role of "communicator") placed his or her fingers on top of those of the subject. Subjects were given headphones with which they listened to questions of varying difficulty. Confederates were given headphones as well, and subjects were led to believe that the confederates would be hearing the same questions, although in fact the confederates heard nothing. Subjects were told to detect subtle, unconscious movements in the confederate's fingers following each question and press the corresponding key in order to answer on the confederate's behalf. It was found that subjects answered easy questions well above chance levels. If they had performed the task strictly according to the instructions, however, they should have performed at chance. Therefore, subjects must have been directing their own key presses. Nonetheless, they attributed a significant causal role for the key presses to the confederate. The degree to which subjects answered easy questions correctly was not correlated with the degree to which they attributed causal responsibility to confederates, suggesting that the generation of action and attribution of action to an agent are independent processes.

To summarize, although theorists have speculated that the awareness of intention may play some role in allowing us to cancel or edit our actions, considerable doubt has been cast by recent empirical evidence.

## EXCLUSION AND INHIBITION

Another kind of situation that seems to require conscious deliberation involves the need to avoid a particular action or response. This is related to "vetoing" as described above, except that the action being inhibited is not necessarily self-paced, and may be specified externally. One example would be to perform stem completion while avoiding a particular word. So for instance, the experimenter may ask the subjects to produce any word starting with letter D (i.e., completing a "stem"), but avoid the word "dinner." So subjects can produce "dog," "danger," "dear," etc., but if they produce the word "dinner," it would be counted as an error. This is called the exclusion task (Jacoby, Lindsay, & Toth, 1992).

One interesting aspect of the exclusion task is that people can perform well only if they clearly see and remember the target of exclusion (i.e., the word "dinner" in the foregoing example). If the target of exclusion is presented very briefly and followed by a mask, such that it was only very weakly perceived, people may fail to exclude it (Debner & Jacoby, 1994; Merikle, Joordens, & Stolz, 1995). In fact, they tend to produce exactly the word they should be avoiding with higher likelihood than if they were not presented with the word at all. It has been argued that this exclusion failure phenomenon is the hallmark of unconscious processing (Jacoby et al., 1992). The weak perception of the target probably produced a representation for the word, but because the signal is not strong enough to reach the level of conscious processing, subjects are unable to inhibit the corresponding response.

In addition to the intuitive appeal, the notion that consciousness is required for exclusion is also supported by a case study of a blindsight patient (Persaud & Cowey, 2007). Subject GY has a lesion to the left primary visual cortex (V1), and reports that most of his right visual field is subjectively blind. However, in forced-choice situation he can discriminate simple stimuli well above chance level in his "blind" field (Weiskrantz, 1997, 1999). In one study he was required to perform an exclusion task (Persaud & Cowey, 2008), i.e., to say the location (up or down) where the target was *not* presented. Although he could do this easily in the normal field, he failed the task when stimuli were presented to his blind field. Note that he was significantly worse than chance in the blind field, as if the unconscious signal drove the response directly and inflexibly, defying exclusion control. This seems to support the account that consciousness is required for exclusion.

However, the notion that flexible control or inhibition of perceptual signal requires consciousness is not without its critics (Snodgrass, 2002; Haase & Fisk, 2001; Visser & Merikle, 1999). One problem becomes clear when we consider the motion distractor example above. "Conscious signal" here seems to be equated with "strong signal," driven by larger motion strength in the stimuli. Obviously, signals have to be strong enough to reach the prefrontal cortex in order to trigger the associating executions functions. Do unconscious stimuli fail to be excluded because we are not conscious of them, or is it just because the signal is not strong enough? Or, are the two explanations one and the same? Not all studies are subject to this argument. For instance, in the blindsight study mentioned above (Persaud & Cowey, 2008), the subject failed to exclude in the blindfield even when the contrast level would give a performance that was similar to that in the normal visual field. So if we take forced-choice performance as an index of signal strength, the signal from the blindfield was not weak in this sense. However, in most other cases we often take awareness to be the same as good performance. Are we justified in doing so?

Other researchers have reported evidence that seems to support unconscious inhibition. For instance, in one study (Snodgrass & Shevrin, 2006) people were asked to detect visually presented words. In certain conditions, some subjects showed detection performance that was significantly *worse* than chance. These words were presented so briefly that typically detection performance would be near chance. We usually take chance-level as the objective threshold for conscious perception. Below chance-level performance could be taken as evidence that the subjects did not consciously perceive the words. And yet, if they had no information at all regarding the words, performance should just be exactly at chance rather than below. It seems that these subjects were actively suppressing the words.

These are unusual cases and are somewhat hard to interpret. We take chance-level as the objective threshold for conscious perception because when people perform at chance, it indicates that they do not have the explicit information regarding the target of perception. However, if people perform significantly below chance, it means that somehow they have the information regarding the detection, which violates the very logic we adopt to label perception unconscious. But in any case, the stimuli were supposed to be really weak, and it is intriguing that some subjects seem to be automatically suppressing the words. Are we to take these somewhat unusual cases as evidence to reject the notion that exclusion or inhibition requires consciousness? It seems that, logically, if we claim that a certain function *requires* consciousness, we should predict there will never be a case where one could perform such function unconsciously. How seriously are we to take this logic and reject functions as requiring consciousness by a single experiment? We will return to this argument in the last section of the chapter.

## TOP-DOWN COGNITIVE CONTROL

So far we have discussed acts of volition that are relatively simple, like starting a motor movement, or avoiding a particular action. Sometimes we also voluntarily prepare for a set of rules or action plans in order to satisfy a more abstract goal in mind. For instance, a telephone ring may usually trigger a particular action, e.g., to pick up the phone. However, when one visits friends at their homes, one may deliberately change the mapping between the stimulus (telephone ring) and action, i.e., it would be more appropriate to sit still, or ask the host to pick up the phone, rather than picking it up oneself. This volitional change of stimulus-response contingency is an example of top-down cognitive control. It has been suggested that top-down cognitive control may require consciousness (Dehaene & Naccache, 2001). The idea is that unconscious stimuli can trigger certain prepared actions, as demonstrated in studies in subliminal priming (Kouider & Dehaene, 2007). However, the preparation or setting up of the stimulus-response contingency may require consciousness.

However, recent studies suggest that this might not be true, in the sense that unconscious information seems to be able to influence or even trigger top-down cognitive control too (Mattler, 2003; Lau & Passingham, 2007). In one study subjects had to prepare to do a phonological or semantic judgment, based on the orientation

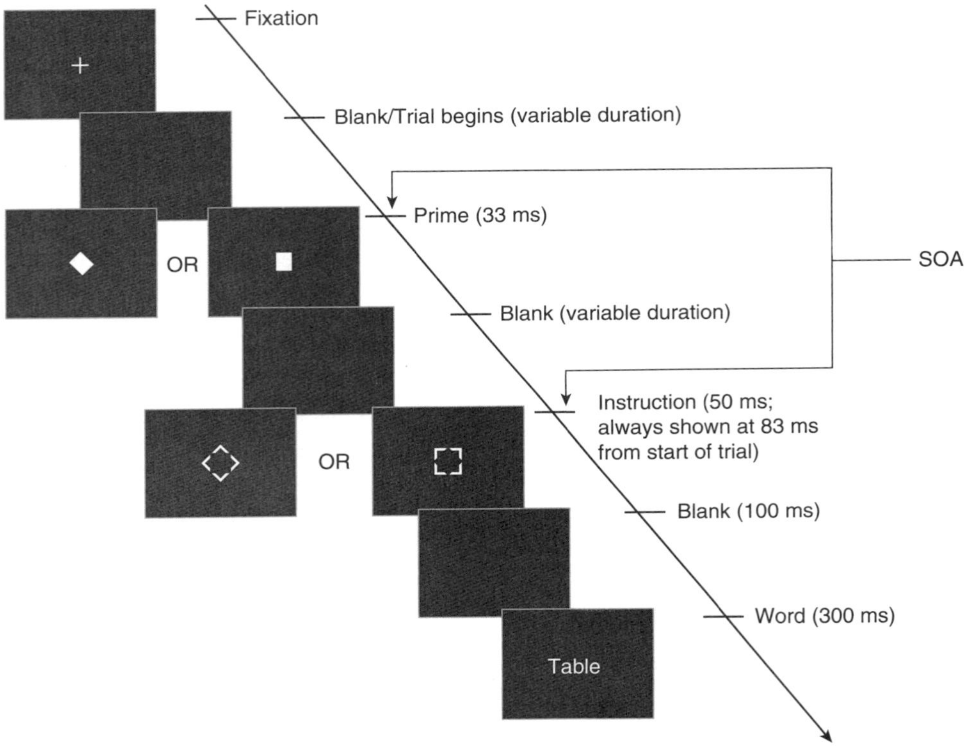


**Figure 10.3** Experimental paradigm of Lau and Passingham (2007). Subjects view briefly presented words and perform either a phonological task (is the word one syllable or two syllables?) or a semantic task (does the word name something concrete or abstract?). Before word presentation, subjects are instructed which task to perform on a given trial by a visual symbol (a square for the phonological task, or a diamond for the semantic task). The symbolic instruction itself acts as a metacontrast mask for an earlier prime, also a square or a diamond. Because the prime is briefly presented and masked, it is not consciously perceived. On half of trials, the prime is congruent with the instruction and on the other half, incongruent. Behavioral and imaging results suggest that the unconscious primes affected top-down task switching. When primes were incongruent with instructions, accuracy fell, reaction time increased, and brain regions corresponding to the task indicated by the prime were partially activated (all relative to the prime-congruent condition). But when the stimulus onset asynchrony (SOA) between prime and instruction was lowered, such that primes became visible, the priming effect was not evident. This double dissociation suggests that the interference of incongruent primes on task switching cannot be attributed to conscious processing. (Figure adapted from Lau and Passingham, 2007).

of a figure they saw (Fig. 10.3). In every trial, if they saw a square, they had to prepare to judge whether an upcoming word has two syllables (e.g., "table") or not (e.g., "milk"). If they saw a diamond, they had to prepare to judge whether an upcoming word refers to a concrete object (e.g., "chair") or an abstract idea (e.g., "love"). In other words, they had to perform top-down cognitive control based on the instruction figure (square or diamond). However, before the instruction figure was presented, there was an invisible prime figure, which could also be a diamond or a square. It was found that the prime could impair subjects' performance when it suggested the alternative (i.e., wrong) task to the subjects (incongruent condition). One could argue that this was only because the prime distracted the subjects on a perceptual level, and did not really trigger cognitive control. However, the experiment was performed in the fMRI scanner, and the brain recordings suggest that when being primed to perform the wrong task, subjects used more of the wrong neural resources too (Lau & Passingham, 2007). That is, areas that are more sensitive to phonological or semantic processing showed increased activity when the explicit instruction figure made subjects perform the phonological and semantic tasks respectively. The invisible primes also seem to be able to trigger activations in task sensitive areas. This suggests that they can influence or exercise top-down cognitive control.

Another study examines how unconscious information affects our high-level objectives by focusing on how the potential reward influences our level of motivation (Pessiglione et al., 2007). Subjects squeezed a device to win a certain amount of money. The harder they squeezed, the more money they would win. However, the size of the stake in question for a particular trial was announced in the beginning by presenting the photo of a coin. The coin could either be a British pound (~2 U.S. dollars) or a penny (~2 U.S. cents), and it signified the monetary value of the maximal reward for that trial. Not surprisingly, people squeezed harder when the stakes were high, but interestingly, the same pattern of behavior was observed even when the figure of the coin was masked such that subjects reported not seeing it. This suggests that unconscious information can influence our level of motivation as well.

If unconscious information alone is sufficient to exercise all these sophisticated top-down control functions, why do we need to be conscious at all?

## HOW TO FIND THE TRUE FUNCTION OF CONSCIOUSNESS?

The foregoing is not meant to be an exhaustive review of all studies on the potential functions of consciousness. We select some examples from a few areas that are particularly related to volition, and discuss what role consciousness may play. It may, of course, be that there are other psychological functions that require consciousness.

Yet, one cannot help but feel that there seems to be some inherent limitation to this whole enterprise of research. If we claim that a certain function requires consciousness, strictly speaking, the interpretation could be that the function should never be able to be performed unconsciously. Of course, one could make the weaker claim that a certain function is usually or most suitably performed consciously, and when consciousness fails, unconscious processing can act as a backup. This is similar to arguing that one function of having legs is to facilitate locomotion; if we lose our legs, we could still move around, albeit poorly. However, let us assume that one is to make the stronger prediction that such functions should never be able to be performed unconsciously. In principle, it would only take a single experiment to falsify that. This explains why this review may seem biased in that we focus on studies that show the power of the unconscious, rather than studies demonstrating what functions definitely require consciousness. In principle, falsifying the claim that a certain function requires consciousness is straightforward. But this is not the case for demonstrating functions that would always require consciousness.

One can, of course, try to show that subjects could normally do a task if the relevant information is consciously perceived. And then one tries to "knock-out" the conscious perception for such information, and try to show that the task could no longer be performed, or that it is performed at an additional cost, i.e., slower or with more errors. But how would one know that in "knocking-out" the conscious perception, one does not "knock-out" too much? One typically suppresses conscious perception by visual masking, by using brief presentation, by distracting the subject, by applying transcranial magnetic stimulation, by pharmacological manipulations, etc. But all of these could potentially impair the unconscious as well as the conscious signal. Maybe in cases where the perception has been rendered unconscious, the signal is just no longer strong enough to drive the function in question? This would mean that, in principle, it would be possible for a future study to find the optimal procedure or setup to just render the information unconscious, without reducing the signal strength too much. And in that case the subjects may be able to perform the task in question. That would falsify our claim.

This means that in looking for functions that require consciousness, we need to adopt some different strategies. One potentially useful approach is to try to demonstrate something akin to a "double dissociation." When conscious perception is suppressed, we often find that a sophisticated function (e.g., top-down cognitive control) can no longer be performed, though some simpler function (e.g., priming for a prepared motor response) may still be activated by unconscious information. From the foregoing discussion, one could see that this may not be as surprising or informative as it seems. It could be just that the unconscious signal is just too weak to drive the relatively sophisticated function. A demonstration of the opposite would, however, be much more convincing: If after suppression of conscious perception, the subjects can still perform a rather sophisticated function, but fail to perform a simple function, that would suggest that the simple function really requires consciousness. In this case, it could not be that the suppression of conscious perception has taken away too much of the signal strength, because if that were the case then the subjects should not be able to perform the relatively sophisticated function (Fig. 10.4). Understanding this "double dissociation" approach helps us to see the logic behind how we could deal with signal strength as a confounding variable. However, one problem is that it is unclear what is the most convincing way to define "sophisticated/complicated" functions versus "simple" functions.

An alternative approach may be to directly match for signal strength between the conscious and the unconscious conditions. This might seem difficult because conscious signals may seem to be strong in general. However, as discussed above, blindsight subjects can perform forced-choice discrimination on visual stimuli well above chance, even when they claim that conscious awareness is missing. Forced-choice performance is often taken as an objective estimate of signal strength; the detection theoretical measure d′ is mathematically just the signal-to-noise ratio. In blindsight subject GY, where only half of the visual field lacks awareness, we can imagine presenting weak stimuli to the normal visual field such that forced-choice performance would match that in the blind field (Weiskrantz, Barbur, & Sahraie, 1995). This way we can test if certain functions cannot be performed based on information presented to the blind field, which may shed light on when consciousness is required.

One may argue that blindsight patients are rare and the way their brains process visual information may not generalize to intact brains. However, there are other paradigms in which one could match for forced-choice performance in normal subjects, and yet produce a difference in the level of conscious awareness. For instance, in one study (Lau & Passingham, 2006) metacontrast masking was used to create similar conditions where forced-choice discrimination accuracy for the visual targets were matched, and yet the subjective reports of how often subjects saw the identity of the targets differed (Fig. 10.5). One could imagine presenting these stimuli to subjects and seeing if they drive a certain function with different effectiveness. If the subjects perform better in the condition where subjective conscious awareness of the stimuli is more frequent, one could argue that

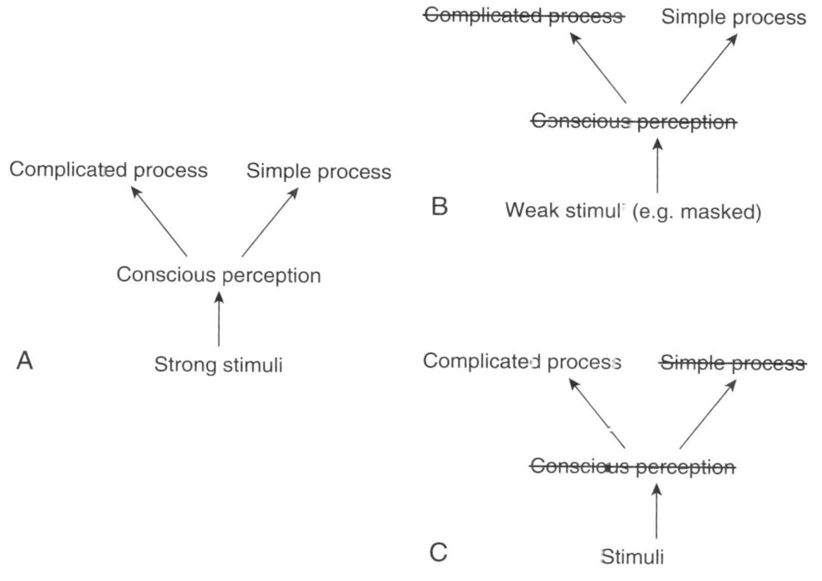


**Figure 10.4** (**A**) The normal situation for conscious perception. Stimuli are strong enough to drive processes of different complexity. (**B**) A typical situation for unconscious perception. Stimuli are weak such that complicated processes are no longer activated, though simple processes can still be triggered. It could be argued that this is not surprising as we may expect that complicated processes require a stronger signal. (**C**) A potentially more informative situation. If one could find a stimulus that is not consciously perceived, but yet is sufficiently strong to trigger a complicated process, then the relatively simple process that the stimulus does not drive would seem to critically depend on consciousness.

this function is likely to depend critically on consciousness.

## CONCLUSION

Acts of volition are accompanied by a sense of conscious effort or intention. The fact that we feel the conscious effort is not in doubt. What is less clear is whether the processes underlying the conscious experience directly contribute to the execution of the actions, in a way that is not accomplished by unconscious processes just as effectively. The general picture seems to be that many sophisticated functions can be performed unconsciously or driven by unconscious information.

Does this mean that consciousness has no special function at all? The answer is not yet clear. It is likely that some psychological functions do require consciousness. That is, there may be some functions that can only be performed poorly with unconscious information. Or, there may even be functions that can never be performed unconsciously. But experiments have not yet been able to convincingly pin them down.

They will have to overcome the following problem. If we assume that conscious perception is always accompanied by stronger and longer-lasting signals that are more effective than unconscious signals in propagating themselves throughout the brain, then consciousness would certainly be associated with the functions of these strong signals. However in studies of blindsight (Weiskrantz et al., 1995) as well as in normals (Lau & Passingham, 2006) it has been shown that signal strength as indicated by forced-choice performance is not always one and the same as conscious awareness. Therefore, future studies may need to focus on identifying the functions that really cannot be performed unconsciously, even when the signal strength is sufficiently strong. This may help to reveal the true function of consciousness.

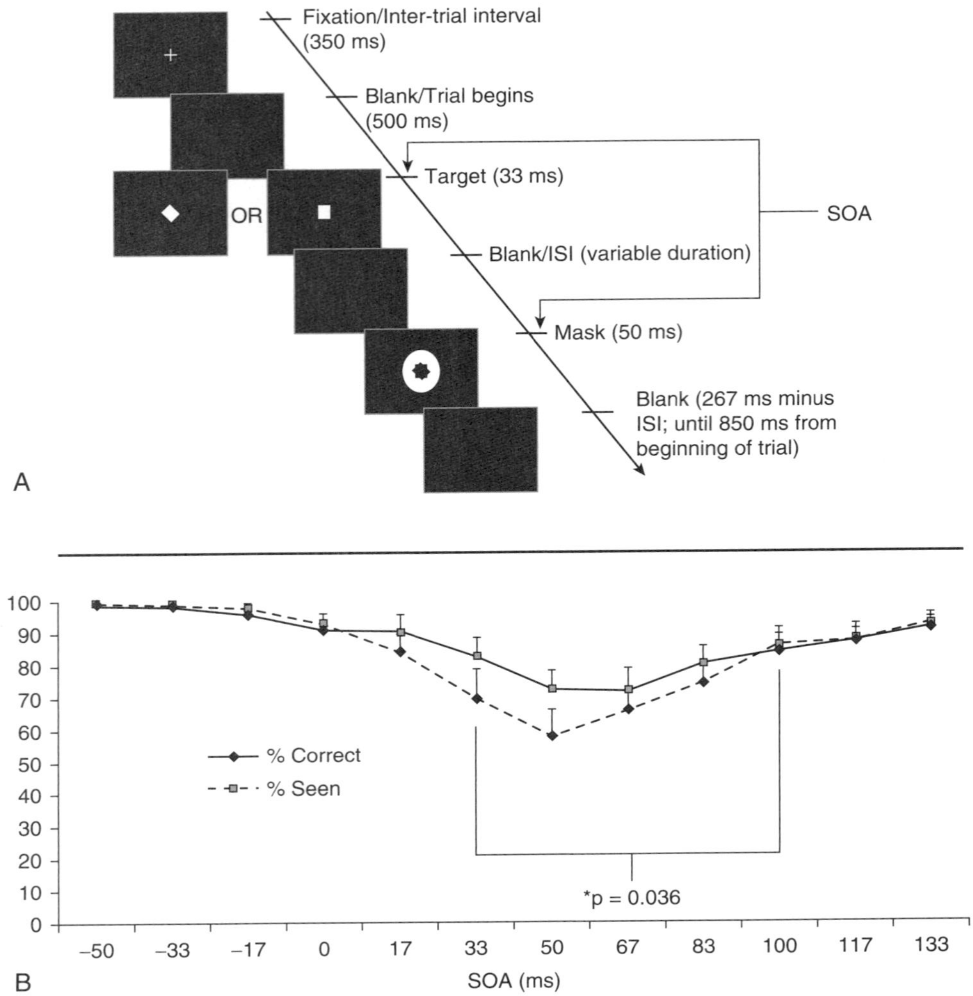


**Figure 10.5 Inducing relative blindsight in normal observers using metacontrast masking.** (**A**) Metacontrast masking paradigm. The subject is presented with a visual target (in this case, either a square or diamond). Afterward, a metacontrast mask is presented. The mask differentially affects discrimination accuracy and visual awareness of the target as a function of stimulus onset asynchrony (SOA). (**B**) Discrimination accuracy and visual awareness as a function of metacontrast mask SOA. The metacontrast mask creates a characteristic U-shaped function of performance vs. SOA. At shorter and longer SOAs, discrimination accuracy is high, but it dips at intermediate SOAs. The same is true for visual awareness, but the shape of the awareness masking function is not perfectly symmetrical with respect to the performance masking function. That is, there are certain SOAs at which forced choice performance is matched, but visual awareness differs significantly (e.g. as illustrated in the SOAs of 33 ms and 100 ms). Such performance-matched conditions could be used to investigate the functions of consciousness. If some task can be performed better in the condition of higher subjective visibility, it can plausibly be said to require visual awareness. Because forced-choice discrimination accuracy is matched across the two conditions, the superior performance of the task in the high visibility condition cannot be attributed to a difference in signal strength. (Figure adapted from Lau and Passingham, 2006).

## ACKNOWLEDGMENTS

The authors thank David Rosenthal and Uriah Kriegel for comments.

## REFERENCES

Ball, T., Schreiber, A., Feige, B., Wagner, M., Lücking, C. H., & Kristeva-Feige, R. (1999). The role of higher-order motor areas in voluntary movement as revealed by high-resolution EEG and fMRI. *NeuroImage, 10*(6), 682–694.

Brass, M., & Haggard, P. (2007). To do or not to do: The neural signature of self-control. *The Journal of Neuroscience: The Official Journal of the Society for Neuroscience, 27*(34), 9141–9145.

Cunnington, R., Windischberger, C., Deecke, L., & Moser, E. (2003). The preparation and readiness for voluntary movement: A high-field event-related fMRI study of the Bereitschafts-BOLD response. *NeuroImage, 20*(1), 404–412.

Debner, J. A., & Jacoby, L. L. (1994). Unconscious perception: Attention, awareness, and control. *Journal of Experimental Psychology: Learning, Memory, and Cognition, 20*(2), 304–317.

Dehaene, S., & Naccache, L. (2001). Towards a cognitive neuroscience of consciousness: Basic evidence and a workspace framework. *Cognition, 79*(1–2), 1–37.

Erdler, M., Beisteiner, R., Mayer, D., Kaindl, T., Edward, V., Windischberger, C., et al. (2000). Supplementary motor area activation preceding voluntary movement is detectable with a whole-scalp magnetoencephalography system. *NeuroImage, 11*(6), 697–707.

Gomes, G. (2002). The interpretation of Libet's results on the timing of conscious events: A commentary. *Consciousness and Cognition, 11*(2), 221–230; discussion 308–313, 314–325.

Haase, S. J., & Fisk, G. (2001). Confidence in word detection predicts word identification: Implications for an unconscious perception paradigm. *The American Journal of Psychology, 114*(3), 439–468.

Haggard, P., & Eimer, M. (1999). On the relation between brain potentials and the awareness of voluntary movements. *Experimental Brain Research. Experimentelle Hirnforschung. Expérimentation cérébrale, 126*(1), 128–133.

Jacoby, L. L., Lindsay, D. S., & Toth, J. P. (1992). Unconscious influences revealed: Attention, awareness, and control. *The American Psychologist, 47*(6), 802–809.

Joordens, S., van Duijn, M., & Spalek, T. M. (2002). When timing the mind one should also mind the timing: Biases in the measurement of voluntary actions. *Consciousness and Cognition, 11*(2), 231–240; discussion 308–313.

Klein, S. (2002). Libet's research on the timing of conscious intention to act: A commentary. *Consciousness and Cognition, 11*(2), 273–279; discussion 304–325.

Kornhuber, H., & Deecke, L. (1965). Hirnpotentialänderungen bei Willkurbewegungen und passiven Bewegungen des Menschen: Bereitschaftspotential und reafferente Potentiale. *Pflügers Archive, 284*, 1–17.

Kouider, S., & Dehaene, S. (2007). Levels of processing during non-conscious perception: A critical review of visual masking. *Philosophical Transactions of the Royal Society of London: Series B, Biological Sciences, 362*(1481), 857–875.

Lau, H. C., & Passingham, R. E. (2006). Relative blindsight in normal observers and the neural correlate of visual consciousness. *Proceedings of the National Academy of Sciences of the United States of America, 103*(49), 18763–18768.

Lau, H. C., & Passingham, R. E. (2007). Unconscious activation of the cognitive control system in the human prefrontal cortex. *The Journal of Neuroscience: The Official Journal of the Society for Neuroscience, 27*(21), 5805–5811.

Lau, H. C., Rogers, R. D., Haggard, P., & Passingham, R. E. (2004). Attention to intention. *Science, 303*(5661), 1208–1210.

Lau, H. C., Rogers, R. D., & Passingham, R. E. (2006). On measuring the perceived onsets of spontaneous actions. *The Journal of Neuroscience: The Official Journal of the Society for Neuroscience, 26*(27), 7265–7271.

Lau, H. C., Rogers, R. D., & Passingham, R. E. (2007). Manipulating the experienced onset of intention after action execution. *Journal of Cognitive Neuroscience, 19*(1), 81–90.

Libet, B. (1985). Unconscious cerebral initiative and the role of conscious will in voluntary action. *Behavioral and Brain Sciences, 8*, 529–566.

Libet, B., Gleason, C. A., Wright, E. W., & Pearl, D. K. (1983). Time of conscious intention to act in relation to onset of cerebral activity (readiness-potential): The unconscious initiation of a freely voluntary act. *Brain: A Journal of Neurology, 106*(3), 623–642.

Libet, B., Wright, E. W., & Gleason, C. A. (1982). Readiness-potentials preceding unrestricted "spontaneous" vs. pre-planned voluntary acts. *Electroencephalography and Clinical Neurophysiology, 54*(3), 322–335.

Libet, B., Wright, E. W., & Gleason, C. A. (1983). Preparation- or intention-to-act, in relation to pre-event potentials recorded at the vertex. *Electroencephalography and Clinical Neurophysiology, 56*(4), 367–372.

Mattler, U. (2003). Priming of mental operations by masked stimuli. *Perception & Psychophysics, 65*(2), 167–187.

McDonald, J. J., Teder-Sälejärvi, W. A., Di Russo, F., & Hillyard, S. A. (2005). Neural basis of auditory-induced shifts in visual time-order perception. *Nature Neuroscience, 8*(9), 1197–1202.

Merikle, P. M., Joordens, S., & Stolz, J. A. (1995). Measuring the relative magnitude of unconscious influences. *Consciousness and Cognition, 4*(4), 422–439.

Miller, J., & Trevena, J. A. (2002). Cortical movement preparation and conscious decisions: Averaging artifacts and timing biases. *Consciousness and Cognition, 11*(2), 308–313.

Nikolov S, Rahnev DA, Lau H (in review) Probabilistic Model of Onset Detection Explains Paradoxes in Human Time Perception.

Persaud, N., & Cowey, A. (2008). Blindsight is unlike normal conscious vision: Evidence from an exclusion task. *Consciousness and Cognition, 17*(3), 1050–1055.

Pessiglione, M., Schmidt, L., Draganski, B., Kalisch, R., Lau, H., Dolan, R. J., et al. (2007). How the brain translates money into force: A neuroimaging study of subliminal motivation. *Science, 316*(5826), 904–906.

Romo, R., & Schultz, W. (1987). Neuronal activity preceding self-initiated or externally timed arm movements in area 6 of monkey cortex. *Experimental Brain Research. Experimentelle Hirnforschung. Expérimentation cérébrale, 67*(3), 656–662.

Searle, J. R. (1983). *Intentionality: An Essay in the Philosophy of Mind* (p. 278). Cambridge, UK: Cambridge University Press.

Shima, K., & Tanji, J. (1998). Both supplementary and presupplementary motor areas are crucial for the temporal organization of multiple movements. *Journal of Neurophysiology, 80*(6), 3247–3260.

Shore, D. I., Spence, C., & Klein, R. M. (2001). Visual prior entry. *Psychological Science: A Journal of the American Psychological Society/APS, 12*(3), 205–212.

Sirigu, A., Daprati, E., Ciancia, S., Giraux, P., Nighoghossian, N., Posada, A., et al. (2004). Altered awareness of voluntary action after damage to the parietal cortex. *Nature Neuroscience, 7*(1), 80–84.

Snodgrass, M. (2002). Disambiguating conscious and unconscious influences: Do exclusion paradigms demonstrate unconscious perception? *The American Journal of Psychology, 115*(4), 545–579.

Snodgrass, M., & Shevrin, H. (2006). Unconscious inhibition and facilitation at the objective detection threshold: Replicable and qualitatively different unconscious perceptual effects. *Cognition, 101*(1), 43–79.

Soon, C. S., Brass, M., Heinze, H., & Haynes, J. (2008). Unconscious determinants of free decisions in the human brain. *Nature Neuroscience, 11*(5), 543–545.

Tanji, J., & Shima, K. (1996). Supplementary motor cortex in organization of movement. *European Neurology, 36*(Suppl. 1), 13–19.

Thaler, D., Chen, Y. C., Nixon, P. D., Stern, C. E., & Passingham, R. E. (1995). The functions of the medial premotor cortex: Vol. 1. Simple learned movements. *Experimental Brain Research. Experimentelle Hirnforschung. Expérimentation cérébrale, 102*(3), 445–460.

Trevena, J. A., & Miller, J. (2002). Cortical movement preparation before and after a conscious decision to move. *Consciousness and Cognition, 11*(2), 162–190; discussion 314–325.

Tsushima, Y., Sasaki, Y., & Watanabe, T. (2006). Greater disruption due to failure of inhibitory control on an ambiguous distractor. *Science, 314*(5806), 1786–1788.

Visser, T. A., & Merikle, P. M. (1999). Conscious and unconscious processes: The effects of motivation. *Consciousness and Cognition, 8*(1), 94–113.

Wegner, D. M. (2002). *The illusion of conscious will.* Cambridge, MA: MIT Press.

Wegner, D. M., Fuller, V. A., & Sparrow, B. (2003). Clever hands: Uncontrolled intelligence in facilitated communication. *Journal of Personality and Social Psychology, 85*(1), 5–19.

Weilke, F., Spiegel, S., Boecker, H., von Einsiedel, H. G., Conrad, B., Schwaiger, M., et al. (2001). Time-resolved fMRI of activation patterns in M1 and SMA during complex voluntary movement. *Journal of Neurophysiology, 85*(5), 1858–1863.

Weiskrantz, L. (1986). *Blindsight: A Case Study and Implications* (p. 187). Oxford: Oxford University Press.

Weiskrantz, L. (1997). *Consciousness Lost, Found: A Neuropsychological Exploration* (1st ed., p. 304). New York: Oxford University Press.

Weiskrantz, L., Barbur, J. L., & Sahraie, A. (1995). Parameters affecting conscious versus unconscious visual discrimination with damage to the visual cortex (V1). *Proceedings of the National Academy of Sciences of the United States of America, 92*(13), 6122–6126.

# CHAPTER 11

## Neuroscience, Free Will, and Responsibility

*Deborah Talmi and Chris D. Frith*

Materialists believe that everything, including the human psyche, is made of matter. Reductionists believe that the behavior of complex, large-scale systems such as the mind and the brain can be fully explained in terms of the simpler units of which they are composed such as neurons, molecules, and atoms. (Hard) determinists believe that, given a complete knowledge of the past state of the universe (i.e., the location and velocity of all the particles in it) then, by using the laws of physics and other sciences, it is, in principle, possible to predict the future state of the universe. Given these beliefs, all the choices we make are predetermined by our past history, and so the human experience of free will must be an illusion.

This is a very difficult conclusion to accept. First, it is strongly contradicted by our subjective experience. For example, we frequently have the vivid experience of a strong urge to perform some action which we are successfully able to suppress. This feels like the exertion of free will. Second, as we shall discuss below, the denial of this experience has worrying implications for the idea of individual responsibility, which is so closely linked to the idea of free will.

The problem of free will has a very long history, but has recently emerged in an acute form for cognitive neuroscience. This discipline is directly concerned with the relationship between the mind and the brain. Most neuroscientists accept the doctrine of materialism, believing that our mental life emerges from the physical activity of the brain without the need of any additional purely mental processes. There is less agreement concerning reductionism. There are cogent arguments suggesting that complex physical systems may exhibit behavior that *cannot* be understood solely on the basis of the laws governing their microscopic constituents (e.g., Gu, Weedbrook, Perales, & Nielsen, 2008). However, many neuroscientists would accept a softer form of reductionism, believing that mental activity can be understood in terms of neural activity, if not in terms of atoms or molecules. Given this attitude, determinism can be framed as an empirical question: Is it possible to predict peoples' actions on the basis of neural activity that precedes their conscious decisions? If so, then free will is an illusion.

In the current zeitgeist, such work is having a considerable impact on public discussions concerning human nature and responsibility. In legal cases jurors now expect forensic scientists to be able to show definitively who committed the crime from DNA, fingerprinting, and detailed crime scene investigations. This is known as the CSI effect from the popular TV series of the same name (Schweitzer & Saks, 2007). In the same vein there is increasing expectation that brain scientists, aided by the brightly colored brain images loved by the media, can reveal whether or not the accused was responsible for his actions. A more extreme version of this approach (e.g., Singer, 2007) would hold that no one is responsible for their action since all is predetermined by the brain. This view has major implications for legal systems (e.g., Kawohl & Habermeyer, 2008) since, in nearly all such systems, guilt depends upon intentions rather than actions and a major distinction is made between intended and unintended actions. However, the view may also have a larger impact on society. As we shall see, the belief that we are all responsible for our actions seems to be critical for cooperative and moral behavior.

In this introduction we have demonstrated the relevance of neuroscience to the free will debate. We shall now consider in more detail the psychological process that we call free will. Finally, we will consider why claims about the illusory nature of free will might have a dangerous impact on moral behavior.

## 1. LIBET'S SUBVERSION OF FREE WILL

The experiment carried out by Libet and colleagues (Libet, Gleason, Wright, & Pearl, 1983) was probably the first to address the question: Can the decision to act be predicted by preceding brain activity? The answer was, yes, and the result has been widely interpreted as showing that our experience of free will may be an illusion. In that experiment participants were asked to move a finger when they "had the urge to do so," note the position of a clock's hand "when they first felt this urge to move," and report this position some time later. The critical finding was that the brain activity, as measured by EEG, began preparing for the action about 1 second before the movement, long before participants felt the urge to move their finger, which they reported to be, on average, ~200 ms before the movement (see detailed review in Haggard, 2008). An action, that was consciously felt to be freely willed, was in fact predetermined. More recently Haynes and his colleagues (Soon, Brass, Heinze, & Haynes, 2008), using fMRI, have reported that patterns of brain activity can be used to predict a decision (left or right finger movement) up to 10 seconds before subjects are aware of making their "free choice." So, does this evidence from neuroscience show that our decisions are predetermined and our experience of free will is an illusion?

One way to characterize the result of Libet's experiment is that it reveals a discrepancy between the subjective experience of a decision and the "true" cause of that decision. This is not just an isolated instance where experimental participants report a subjective experience of a decision that the experimenter knows to be discrepant with reality. There is ample evidence to show that verbal reports derived from introspection often have little relation to the cognitive processes that caused the experience (Nisbett & Wilson, 1977). When asked for the reasons for their decisions, participants often resort to post-hoc rationalization on the basis of their own theory of decision-making. In the "mere exposure effect" (Bornstein, 1989), for example, participants believe they are choosing between stimuli on the basis of preference, but this preference is determined by familiarity with the stimuli. More recently Johansson, Hall, Sikström, and Olsson (2005) asked participants to select the more attractive of two faces and then justify their decision. On 20% of these trials a double-card ploy was used to switch pictures so that the picture the subjects were asked to justify was not the one they had just chosen. On ~75% of trials this switch was not detected, so that participants were giving justifications for choices that they had not actually made.

Libet's results have been interpreted as a distilled example for people's illusion that they are taking a freely chosen action, when in fact their action has been predetermined. The predetermination in the Libet experiment originated from participants' own brains, while in other studies, it was a result of experimental manipulations.

However, if we are to understand the implications of the Libet experiment, a conceptual analysis of the task is required. We take up this challenge next.

## 2. THE PSYCHOLOGY OF FREE WILL

Our conceptual perspective on two contrasting cognitive processes has previously been applied in many fields of psychology: attention (controlled vs. automatic, Shiffrin & Schneider, 1977), judgment (system 1 vs. system 2, Kahneman & Frederick, 2002), control of action (willed vs. automatic, Norman & Shallice, 1986), and social psychology (Chaiken & Trope, 1999;

and most recently, controlled vs. automatic, Lieberman, 2007). Here we shall use the terms "type 1" and "type 2" for these two types of process. Different fields have their own unique conceptualization of these two processes, as has been recently reviewed in detail (Evans, 2008; Sloman, 1996. However, most portray type 1 processes as fast, automatic, and unconscious. These processes are believed to occur in dedicated, domain-specific modules. The limited domain of these computations and their mandatory nature allow their computation to be carried out quickly. Fodor (1983) proposed modules for perception, in the posterior neocortex; others suggested that memory encoding and retrieval may also be modular (Moscovitch, 1992). The essential feature of type 1 processes is that they are informationally encapsulated, so that their inner workings are "cognitively impenetrable" (Pylyshyn, 1999), and only their output is available.

Type 2 processes are domain general control processes that are slow, deliberate, and conscious. Because we can only be conscious of a limited number of items (Cowan, 2000) at any one time, perhaps only one (McElree, 2001; Oberauer, 2002), type 2 processes are slower and serial in nature. In consequence, type 2 processes are less good than type 1 processes at making decisions in which many different factors must be considered simultaneously (Dijksterhuis, Bos, Nordgren, & van Baaren, 2006) or when actions need to be carried out in a precisely timed manner. However, type 2 processes can, to some extent, override and control the effects of type 1 processes. Norman & Shallice (1986) defined "will" as the "direction of action by deliberate conscious control" (p. 15), the quantity of which amounts to the degree of schema inhibition or activation required for goal attainment.

Type 1 processes allow experience to change the way modules process incoming information. Posterior neocortical modules store unimodal memories of items and association between items. This means that having seen a line drawing once, it is easier to recognize a scrambled version of it the second time around (Warrington & Weiskrantz, 1970). Similarly, having read the word "news" next to the word "stand," we store an association between these two words and find it easier to process the second word after we read the first word at another occasion. Structures in the medial temporal lobe can bind multimodal information into a single memory trace. One of these structures is the hippocampus, which is able to store attended information. When a cue is presented it may automatically trigger the memory trace and result in the recollection of the entire event, and may change perception and behavior in sometimes nonconscious ways (Moscovitch, 2008). Subcortical structures such as the amygdala and the striatum can store the association between aversive or appetitive reinforcers and a preceding neutral cue (Cardinal, Parkinson, Hall, & Everitt, 2002), so that the neutral cue acquires a valence and can later bias instrumental responding (Balleine & Dickinson, 1998). The basal ganglia store procedural and motor skills (Knowlton, Mangels, & Squire, 1996).

To use another conceptual framework for these ideas, type 1 processing changes the brain's priors, and influences the way it will process new information. Without priors, it is difficult to make sense of incoming information: for instance, without relevant contextual knowledge, it is difficult to comprehend prose passages (Bransford & Johnson, 1972). Prior experience allows us to make sense of the present and make accurate predictions about the future. This adaptive mechanism also has disadvantages. For example, because of the rarity of targets, airport workers screening baggage develop a "prior" that targets would be absent. This increases the number of missed targets (Wolfe, Horowitz & Kenner, 2005). When the predictions are not accurate, the brain's priors will be changed appropriately, allowing a continual updating of our model of the world.

Experience also changes the degree to which type 2 processes are recruited or are available to carry out particular tasks. First, cognitive processes that initially relied on deliberate and conscious control become habitual and automatic with practice. These include procedural skills (playing the piano), cognitive skills (playing chess, memorizing poems, driving), and higher mental processes such as evaluation, emotion, goal pursuit, and social behavior (reviewed in Bargh & Chartrand, 1999). As a result, type 2 processes that were previously allocated to certain tasks can be utilized in other ways. This means that experts have a large amount of stored information, schemas, and habits they can draw on confidently, while using scarce controlled processes in a more efficient manner. We are all experts in living, and can draw on a variety of encapsulated type 1 processes that have been shaped by lifelong experience. This is what we call "intuition". Second, the availability of type 2 processes is also influenced by experience more directly, as Baumeister has demonstrated in a series of experiments. In these experiments, participants' ability to exert type 2 control over the "decision" reached by type 1 processes was taxed by requiring them to exert control in another task. This requirement made participants more likely to succumb to temptation in the second task. In one experiment (Baumeister, Bratslavsky, Muraven, & Tice, 1998), participants had to sit next to a bowl of tasty cookies and not eat any, while a control group sat next to a bowl of radishes. Subsequently the experimental group spent much less time trying to solve impossible word puzzles relative to the control group. The experimental group complained of more mental fatigue, presumably due to the effort of self-control they had had to exert. Experience changes type 2 processes in two ways, according to Baumeister's "strength" model of will power: he conceives of will as a muscle, which can fatigue, but importantly can also be strengthened with exercise.

Of most relevance to the problem of free will are the processes associated with decision making. Tversky and Kahneman (1974) have described a large number of decision-making heuristics that could correspond to type 1 processes (Kahnmenan & Frederick, 2002). The "affect heuristic" (Slovic, Finucane, Peters, & MacGregor, 2002) is applied to situations where participants need to decide between two options. The affect tags associated with one of the options, namely, encapsulated, type 1 modular computations acquired through previous experience with this option, are summarized as a single "goodness" or "badness" judgment, and bias choice. For example, a woman who had her honeymoon in a rose-colored villa might, years later, select rose-colored rather than lilac linen because rose activates the honeymoon associations, making her feel happier, even if she doesn't consciously think about these positive memories when shopping for linen. The field of moral decision talks of "emotional" reasoning, a type 1 process depending on "gut feelings" that are thought of as a combination of hard-wired and experience-based stimulus driven reactions, e.g., aversion to hurting a conspecific.

To counter such heuristics and intuitions, people can decide to follow formal rules of reasoning, a typical type 2 process. This happens when we actively attend to the situation, in which case type 1 and type 2 will be processing the incoming information simultaneously, evident in implicit learning paradigms (Foerde, Knowlton, & Poldrack, 2006). When we are not attending the situation type 1 processes occur quickly and are obligatory, but type 2 processes may not be deployed (Norman & Shallice, 1986), unless type 1 processes activate relevant stored representations, which may act as an interrupt signal and engage type 2 processes (Damasio, 1996; Norman & Shallice, 1986). Type 2 processes can then modulate type 1 processes (Shallice & Burgess, 1996), e.g., to allow people to draw on prior experience in a deliberately controlled fashion, instead of a stimulus-driven one (Burgess, Gilbert, & Dumontheil, 2007).

On the basis of these ideas we propose a distinction between the "philosophical" concept of free will and free will as a psychological concept. According to our conceptual framework, people claim to have free will for at least two reasons. First, we judge that we would be able to exert type-2 control over type-1 dependent urges if we choose to do so. This feeling arises whenever we have consciously considered various possible options before making a decision. This judgment is often accurate: for example, dieters often are able to avoid eating fatty foods even when they have a strong urge to eat them. However, like any judgment, the judgment here could also be mistaken. For example, smokers often assume they would be able to quit if they only choose, but fail when they actually try.

The second reason people claim to have free will is because our sense of self is based on the stored information and predictions in our brain, so that our subjective intuitions and urges, which are type 1 processes, reflect what really matters to us as unique human beings. In that sense, the feeling we have about an option, or an urge to act in a particular way, reflects our individual history; when, upon introspection, we decide to act as our urges have indicated, the decision seems *right* for us. This, to us, may be the difference between the experiential feeling of freely willed action that accompanies behavior in response to type 1 processes, and the feeling a behavior occurred "by itself" in response to external stimulation (Penfield, 1958, see discussion in Bargh & Ferguson, 2000). In this sense, people feel free to act in a manner that seems right to them, even though they cannot, at will, feel differently than they do. It is hard work to change the way we feel about ourselves, requiring help from techniques such as cognitive behavior therapy.

Psychological free will has little to do with the philosophical dilemma of free will. The strong feeling that we have free will does not prove that we have it (Langer, 1975). Critically, type 1 and type 2 processes are both caused—by our genetic endowment, our previous history, and our current circumstances (Bargh & Ferguson, 2000).

So far our considerations concern the subjective, first-person experience of free will. The situation looks rather different from the third-person perspective. When we look for evidence of free will in the behavior of others we put much more weight on determinism. We think that other people demonstrate free will if we cannot predict their actions from what we know about their current circumstances and their previous history. This approach leads to many problems. For example, random behavior is not predictable, but is neither rational nor is it typically advantageous (except when playing games, such as rock-paper-scissors, van den Nouweland, 2007). It also does not seem right that doing the right (predictable) thing given the circumstances should be perceived from the third-person perspective as an example of a lack of free will, while doing the wrong thing is an example of free will. Likewise, actions that strongly suppress urges, such as dying for one's beliefs, can be seen as extreme examples of free will if we share the belief in question, while the same action can be explained away as brain washing, if we do not share the belief. Unfortunately, as we shall see below, it is this idea of free will as being unpredictable that has a major role in the design of experiments on free will.

## 3. THE LIBET EXPERIMENT UNPACKED

The Libet experiment explicitly engages type 2 processes because participants are asked to continuously and consciously monitor their decisions to act in order to report the time at which the decisions occur. At the same time type 1 processes will be generating a continuously fluctuating level of endogenous urge to lift the finger, which will also be monitored. Participants, therefore, have to use type 2 processes to come up with a strategy for when to allow these endogenous automatic urges to be translated into action. Furthermore, the participants are faced with a complex social situation. The experimental instructions state that the participants should move their finger whenever they have the urge to do so. But, given the social situation, these instructions are more complex than they first appear. Having agreed to take part in the experiment the participant will strive to please the experimenter by reading his or her implicit expectations. First, the instructions convey a strong implicit message that the participant *should* have an urge to move their finger during the course of the experiment, and that they should have more than one such urge. Second, the instructions convey the message that there is a particular temporal pattern of finger movement that is "correct." The participants were instructed to "let the urge happen on its own at any time" implying that movements at some particular time would not be right. We have previously argued (Roepstorff & Frith, 2004) that the instructions can be unpacked to mean that participants should perform "*as if* they had free will." To do this appropriately, participants should use their folk theories on free will.

In this particular case, it is clear that the temporal pattern of finger movement should be unpredictable to the experimenter. In terms of the pattern of brain activity, the similarity between experiments in which subjects are asked to choose responses freely and those where they are explicitly asked to choose randomly is striking (Jahanshahi, Dirnberger, Fuller, & Frith, 2000). In both cases the same type 2 processes are involved. As we have argued, type 2 control of action in willed action experiments ultimately comes from the experimenter, or more exactly, from the interaction between participant and experimenter. Control does not solely reside with the participant (Roepstorff & Frith, 2004). In this sense the will of the participant is not completely free.

The physiological finding in Libet's study could now be interpreted in line with the conceptual analysis above. Nonspecific type 1 processes, such as environmental and internal variations in arousal, could supply particular "urges" to move the finger. To please the experimenter, participants would be responsive to these type 1 processes, but only when they conform to the temporal pattern type 2 processes have designated as appropriate. It is likely that type 1 processes would develop to a full urge to move only when they are appropriate within the framework type 2 processes provide. When such an urge develops, type 2 processes would carry out a final check to ensure movement is appropriate (Haggard, 2008). The two-process framework explains that type 1 processes are earlier than type 2 processes, so that conscious awareness and check of type 1 "decisions" is relatively delayed. This results in a pattern of early brain signal and late reported awareness.

The social situation that we analyzed above does not influence participants' subjective experience that they are acting freely. Participants would feel that their action is freely willed because of the two reasons we proposed above: type 1 processes that generate the local urge to move the finger feel personal and integral; more importantly, participants feel that they are able to control these urges, if they so wish, because they are constantly monitoring and deciding whether or not to follow them. This is not just an illusion, as the Brass & Haggard (2007) experiment shows. Free will here is a strong intuition that obeys its own psychological rules, which has little to do with the philosophical sense of "free will" as physical nondetermination.

## 4. WHY DO CLAIMS ABOUT FREE WILL SEEM SO DANGEROUS FOR MORAL BEHAVIOR?

We suggested in the introduction that the expectation is growing that science may be able to provide evidence in court to determine whether or not someone was responsible for their actions. It is only a small step from this to the idea that neuroscience can show that free will in general is an illusion. This potential raises two important questions. In this section, we tackle the question of whether it would be dangerous for people to believe that there is no free will. In the next section we ask if neuroscientists should worry about this line of research.

Recent research on cooperation within groups has revealed the importance of altruistic punishment (Fehr & Gächter, 2002). In a trust game the group benefits through individuals putting money into the system. However, free riders (or defectors) will appear in such groups. These players benefit from the investments of others while making no investments themselves. The appearance of such behavior reduces cooperation: fewer and fewer individuals continue to invest. Cooperation can be reinstated in such groups by instituting punishment. Players can punish free riders by taking money away from them. This is known as altruistic punishment because the punisher has to pay to apply punishment. When altruistic punishment is introduced, free riding is reduced and cooperation within the group is increased. As a result, the group as a whole benefits.

What has this to do with free will? Free will is relevant because punishment for defection and reward for cooperation is only applied to players who are perceived as making free and deliberate choices. Singer et al. (2006) told subjects in a trust game that some of the players were making their responses on the basis of a sheet of instructions generated by a computer, while others were making free choices. Rewards and punishments were only applied to the players who made deliberate and free choices. Furthermore, patterns of brain activity elicited in the subjects by the players' faces showed that the subjects only developed emotional responses to the players who made free choices. These results demonstrate the importance of our beliefs that people are responsible for their actions for the maintenance of social cooperation.

In terms of our two-process account, we explain these observations as follows. While performing the task subjects will experience the type 1 urge to defect to get a short-term gain. When others defect, subjects will also experience type 1 anger, and the urge to punish the defector. They will also experience their ability to suppress both of these urges and choose either prosocial or economically rational behaviors instead. Punishment, therefore, may arise for two reasons: because of type 2 assumption that the free riders in the group have failed to suppress these selfish urges and that punishment will increase the likelihood that they will suppress these urges in the future, and because of a type 1 urge to punish unfairness. Players who simply respond to instructions do not have the option to suppress their urges and do not cause anger, an emotion thought to be dependent on the attribution of responsibility (Lazarus, 1991).

A direct demonstration of a role for beliefs about free will in causing prosocial behavior is provided by a recent experiment by Vohs & Schooler (2008). In this study one group of subjects were given a passage to read stating that most rational people, including most scientists, now recognize that free will is an illusion. A second group read a control passage about consciousness. Subsequently both groups performed an arithmetic test in which it was rather easy to cheat. People in the group who had previously read the passage claiming that free will was an illusion were significantly more likely to cheat.

It will be important to explore further why subjects with a reduced belief in free will were more willing to give in to the urge to cheat. Our suggestion is as follows. Fairness is a behavior that is initially dependent on type 2 control—e.g., in response to parental instruction. Eventually, repeated adherence to the cognitive norm of fairness, and repeated fair play, render fairness habitual and automatic: we become "not the kind of person who cheats." In a situation where cheating (apparently) cannot be detected it is not fear of punishment or ridicule that deters us. In that situation we may experience both the urge to cheat, and the urge to play fairly. It is a situation that allows us to suppress one of our urges and therefore an occasion where we would feel strongly that we act freely. Which urge we act upon will depend on type 2 processes and how strong each one of the type 1 urges are. However, if we have been told that free will is an illusion, we conclude that type 2 control is not possible and give in to the strongest urge.

## 5. SHOULD NEUROSCIENTISTS WORRY?

We have sketched some preliminary evidence that beliefs about free will have an effect on social and moral behavior. If these results are replicated and extended, one implication seems to be that a definitive demonstration that free will is an illusion could have undesirable effects on human behavior. For now, it is perhaps comforting to acknowledge that we still lack a generally accepted empirical demonstration that free will is an illusion. We have also suggested that the intuition people have about having free will does not in fact correspond to the philosophical dilemma of predetermination, so that even if the "philosophical" free will is shown to be an illusion, the "psychological" free will may not be harmed.

The psychological feeling of free will does, however, rely on people's ability to introspect upon their urges and to have the strong feeling that they can often control these urges. However, psychology, as well as neuroscience, is increasingly revealing the importance of type 1 processes in many kinds of choice behavior, including financial and moral decisions. For example, when confronted with moral dilemmas, subjects will choose the emotional option rather than the more "rational" option that maximizes utility (Greene, Sommerville, Nystrom, Darley, & Cohen, 2001). The danger is that people might relinquish control attempts, using findings from science to justify immoral behavior. The danger is exacerbated with the zeitgeist that emphasizes "listening to your emotions" over analytical contemplation, and cultural relativity over value judgments. In our times personal responsibility and accountability are becoming less fashionable, and "fashionable," in fact, is becoming an important value judgment: what's not "cool" seems also "wrong." The irony here is that type 2 processes are being used to justify abandonment of control by type 2 processes.

Results like this are often presented as unfortunate examples of primitive type 1 processes winning over the more evolved type 2 processes associated with free will. However, it is simplistic to believe that giving in to type 1 processes is always undesirable. In the case of the ultimatum game, the emotional rejection of an unfair offer is a form of altruistic punishment, which could well be the result of a type 1 process and, as we have seen, benefits the group in the context of repeated exchanges. Likewise, the deliberations associated with type 2 processes do not necessarily lead to better behavior. Valdesolo & DeSteno (2008) have shown that moral hypocrisy does not result from giving in to type 1 urges, but is rather the result of type 2 deliberations used to justify bad behavior. Clearly, both type 1 and type 2 processes are morally neutral. Morality is a product of the relationship culture and the brain, not a property of the isolated brain.

To respond to the potential impact of scientific findings on the social moral climate neuroscience could emphasize that our brain frequently engages in balancing the demands of controlled and uncontrolled processes. Neuroscientists could aim to convey a stronger message that people can change both type 1 and type 2 processes to improve well-being. For example, sensitization techniques can help change emotions such as fear; the 'social and emotional aspects of learning (SEAL) program teaches young people to control their emotional urges; and mindfulness training can change the way people respond to these urges even if they let them unfold naturally. It is also important to emphasize that it is a mistake to think that problems in morality can be solved by restricting one's responses just to the outputs of type 1 or just to the outputs of type 2 processes.

Whether or not we have free will, our ability to think about the decisions we are making is a key aspect of human nature. Morality emerges from this ability to deliberate about the different courses of action we might take and to discuss these options with other people. It is the experience of free will that generates the discussions about free will that are such an important legacy of Libet's experiment.

## ACKNOWLEDGMENTS

Deborah Talmi is supported by the Wellcome Trust. CDF is supported by the Danish National Research Foundation and the AHRC CNCC scheme AH/E511112/1.

## REFERENCES

Balleine, B. W., & Dickinson, A. (1998) Goal-directed instrumental action: Contingency and incentive learning and their cortical substrates. *Neuropharmacology, 37*(4–5), 407–419.

Bargh, J. A., & Chartrand, T. L. (1999). The unbearable automaticity of being. *American Psychologist, 54*, 462–479.

Bargh, J., & Ferguson, M. (2000). Beyond behaviourism: On the automaticity of higher mental processes. *Philosophical Bulletin, 126*(6), 925–945.

Baumeister, R. F., Bratslavsky, E., Muraven, M., & Tice, D. M. (1998) Ego depletion: Is the active self a limited resource? *Journal of Personality and Social Psychology, 74*(5), 1252–1265.

Bornstein, R. F. (1989) Exposure and affect: Overview and meta-analysis of research, 1968–1987. *Psychological Bulletin, 106*, 265–289.

Bransford, J. D., & Johnson, M. K. (1972) Contextual prerequisites for understanding: Some investigators of comprehension and recall. *Journal of Verbal Learning and Verbal Behavior, 11*, 717–726.

Brass, M., & Haggard, P. (2007) To do or not to do: The neural signature of self-control. *Journal of Neuroscience, 27*(34), 9141–9145.

Burgess, P. W., Gilbert, S. J., & Dumontheil, I. (2007). Function and localization within rostral prefrontal cortex (area 10). *Philosophical*

*Transactions of the Royal Society of London B, 362,* 887–899.

Cardinal, R. N., Parkinson, J. A., Hall, J., & Everitt, B. J. (2002). Emotion and motivation: The role of the amygdala, ventral striatum, and prefrontal cortex. *Neuroscience and Biobehavioral Reviews, 26*(3), 321–352.

Chaiken, S., & Trope, Y. (Eds.). (1999). *Dual-process theories in social psychology.* New York: Guilford.

Cowan, N. (2000). The magical number 4 in short-term memory: A reconsideration of mental storage capacity. *Behavioral and Brain Sciences, 24,* 87–185.

Damasio, A. R. (1996). The somatic marker hypothesis and the possible functions of the prefrontal cortex. *Philosophical Transactions of the Royal Society, 351*(1346), 1413–1420.

Dijksterhuis, A., Bos, M. W., Nordgren, L. F., & van Baaren, R. B. (2006). On making the right choice: The deliberation-without-attention effect. *Science, 311*(5763), 1005–1007.

Evans, J. S. B. T. (2008). Dual-processing accounts of reasoning, judgment, and social cognition. *Annual Review of Psychology, 59,* 255–278.

Fehr, E., & Gächter, S. (2002). Altruistic punishment in humans. *Nature, 415*(6868), 137–140.

Foerde, K., Knowlton, B. J., & Poldrack, R. A. (2006). Modulation of competing memory systems by distraction. *Proceedings of the National Academy of Sciences, 103,* 11778–11783.

Fodor, J. A. (1983). *Modularity of mind: An essay on faculty psychology.* Cambridge, MA: MIT Press.

Greene, J. D., Sommerville, R. B., Nystrom, L. E., Darley, J. M., & Cohen, J. D. (2001). An fMRI investigation of emotional engagement in moral judgment. *Science, 293*(5537), 2105–2108.

Gu, M., Weedbrook, C., Perales, A., & Nielsen, M. A. (2009). More really is different. *Physica D-Nonlinear Phenomena, 238*(9–10), 835–839.

Haggard, P. (2008). Human volition: Towards a neuroscience of will. *Nature Reviews Neuroscience, 9*(12), 934–946.

Jahanshahi, M., Dirnberger, G., Fuller, R., & Frith, C. D. (2000). The role of the dorsolateral prefrontal cortex in random number generation. *Neuroimage, 12*(6), 713–725.

Johansson, P., Hall, L., Sikström, S., & Olsson, A. (2005). Failure to detect mismatches between intention and outcome in a simple decision task. *Science, 310*(5745), 116–119.

Kahneman, D., & Frederick, S. (2002). "Representativeness Revisited: Attribute Substitution in Intuitive Judgment" in Thomas Gilovich, Dale Griffin, Daniel Kahneman. *Heuristics and Biases: The Psychology of Intuitive Judgment.* Cambridge: Cambridge University Press.

Kawohl, W., & Habermeyer, E. (2008). Free will: Reconciling German civil law with Libet's neurophysiological studies on the readiness potential. *Behavioral Sciences & the Law, 25*(2), 309–320.

Knowlton, B. J., Mangels, J. A., & Squire, L. R. (1996). A neostriatal habit learning system in humans. *Science, 273*(5280), 1353–1354.

Langer, E. J. (1975). The illusion of control. *Journal of Personality and Social Psychology,* 32(2), 311–328.

Lazarus, R. S. (1991). Progress on a cognitive motivational relational theory of emotion. *American Psychologist, 46*(8), 819–834.

Libet, B., Gleason, C. A., Wright, E. W., & Pearl, D. K. (1983). Time of conscious intention to act in relation to onset of cerebral activity (readiness-potential): The unconscious initiation of a freely voluntary act. *Brain, 106,* 623–642.

Lieberman, M. D. (2007). Social cognitive neuroscience: A review of core processes. *Annual Review of Psychology, 58,* 259–289.

McElree, B. (2001). Working memory and focal attention. *Journal of Experimental Psychology: Learning, Memory, and Cognition,* 27(3), 817–835.

Moscovitch, M. (1992). Memory and working-with-memory – a component process model based on modules and central systems. *Journal of Cognitive Neuroscience, 4*(3), 257–267.

Moscovitch, M. (2008). The hippocampus as a "Stupid," domain-specific module: Implications for theories of recent and remote memory, and of imagination. *Canadian Journal of Experimental Psychology-Revue Canadienne De Psychologie Experimentale, 62*(1), 62–79.

Nisbett, R. E., & Wilson, T. D. (1977). Telling more than we can know: Verbal reports on mental processes. *Psychological Review, 84,* 231–259.

Norman D. A, & Shallice, T. (1986). Attention to action: Willed and automatic control of behavior. In R. J. Davidson, G. E. Schwartz, & D. Shapiro (Eds.), *Consciousness and self regulation: Advances in research* (vol. 4, pp. 1–18). New York: Plenum Press.

Oberauer, K. (2002). Access to information in working memory: Exploring the focus of attention. *Journal of Experimental Psychology: Learning, Memory, and Cognition, 28,* 411–421.

Penfield, W. (1958). The excitable cortex in conscious man. Liverpool, England: Liverpool University Press.

Pylyshyn, Z. (1999). Is vision continuous with cognition? The case for cognitive impenetrability of visual perception. *Behavioral and Brain Sciences, 22,* 341–365.

Roepstorff, A., & Frith, C. (2004). What's at the top in the top-down control of action? Script-sharing and 'top-top' control of action in cognitive experiments. *Psychological Research, 68*(2–3), 189–198.

Schweitzer, N. J., & Saks, M. J. (2007). The CSI effect: Popular fiction about forensic science affects public expectations about real forensic science. *Jurimetrics, 47*(3), 357–364.

Shallice, T., & Burgess, P. (1996). The domain of supervisory processes and temporal organization of behaviour. *Philosophical Transactions of the Royal Society, 351*(1346).

Shiffrin, R. M, & Schneider, W. (1977). Controlled and automatic human information-processing: 2, Perceptual learning, automatic attending, and a general theory. *Psychological Review, 84*(2), 127–190.

Singer, T., Seymour, B., O'Doherty, J. P., Stephan, K. E., Dolan, R. J., & Frith, C. D. (2006). Empathic neural responses are modulated by the perceived fairness of others. *Nature, 439*(7075), 466–469.

Singer, W. (2007) Zum Problem der Willensfreiheit. In K. P. Liessmann (Eds.), *Die Freiheit des Denkens* (pp. 111–143). Philosophicum Lech 10. Vienna: Paul Zsolnay Verlag.

Sloman, S. A. (1996). The empirical case for two systems of reasoning. *Psychological Bulletin, 119*(1), 3–22.

Slovic, P., Finucane, M., Peters, E., & MacGregor, D. G (2002). The affect heuristic. In T. Gilovich, D. Griffin, & D. Kahneman, (Eds.), *Intuitive judgment: Heuristics and biases.* Cambridge, UK: Cambridge University Press.

Soon, C. S., Brass, M , Heinze, H. J., & Haynes, J. D. (2008). Unconscious determinants of free decisions in the human brain. *Nature Neuroscience, 11*(5), 543–545.

Tversky, A., & Kahneman, D. (1974). Judgment under uncertainty: Heuristics and biases. *Science, 185,* 1124–1131.

Valdesolo, P., & DeSteno, D. (2008). The duality of virtue: Deconstructing the moral hypocrite. *Journal of Experimental Social Psychology, 44*(5), 1334–1338.

van den Nouweland, A. (2007). Rock-paper-scissors: A new and elegant proof. *Economics Bulletin, 3*(43). 1–6.

Vohs, K. D., & Schooler, J. W. (2008). The value of believing in free will: encouraging a belief in determinism increases cheating. *Psychological Science, 19*(1). 49–54.

Warrington, E. K., & Weiskrantz, L. (1970). Amnesic syndrome: Consolidation or retrieval? *Nature, 228,* 628–630.

Wolfe, J. M., Horowitz, T. S., & Kenner, N. M (2005). Cognitive psychology: Rare items often missed in visual searches. *Nature, 435,* 439–440.

# CHAPTER 12

## Bending Time to One's Will

*Jeffrey P. Ebert and Daniel M. Wegner*

During the course of a day, a person might perform hundreds of actions and observe countless events. Even before sitting down for breakfast, it is possible to scramble eggs, put bread in the toaster, pour cream into coffee, and whistle a duet with the friendly bird outside. While performing these and other actions, one's senses are bombarded with information about surrounding events: eggs curdling, cream swirling in coffee, a squirrel leaping past the bird, ruffling its feathers and song, the local news reporting on a house fire, and . . . is that the smell of burning toast? Despite all these channels on the mind's TV, one usually has little difficulty keeping track of the events for which one is, and is not, responsible. How does the mind pull off this nifty feat? What factors does it consider when determining authorship for events, and what does this experience of authorship *feel* like?

Time is an important factor in determining authorship. If one comes across an empty soda can in the road and gives it a good kick, the typical empty soda can response is to take off without hesitation, skid for a bit, and arrive at a new resting place somewhere down the road, a little worse for the journey. Under these circumstances, one would experience an unmistakable sense of authorship for the can's movement, and perhaps a touch of pride ("*I* did that"). But what if, upon receiving the kick, the can just stood there for a minute (wondering, maybe, how it got into this situation), and only after this delay did it make the trip down the road? It is a safe bet that one's experience of authorship would be diminished, along with any pride.

For physical events, causes are usually followed soon after by their effects (Michotte, 1963), and so the mind expects one's actions to be followed promptly by the events they cause. Any gap between action and event therefore lessens the feeling of having caused the event—making temporal proximity one of the most important indicators of authorship. But this is only half the story. Just as perceiving a brief delay between action and event can lead to a determination of authorship, a determination of authorship can lead to perceiving a brief delay between action and event (Haggard, Clark, & Kalogeras, 2002). Consider, again, the person who approaches a soda can and gives it a kick. Ordinarily, a split-second later the can would fly forward through the air, and personal authorship for the can's movement would be inferred. Now, imagine instead that a split-second after the kick, the streetlight turned on. Delusional individuals aside, most people would dismiss this as coincidence and not infer authorship. We proposed that, with authorship more plausible for the can's movement than for the light's turning on, the delay between kicking and the can's moving would *feel* briefer than the delay between kicking and the light's turning on. The logic is thus: The mind knows that causes are temporally bound to their effects, and so when authorship is inferred, the perception of time is warped to match this inference, such that one's action and inferred effect are perceived to be especially close in time.

This dual proposal that perceived temporal proximity of actions and events is both a key indicator of authorship and a significant part of its phenomenology ultimately rests on the work of Benjamin Libet, whose discoveries challenged two long-held, commonsense views: first, that conscious will causes actions; and second, that the conscious experience of time is objective, with events perceived as they happen and without filter. Building on the research of Libet and others, we first show that conscious will, and authorship more generally, is less a cause of events than an *experience* one has when the mind determines an event should be ascribed to the self—and that time plays a key role in such determinations. We then show that this experience of authorship involves a subjective bending of time, such that actions and events are perceived to be temporally closer to each other when authorship is inferred.

## CONSCIOUS WILL AND THE INFERENCE OF AUTHORSHIP

In an experiment by Libet, Gleason, Wright, and Pearl (1983), participants were asked to voluntarily choose when to move their finger, and then report the position of a dot on a clock face when they first were aware of intending to move. On each trial, scalp recordings monitored cerebral activity for a readiness potential (RP) known to precede voluntary actions. This RP was found to precede finger movements by at least 550 ms—a finding that by itself is not surprising, as brain activity of *some* kind had to cause the fingers to move. However, it was also found that participants' conscious intentions preceded the finger movements by a mere 200 ms or less—placing conscious intentions several hundred ms *after* the start of the RP. In other words, brain activity involved with preparing the act began hundreds of ms before any hint of willing the act appeared in the person's conscious experience. As Libet et al. (1983) wrote, "the brain evidently 'decides' to initiate or, at the least, prepare to initiate the act at a time before there is any reportable subjective awareness that such a decision has taken place" (p. 640).

For those believing that conscious will causes action, this was bad news. Conscious will, supposed to be the initiator of voluntary behavior, the Prime Mover of the mind, was found to *trail*—and by quite a substantial margin—brain activity known to trigger voluntary behavior. A straightforward interpretation of these results is that unconscious processes drive behavior, with conscious thought merely coming along for the ride. This view is the starting point for the theory of apparent mental causation.

### Apparent Mental Causation

Wegner and Wheatley (1999) and Wegner (2002) offered a theory of apparent mental causation—beginning with the idea that conscious will is an experience, akin to sensing the color red or feeling joy on a spring day. This experience arises from interpreting one's thought as the cause of an action, independent of whether or not such a causal link actually exists. The notion that conscious will is independent of causal forces was suggested by the existence of motor automatisms, such as Ouija-board spelling, and certain neuropsychological disorders, such as alien hand syndrome, in which seemingly voluntary actions feel unwilled and unintended. Because the experience of conscious will appears separable from the processes that cause action, how the mind creates this experience requires its own explanation.

Drawing on Michotte's (1963) research on how people perceive causality for physical events, Wegner and Wheatley (1999) hypothesized that conscious will should be strongest when one's thought: a) is consistent with an action (consistency); b) occurs before the action (priority); and c) is not accompanied by other potential causes of the action (exclusivity). So, if one thinks about kicking a soda can right before doing so, and no one else is around to tug on one's leg, the act of kicking should feel strongly willed. Several experiments have examined how consistency, priority, and exclusivity affect the experience of will; let us consider some evidence for each.

#### Consistency

An experiment by Wegner and Wheatley (1999) found that participants who were primed with a thought (e.g., the word "swan" spoken over headphones) that was consistent with a subsequent action (e.g., stopping a computer mouse such that the cursor landed on a swan) felt as though they had willed the action—even though the action had been caused by someone else (a confederate of the experimenter) (see also Aarts, Custers, & Wegner, 2005; Pronin, Wegner, McCarthy, & Rodriguez, 2006; Wegner, Sparrow, & Winerman, 2004).

### Priority

In this same experiment, the timing of the consistent prime in relation to the action was found to matter for the experience of will. When the prime occurred 5 s or 1 s before the action, participants reported that they had willed the action; in contrast, when the prime occurred 30 s before or 1 s after the action, participants reported that the action felt unwilled. For a thought to enhance the experience of will, it must therefore occur immediately prior to the action (see also Wegner et al., 2004).

### Exclusivity

An experiment by Wegner, Fuller, and Sparrow (2003) found that participants who pressed keys to answer a series of easy yes-no questions attributed much of their correct responding to another person whose hand was placed atop their own. Participants had been instructed to "read the unconscious muscle movements" this person made after each question and to press the keys according to these subtle movements. In actuality, the other person was a confederate who could not hear the questions—meaning that participants attributed their own answers to the influence of someone who could not have possibly helped. So, even though participants were fully responsible for their actions, their experience of will was undermined by the presence of another plausible cause (see also Wegner & Sparrow, 2007).

### Libet Revisited

It is safe to assume that participants in Libet et al.'s (1983) experiment felt their actions to be consciously willed. On each trial, they experienced an action-consistent thought ("I want to move my finger!") just prior (by about 200 ms) to moving their finger, and no alternative causes of this action were readily apparent. This conjunction of thought and action happened over and over again, without exception. Faced with such evidence, participants might reasonably have concluded that their conscious intention to move their finger *caused* the finger to move.

But what is reasonable is not necessarily true. Though the conscious intention that appeared prior to acting may have provided a helpful preview of the action to come (Wegner, 2008), the decision to act was made earlier, by a process outside of conscious awareness.

### Authorship Processing

The theory of apparent mental causation describes how actions and thoughts are linked to the self, and is therefore one part of a more general description of authorship processing, "the set of mental processes that monitors indications of authorship to judge whether an event, action, or thought should be ascribed to self as a causal agent" (Wegner & Sparrow, 2004, p. 1201). To feel as though one has personally authored an external event (e.g., a soda can's traveling down the road), the event must be causally linked to an action one performed (e.g., kicking the can), ideally an action that felt willed (e.g., a kick performed freely and with forethought).

To determine authorship for events, the mind again relies on the trusted indicator's consistency, priority, and exclusivity. So, feelings of authorship for an event should be greatest when the event is consistent with one's immediately prior action and has no other potential causes. One would thus have strong feelings of authorship for a soda can's trip down the road if the can traveled in a direction consistent with one's kick, which was performed just prior to the can's movement, with the kick's exclusivity as a potential cause unchallenged by the presence of, say, a strong wind or that meddling squirrel again.

## BENDING TIME

We have seen how the mind relies on certain indicators, including the briefness of the delay between one's action and an event, to determine authorship. But what if the link between indicators and authorship is bidirectional? What if, upon determining that an event was authored by oneself, certain authorship indicators are accentuated, including the briefness of the delay between action and event? This notion, far-fetched at first glance, gains plausibility when one considers research on: a) the subjective antedating of sensory experience (Libet, 2004; Libet, Wright, Feinstein, & Pearl, 1979); b) the "idealized" perceptions that occur during authorship processing (Preston & Wegner, 2005); and c) a recently discovered phenomenon known as "intentional binding" (Haggard et al., 2002).

### Subjective Antedating of Sensory Experience

Libet et al. (1979) discovered that it can take up to 500 ms of activation in the sensory cortex before one becomes consciously aware of a sensory signal—yet one does not experience this delay. Instead, the subjective experience seems to be "antedated" to around the time when the signal first arrived at the cortex. Libet (2004) gave the example of driving a car down a city street when, suddenly, a boy runs in front of the car. In this situation, it is possible to brake quickly—perhaps in as little as 150 ms—to avoid hitting the boy. But conscious awareness of the boy takes longer—perhaps as much as 500 ms—indicating that any decision to brake must be made entirely unconsciously. But because subjective experience is antedated, the driver consciously perceives the boy first, the brakes being applied second—even though the boy does not reach conscious awareness until *after* the brakes are applied.

These findings imply that the sense of time is both subjective and reconstructive, with the mind reordering events as needed to preserve causal priority and provide a coherent description of the world in conscious awareness—prerequisites for a mental system that temporally binds actions and effects together in consciousness. Moreover, a related finding that the perception of an event may be altered by a subsequent event occurring up to 500 ms later (Libet et al., 1979) suggests the existence of a brief window during which the perceived timing of one's action may be altered by its effect.

### Authorship and Idealized Perceptions

It may be that the experience we have of authoring our actions is part of a mental system that constructs an ideal causal account of action. Preston and Wegner (2005) proposed that humans see themselves as ideal agents for whom thought, will, and action are always aligned with each other and with achieving optimal outcomes. In a given situation, any one of these components may be absent or difficult to detect, but because we idealize our own agency every component is nevertheless perceived to be present. So, when will and action are present, thought is inferred (intention confabulation); when thought and action are present, will is inferred (apparent mental causation); and when thought and will are present, action is inferred (action misperception).

Most relevant for present purposes is action misperception. Preston and Wegner (2003) conducted an experiment in which participants fired foam bullets from a toy gun at a target 10 ft away, and were asked to judge how close they came to hitting the bull's-eye after each shot. Thought was manipulated on different trials by projecting onto the bull's-eye the face of a famous person who was either widely disliked (e.g., Adolf Hitler) or widely liked (e.g., Mahatma Gandhi). Conscious will, which had been found to be greater when a countdown was provided prior to action, was manipulated by having the experimenter either count down to firing ("3–2–1–Go!") or not ("Go!"). Controlling for actual distance from the bull's-eye, participants judged their shots to be more on-target when given a countdown and firing at a disliked face. These results suggest that when a determination of authorship is made, the mind engages in a bit of perceptual trickery, exaggerating authorship indicators in the service of maintaining one's image as an ideal agent. In reality, the bullet might have grazed Hitler's uniform, but to the person pulling the trigger, the bullet found its mark.

Given this penchant for authors to subjectively rewrite history, it wouldn't be surprising to find that individuals also perceive actions and their effects as closer in time when personal authorship is implicated. In the scenario just described, the time between when the trigger is pulled and the bull's-eye is hit should feel briefer if the target is Hitler than if it is Gandhi, all else equal, because the sense of authorship is greater in the first case.

### Intentional Binding

A straightforward way to test for temporal binding of actions to effects is to examine their perceived timing. Haggard et al. (2002) conducted a clever experiment, based on Libet's time judgment paradigm (Libet et al., 1983), in which participants were told to press a key when they felt the urge to do so, and an auditory tone was played shortly after they acted. Participants were asked to judge, in separate blocks, either the time of their keypress or the time of the subsequent tone, by referring to a clock hand.

The main results showed that participants' judgments of when their action occurred were shifted forward in time (toward the tone), while judgments of when the tone occurred were shifted backward in time (toward the action), relative to judgments made in baseline blocks where action and tone occurred alone. Critically, these perceptual shifts did not occur when transcranial magnetic stimulation (TMS) was used to induce the participant to make an involuntary keypress, suggesting that binding happens only for voluntary actions. Calling this phenomenon "intentional binding," Haggard et al. (2002) proposed that the "brain contains a specific cognitive module that binds intentional actions to their effects to construct a coherent conscious experience of our own agency" (p. 385).

Since then, several experiments have supported this view, while suggesting that binding is sensitive to two different kinds of authorship indicators: those that are internal to the individual and involved in controlling actions and predicting their effects (Blakemore, Wolpert, & Frith, 2000; Haggard & Clark, 2003), and those that are external to the individual and retrospective in nature, such as characteristics of the event occurring after one's action (Moore & Haggard, 2008). Demonstrating the importance of internal, predictive indicators, it has been found that binding is weak (Engbert, Wohlschläger, Thomas, & Haggard, 2007) or nonexistent (Engbert, Wohlschläger, & Haggard, 2008) when observing another person's finger pressing a key, or when one's own finger is involuntarily made to press a key by a motor attached to the key (Engbert et al., 2008). Demonstrating the importance of external, retrospective indicators, it has been found that under circumstances in which actions are unreliably followed by tones, an action is perceived as shifted forward in time only when the tone does occur—information that can be known only after the fact (Moore & Haggard, 2008). That binding is sensitive to a variety of authorship indicators supports the hypothesis that when the mind infers authorship for an event, it also shapes the perception of action and event, such that they seem temporally closer.

## TESTING THE AUTHORSHIP-BINDING LINK

Still, evidence for this authorship-binding link has been indirect. Previous research has not administered corroborating measures of perceived authorship, so it isn't clear that temporal binding occurs alongside the experience of authorship. Moreover, key authorship indicators, such as the degree of consistency between actions and events, have not been manipulated to examine their effects on binding. Seeking a more direct test of the hypothesis, we conducted a series of experiments (Ebert, 2008; Ebert & Wegner, 2010) examining binding in relation to previous research on authorship processing. In each experiment, participants performed actions that were followed a brief while later by events. Across experiments, various authorship indicators were manipulated, and their effects on both binding and self-reported authorship were measured. In some experiments we also included measures of clinically relevant variables known to involve a distorted sense of authorship, such as depression, to see if they would predict binding effects.

If the authorship-binding hypothesis is correct, indicators that affect the sense of authorship should affect binding in similar ways, and clinically relevant variables should moderate these effects. For instance, consider the degree of consistency between actions and events. After kicking a can, it might obligingly shoot forward in the same direction as one's foot (consistent event), or it might careen wildly off course, landing, say, in the bed of a passing truck (inconsistent event). Authorship for the can's movement should be greater when this movement is consistent with one's action, and binding should be greater as well. What about someone who is depressed, though? To the extent that depressed individuals generally have low expectations that their actions will bring about successful outcomes ("Knowing me, when I kick this can it'll probably veer off and hit somebody's passing car"), among depressed participants, whether an event is consistent or inconsistent with one's action should matter little for one's experience of authorship and binding.

### The Push/Pull Paradigm

Our research was conducted within a naturalistic "push/pull" paradigm, in which participants experienced action-event sequences that resembled those they might encounter in their daily lives, such as pulling on a door handle and watching the door open, or pushing a ball and watching it go away. The acts of pulling and pushing are imbued with bodily significance (Niedenthal, Barsalou, Winkielman, Krauth-Gruber, & Ric, 2005), implying both an orientation toward whatever is acted upon and a specific expected outcome of the action. Pulling corresponds to an approach orientation toward an object and is undertaken with the expectation that the object will come closer, whereas pushing corresponds to an avoid orientation and is undertaken with the expectation that the object will move away (Cacioppo, Priester, & Berntson, 1993; Chen & Bargh, 1999). Because the push/pull paradigm simulates everyday actions and events, we believe results obtained with it are of relatively high external validity.

In each experiment, participants completed a series of trials on which they saw a picture of an everyday object (e.g., an apple) and pushed or pulled on a joystick in response. This action was followed by a brief delay (in most experiments, 100 ms, 400 ms, or 700 ms), after which the object appeared to move either away from or toward the participant (the event). Participants then estimated the length of the delay between their action and the object's movement, and these interval estimates served as the measure of binding (see Engbert et al., 2008; Engbert et al., 2007; Moore, Wegner, & Haggard, 2009). Participants also reported the degree to which they felt that their action had caused the object to move, which served as the measure of authorship.

The authorship indicators that were manipulated and the clinically relevant variables that were measured are now described, along with key results for each.

### Manipulated Authorship Indicators

Across several experiments, a variety of authorship indicators were manipulated to examine their effect on binding. Specifically, we manipulated whether the object moved in the same direction as the participant's action (action-event consistency), whether participants pulled for desirable objects and pushed for undesirable ones (thought-action consistency), and whether participants freely chose to push or to pull (free choice).

#### Action-Event Consistency

If, upon being kicked, a soda can moves forward in the same direction as one's foot, the experience of authorship should be greater than if the can veers off to the side. Almost by definition, one of the strongest indicators of authorship is whether or not an event is consistent with one's prior action. Although what is considered consistent is likely to vary as a function of the individual's current situation and past experience with actions and their outcomes (Wegner & Sparrow, 2004), our research took advantage of a natural kind of consistency that exists between certain actions and events. Specifically, after pushing in response to an object, a consistent event would be the object's moving away (and an inconsistent event would be the object's moving closer), whereas after pulling, a consistent event would be the object's moving closer (and an inconsistent event would be the object's moving away).

In several experiments, we found that participants judge the delay between consistent actions and events to be briefer than the delay between inconsistent actions and events (Ebert, 2008; Ebert & Wegner, 2010). These effects of consistency on binding were mirrored by large effects of consistency on self-reported authorship; in addition, in most of these experiments, the more consistency increased a given participant's self-reported authorship, the more it increased his or her binding.

When asked at the end of the experiment whether they felt that the delay was briefer for trials on which the object moved in the same direction as their action, briefer for those on which the object moved in the opposite direction, or if it made no difference, many participants said that the delay felt briefer when the object moved in the same direction. In other words, participants reported some awareness of the effect consistency had on binding, presumably because the effect was big enough that over the course of the experiment participants noticed that the delay for consistent trials felt briefer. Critically, a regression analysis indicated that the effect of consistency on binding would have obtained even if subjects had been completely unaware of it (cf. Greenwald, Klinger, & Schuh, 1995)—that the effect does not *depend* on participants' awareness.

### Thought-Action Consistency

Thinking about kicking the soda can before doing so—compared to, say, thinking about how much one likes soda—should lead to greater feelings of authorship when the can speeds away. Several experiments have demonstrated the importance of thought-action consistency for the experience of authorship (Aarts et al., 2005; Wegner et al., 2004; Wegner and Wheatley, 1999), but ours was the first to test whether this authorship indicator affects binding (Ebert, 2008). In this experiment, thoughts were manipulated by presenting participants with either a normatively desirable object (e.g., a slice of pizza) or undesirable object (e.g., a moldy strawberry) on each trial. It was assumed that desirable objects would generally trigger thoughts about pulling, whereas undesirable objects would trigger thoughts about pushing. Actions were manipulated independently of thoughts by cueing participants on each trial either to push or to pull. Thus, half the trials involved thought-action consistency (pulling for desirable objects or pushing for undesirable objects), and half involved inconsistency (pushing for desirable objects or pulling for undesirable objects).

Unexpectedly, thought-action consistency was not found to significantly increase either self-reported authorship or binding in the sample overall. However, across participants the correlation between authorship and binding effects was positive and significant. In other words, among those for whom thought-action consistency did increase authorship, it also increased binding—again suggesting a link between feelings of authorship and binding. The lack of any main effects of consistency might have owed to the cued nature of actions performed in this experiment. Critical for the experience of authorship may be the sense that one is freely choosing how to act.

### Free Choice

If one freely chooses to kick the soda can, the experience of authorship should be greater than if one is ordered to do so. To fully own an action and its consequences, the actor must be the one calling the shots; indeed, authorship is greatest under conditions of free choice, and diminished when one's actions are dictated by another (Milgram, 1974; Wegner & Sparrow, 2004).

To examine the effects of choice on binding, we conducted an experiment with two counterbalanced blocks, one in which participants were cued how to act on each trial (i.e., a prompt appeared telling them whether to push or to pull), and one in which they were prompted to choose (Ebert, 2008). We found that participants judged the delay between actions and events to be briefer under conditions of free choice. A regression analysis indicated that this effect of choice on binding did not depend on participants' awareness of the effect (cf. Greenwald et al., 1995).

Somewhat surprisingly, no effect of choice was found for self-reported authorship. Though this null result could indicate that there are circumstances in which an authorship indicator may affect binding without affecting authorship, we offer a different explanation: the authorship measure we used was ill-suited for detecting an effect of choice. This measure, with its wording focused on the mechanical, causal link between action and event, is not geared toward aspects of authorship having to do with intentionality ("I wanted the object to do that") or personal responsibility ("I'm responsible for what happened to the object")—aspects on which freely chosen actions differ the most from cued actions.

### Delay between Action and Event

As we discussed earlier, authorship should be greatest when a soda can moves right after it is kicked. In accord with past research (Michotte, 1963; Wegner et al., 2004; Wegner & Wheatley, 1999), our experiments have indeed found that briefer delays between action and event lead to an increase in self-reported authorship for the event (Ebert, 2008; Ebert & Wegner, 2010). Unfortunately, the nature of the push/pull paradigm is such that it is difficult to assess the effect of delay on binding, and delay was not manipulated for this purpose. However, previous research using other methods has found that delay is a key moderator, with greater binding effects observed at briefer delays (Haggard et al., 2002). It is therefore worth noting that in our experiments examining action-event consistency, the greatest effects of consistency on binding were found at the briefest delays (Ebert, 2008; Ebert & Wegner, 2010). In fact, these effects were nonsignificant at the longest delay examined (700 ms)—in line with Libet et al.'s (1979) suggestion that there is at most a 500-ms window during which the conscious perception of an event may be altered by a subsequent event. Self-reported authorship, on the other hand, *was* affected by action-event consistency at the longest delay, suggesting that self-reports and binding measure unique aspects of authorship (Ebert & Wegner, 2010).

### Summary of Authorship Indicators Results

Across several experiments, the presence of key authorship indicators was found to increase binding. In addition, these indicators (with the exception of free choice) were found to increase self-reported authorship, and their effects on self-reported authorship were often correlated with their effects on binding. These findings provide some of the strongest evidence yet linking binding to authorship. Because the results were obtained within the naturalistic push/pull paradigm, they also bolster claims about the external validity of binding effects.

### Clinically Relevant Variables

When all goes well, the mind considers a variety of authorship indicators, presumably in proportion to how diagnostic they are, to arrive at a reasonably accurate judgment about whether an event should be attributed to the self. But several clinically relevant tendencies are marked by a distorted sense of authorship—too much or too little—including depression, narcissistic personality, and schizotypal personality. Could it be that individuals exhibiting a distorted sense of authorship overweight or underweight particular authorship indicators, leading them to take credit for events that they did not author or to dismiss those that they did?

To address this question, we looked at whether depression, narcissistic personality, and schizotypal personality would moderate the effects of authorship indicators on binding (Ebert, 2008). Here, we focus on the correlations obtained between each of these clinically relevant variables and the effect of action-event consistency on binding. A positive correlation between a given clinically relevant variable and this binding effect would suggest that those exhibiting the clinical tendency are relatively sensitive to action-event consistency, whereas a negative correlation would suggest relative insensitivity to consistency. Such correlations would thus help to explain, in terms of sensitivity to a key authorship indicator, why certain clinical tendencies are accompanied by heightened or diminished feelings of authorship.

Each of the clinically relevant variables is now described, along with any correlation that was found with the effect of action-event consistency on binding.

### Depression

Experiencing a loss of control is one of the core symptoms of depression (American Psychiatric Association, 1994), and the prominent learned helplessness theory traces depression to the individual's belief that he or she is powerless to overcome negative circumstances (Seligman, 1975). Likewise, depressed individuals have low expectations that their actions will lead to successful outcomes, and may even come to expect outcomes inconsistent with their actions (Alloy & Abramson, 1979; Aarts, Wegner, & Dijksterhuis, 2006). When a depressed individual kicks a can, authorship should not vary much as a function of what the can does next, whether it flies forward in a straight line or dribbles awkwardly into the gutter.

It was therefore predicted that relatively depressed individuals (as measured by the Beck Depression Inventory-II; Beck, Steer, & Brown, 1996) would be insensitive to action-event consistency and exhibit weaker effects of this indicator on binding. In fact, this was what we found in one experiment (Ebert, 2008). It is worth noting that, because events were consistent with actions only half the time in the context of this experiment, a rational case could be made for *not* expecting a consistent event. Thus, the behavior of relatively depressed participants was in keeping with the view that depressed individuals have a soberingly realistic sense of agency in situations marked by low control (Alloy & Abramson, 1979).

### Narcissistic Personality

A narcissistic personality is characterized by exaggerated feelings of power and self-efficacy (DSM-IV). In this sense, narcissism is the opposite of depression, with narcissistic individuals expecting their actions to lead to successful outcomes—and perhaps dismissing inconsistent outcomes as having not been caused by them. When a narcissistic individual kicks a can, authorship should be high if the can's movement is consistent with the kick ("Look—just as I had planned!") and low if it is inconsistent ("Who did *that*?").

It was therefore predicted that relatively narcissistic individuals (as measured by the 37-item version of the Narcissistic Personality Inventory; Emmons, 1987), would be particularly sensitive to action-event consistency and exhibit stronger effects of this indicator on binding. This prediction was borne out in one of our experiments (Ebert, 2008).

### Schizotypal Personality

Individuals with schizophrenia may experience two kinds of distorted authorship, one in which they attribute the consequences of their own actions to others, and one in which they experience authorship over events they did not cause (Haggard, Martin, Taylor-Clarke, Jeannerod, & Franck, 2003). Both distortions might be traceable to deficits in awareness of one's intended actions, awareness that normally arises as part of a predictive "forward model" when actions are planned and carried out (Franck et al., 2001; Frith, 1992; Blakemore et al., 2000). In our research, we examined schizotypal personality, a nonclinical manifestation of some of the same tendencies found in schizophrenia. When a schizotypal individual kicks a can, he or she may have only a faint idea of what the can will do next, and so authorship should not vary as a function of how the can moves.

It was predicted that, due to a deficit in anticipating the outcomes of their actions, relatively schizotypal individuals (as measured by the Schizotypal Personality Questionnaire-Brief; Raine & Benishay, 1995) would be insensitive to action-event consistency and exhibit weaker effects of this indicator on binding. The results of one of our experiments supported this prediction (Ebert, 2008).

## Summary of Clinically Relevant Results

Individuals who scored high on certain clinically relevant variables known to involve a distorted sense of authorship were found to be particularly over- or under-sensitive (depending on the variable) to a key authorship indicator. Specifically, relatively depressed individuals exhibited weak effects of action-event consistency on binding, whereas relatively narcissistic individuals exhibited strong effects—suggesting that the former have lower expectations that their actions will lead to consistent events than do the latter. Relatively schizotypal individuals exhibited weak effects of action-event consistency on binding, perhaps owing to a deficit in anticipating the outcomes of their actions.

Though suggestive, these results should be interpreted with caution. First, participants were sampled from a nonclinical, student population, so generalizing the results to individuals diagnosed with Major Depressive Disorder, Narcissistic Personality Disorder, or schizophrenia would be premature (at the same time, one could argue that sampling from a nonclinical population restricts the range of the clinically relevant variables, thereby *underestimating* the true correlation between each of these variables and binding). Second, it is not clear whether the observed abnormalities in binding are *causes* of the clinical tendencies, or instead effects. In the case of relatively depressed individuals, the observed lack of binding for consistent events could, on the one hand, contribute to their sense of personal inefficacy ("It just didn't feel like I caused the object to come toward me when I pulled"); on the other hand, a sense of personal inefficacy could be the reason they do not expect their actions to lead to consistent events ("When I pulled, I didn't expect the object to come toward me"), which would diminish binding for such events.

To address these issues, future research could sample from clinical populations and examine sensitivity to a wider range of authorship indicators, and longitudinal studies could follow at-risk individuals over time to disentangle which came first: the distorted sense of authorship or the abnormality in binding.

## CONCLUSION

Much is to be gained by focusing on the temporal aspects of authorship. Nearly three decades ago, Libet and colleagues found evidence that conscious will may not cause behavior, by showing that behavioral intentions arrive in consciousness only after unconscious brain activity has set things in motion (Libet et al., 1983). The unconscious causes of one's behavior may remain inscrutable to conscious awareness, but the mind does its best to figure out which events one has authored, and for good reason: Accurate authorship processing enables individuals to evaluate the results of their actions and adjust future behavior accordingly, to discriminate between events that have been caused by themselves rather than by others, and to take responsibility for the consequences of their actions (Wegner & Sparrow, 2004).

The mind appears to make determinations of authorship through a process of causal inference, looking for clues that indicate whether an event should be attributed to the self as causal agent (Wegner, 2002; Wegner & Sparrow, 2004; Wegner & Wheatley, 1999). A key authorship indicator is the temporal proximity between thoughts, actions, and events. Specifically, actions feel willed when they follow on the heels of a consistent thought (Wegner & Wheatley, 1999), and events feel authored when they occur right after a consistent action (Wegner & Sparrow, 2004).

But the link between temporal proximity and authorship appears to go both ways: When the evidence warrants an inference of authorship, one's action and the event are perceived as temporally closer than they otherwise would be. The discovery of "intentional binding"—a shift in the perceived timing of voluntary actions and subsequent events in the direction of each other—first suggested this possibility (Haggard et al., 2002). We have since conducted a series of experiments to further test the hypothesis that binding is a part of the experience of authorship (Ebert, 2008; Ebert & Wegner, 2010).

These experiments employed a naturalistic paradigm, in which action-event sequences resembled those one might encounter in everyday life: flexing and extending one's arm in response to graspable objects, and watching those objects come closer or move away, are basic and common occurrences. Key authorship indicators, such as action-event consistency, were manipulated across experiments, and their effects on self-reported authorship and binding were assessed. In general, these authorship indicators were found to affect binding and self-reported authorship in similar ways. Moreover, the degree to which these indicators affected binding was meaningfully correlated with clinically relevant variables known to involve a distorted sense of authorship.

Together, the results of our experiments support the hypothesis that binding occurs when authorship is inferred—that the mind, in a sense, bends time to one's will.

## ACKNOWLEDGMENTS

This research was supported in part by a Harvard University Dissertation Completion Fellowship to Ebert and NIMH Grant MH 49127 to Wegner.

## REFERENCES

Aarts, H., Custers, R., & Wegner, D. M. (2005). On the inference of personal authorship: Enhancing experienced agency by priming effect information. *Consciousness and Cognition, 14,* 439–458.

Aarts, H., Wegner, D. M., & Dijksterhuis, A. (2006). On the feeling of doing: Dysphoria and the implicit modulation of authorship ascription. *Behaviour Research and Therapy, 44,* 1621–1627.

Alloy, L. B., & Abramson, L. Y. (1979). Judgment of contingency in depressed and nondepressed students: Sadder but wiser? *Journal of Experimental Psychology: General, 108,* 441–485.

American Psychiatric Association. (1994). *Diagnostic and statistical manual of mental disorders* (4th ed.). Washington, DC: Author.

Beck, A. T., Steer, R. A., & Brown, G. K. (1996). *Manual for the Beck Depression Inventory-II.* San Antonio, TX: Psychological Corporation.

Blakemore, S. J., Wolpert, D. M., & Frith, C. D. (2000). Why can't you tickle yourself? *NeuroReport, 11,* R11–R16.

Blakemore, S. J., Wolpert, D. M., & Frith, C. D. (2002). Abnormalities in the awareness of action. *TRENDS in Cognitive Sciences, 6,* 237–242.

Cacioppo, J. T., Priester, J. R., & Berntson, G. G. (1993). Rudimentary determinants of attitudes: 2. Arm flexion and extension have differential effects on attitudes. *Journal of Personality and Social Psychology, 65,* 5–17.

Chen, M., & Bargh, J. A. (1999). Consequences of automatic evaluation: Immediate behavioral predispositions to approach or avoid the stimulus. *Personality and Social Psychology Bulletin, 25,* 215–224.

Ebert, J. P. (2008). *How agency shapes the perception of time.* Doctoral dissertation, Harvard University.

Ebert, J. P., & Wegner, D. M. (2010). Time warp: Authorship shapes the perceived timing of actions and events. *Consciousness and Cognition, 19,* 481–489.

Emmons, R. (1987). Narcissism: Theory and measurement. *Journal of Personality and Social Psychology, 52,* 11–17.

Engbert, K., Wohlschläger, A., & Haggard, P. (2008). Who is causing what? The sense of agency is relational and efferent-triggered. *Cognition, 107,* 693–704.

Engbert, K., Wohlschläger, A., Thomas, R., & Haggard, P. (2007). Agency, subjective time, and other minds. *Journal of Experimental Psychology: Human Perception and Performance, 33*(6), 1261–1268.

Franck, N., Farrer. C., Georgieff, N., Marie-Cardine, M., Dalery, J., d'Amato, T., et al. (2001). Defective recognition of one's own actions in patients with schizophrenia. *American Journal of Psychiatry, 158,* 454–459.

Frith, C. D. (1992). *The cognitive neuropsychology of schizophrenia.* Hove, UK: Lawrence Erlbaum Associates.

Greenwald, A. G., Klinger, M. R., & Schuh, E. S. (1995). Activation by marginally perceptible ("subliminal") stimuli: Dissociation of unconscious from conscious cognition. *Journal of Experimental Psychology: General, 124,* 22–42.

Haggard, P., & Clark, S. (2003). Intentional action: Conscious experience and neural prediction. *Consciousness and Cognition, 12,* 695–707.

Haggard, P., Clark, S., & Kalogeras, J. (2002). Voluntary action and conscious awareness. *Nature Neuroscience, 5,* 382–385.

Haggard, P., Martin, F., Taylor-Clarke, M., Jeannerod, M., & Franck, N. (2003). Awareness of action in schizophrenia. *Cognitive Neuroscience and Neuropsychology, 14,* 1081–1085.

Libet, B. (2004). *Mind time: The temporal factor in consciousness.* Cambridge, MA: Harvard University Press.

Libet, B., Gleason, C. A., Wright, E. W., & Pearl, D. K. (1983). Time of conscious intention to act in relation to onset of cerebral activity (readiness-potential): The unconscious initiation of a freely voluntary act. *Brain, 106,* 623–642.

Libet, B., Wright, E. W., Feinstein, B., & Pearl, D. (1979). Subjective referral of the timing for a conscious sensory experience: A functional role for the somatosensory specific projection system in man. *Brain, 102,* 193–224.

Michotte, A. (1963). *The perception of causality* (T. R. Miles & E. Miles, Trans.). New York: Basic Books.

Milgram, S. (1974). Behavioral study of obedience. *Journal of Abnormal and Social Psychology, 67,* 371–378.

Moore, J., & Haggard, P. (2008). Awareness of action: Inference and prediction. *Consciousness and Cognition, 17,* 136–144.

Moore, J. W., Wegner, D. M., & Haggard, P. (2009). Modulating the sense of agency with external cues. *Consciousness and Cognition, 18,* 1056–1064.

Niedenthal, P. M., Barsalou, L. W., Winkielman, P., Krauth-Gruber, S., & Ric, F. (2005). Embodiment in attitudes, social perception, and emotion. *Personality and Social Psychology Review, 9,* 184–211.

Preston, J., & Wegner, D. M. (2003). Action misperception as a consequence of intention and will to act. Unpublished manuscript.

Preston, J., & Wegner, D. M. (2005). Ideal agency: The perception of self as an origin of action. In A. Tesser, J. Wood, & D. Stapel (Eds.), *On building, defending, and regulating the self* (pp. 103–125). Philadelphia: Psychology Press.

Pronin, E., Wegner, D. M., McCarthy, K., & Rodriguez, S. (2006). Everyday magical powers: The role of apparent mental causation in the overestimation of personal influence. *Journal of Personality and Social Psychology, 91,* 218–231.

Raine, A., & Benishay, D. (1995). The SPQ-B: A brief screening instrument for schizotypal personality disorder. *Journal of Personality Disorders, 9,* 346–355.

Seligman, M. E. P. (1975). *Helplessness: On depression, development, and death.* San Francisco: W. H. Freeman.

Wegner, D. M. (2002). *The illusion of conscious will.* Cambridge, MA: MIT Press.

Wegner, D. M. (2008). Self is magic. In J. Baer, J. C. Kaufman, & R. F. Baumeister (Eds.), *Are we free? Psychology and free will* (pp. 226–247). New York: Oxford University Press.

Wegner, D. M., Fuller, V. A., & Sparrow, B. (2003). Clever hands: Uncontrolled intelligence in facilitated communication. *Journal of Personality and Social Psychology, 85,* 5–19.

Wegner, D. M., & Sparrow, B. (2004). Authorship processing. In M. Gazzaniga (Ed.), *The cognitive neurosciences* (vol. 3, pp. 1201–1209). Cambridge, MA: MIT Press.

Wegner, D. M., & Sparrow, B. (2007). The puzzle of coaction. In D. Ross, D. Spurrett, H. Kincaid, & L. Stephens (Eds.), *Distributed cognition and the will* (pp. 17–38). Cambridge, MA: MIT Press.

Wegner, D. M., Sparrow, B., & Winerman, L. (2004). Vicarious agency: Experiencing control over the movements of others. *Journal of Personality and Social Psychology, 86,* 838–848.

Wegner, D. M., & Wheatley, T. P. (1999). Apparent mental causation: Sources of the experience of will. *American Psychologist, 54,* 480–492.

# CHAPTER 13

## Prospective Codes Fulfilled: A Potential Neural Mechanism of Will

*Thalia Wheatley and Christine E. Looser*

***One of my few shortcomings is that I can't predict the future.***

Lars Ulrich, Metallica

Lars Ulrich was right and wrong. He was right in the way we most often think about the future—as a long stretch of time during which multiply determined events occur. If we could predict this kind of future we would play the lottery every day and avoid embarrassing wardrobe malfunctions. This is clearly not the case. However, converging evidence from neuroscience reveals that our brains do predict the future and do so well, albeit on a much shorter time scale. Bayesian anticipation of likely events appears to be a general principle of brain function. That is, we use information about the probability of past events to predict future events, allowing for a more efficient use of neural resources. While research has begun to show that many systems in the brain code Bayesian predictions, very little work has examined the experiential consequences of this coding. Here we propose that prospective neural facilitation may be fundamental to the phenomenological experience of will.

## THE FEELING OF WILL

The feeling of will is typically associated with having performed an intentional act. Slamming the door to make a point feels willed. Rushing to the airport to make a flight feels willed. Will is the kind of feeling one gets when actions are consciously purposeful. Wegner and Wheatley proposed that this feeling comes from three sources: priority, consistency, and exclusivity (Wegner & Wheatley, 1999). An action feels willed to the degree that one has a prior thought (priority) that is consistent with that action (consistency) and that appears to be the only possible cause of that action (exclusivity). Importantly, these sources of will need not be veridical to action, but can be manipulated independent of action as was illustrated by the following experiment.

### The "I Spy" Study

In this experiment, two people sat across a table from each other with their hands on a large computer mouse. Unbeknownst to the actual subject, their partner was an employee (confederate) of the experiment posing as a participant. On the table, visible to both, was a computer monitor with a screen depicting a variety of objects taken from the children's book *I Spy*. The participant and the confederate were instructed to move the mouse together in sweeping circles and, by doing so, they moved a cursor around the screen. The pair were also instructed to stop moving the mouse approximately every 30 seconds. Finally, both were given headphones and told that they would hear different words, ostensibly as a mild distraction for the task. In reality, the headphones were critical to the experiment. The real subject heard words related to objects onscreen (e.g., "swan . . . monkey"). The confederate heard instructions to force stops on particular objects at particular times. These critical stops occurred at various time intervals after the participant heard a related word. For example, the confederate would force a stop on the swan exactly 5 seconds after the participant heard the word "swan" in their headphones. After each stop the pair rated how much they had intended to make that stop in comparison to their partner.

As the assumption of priority would predict, the amount of time between the preview and the forced act was important to the perception of will. If the preview occurred a few moments before the act, participants mistakenly perceived that they were responsible for (and had intended to perform) the act. If the preview occurred too far in advance (e.g., subjects heard "swan" 30 seconds before the confederate engineered a stop on the swan) or immediately after the stop, subjects did not attribute the act to themselves (see Fig. 13.1).

This study demonstrated that the feeling of will could be evoked by providing people with three bits of information: a preview thought, a consistent act, and the knowledge that the initiating event was exclusive to them. This suggests that will, as a phenomenological experience, can be attributed erroneously whenever stimuli mimic the natural sources of will. Since this study, several other paradigms have demonstrated that the feeling of will can be manipulated independently of action (Banks & Isham, 2009; Choi & Scholl, 2006; Lau, Rogers, & Passingham, 2007; Wegner, Fuller, & Sparrow, 2003; Wegner, Sparrow, & Winerman, 2004). Collectively, these manipulations of will demonstrate the flexibility of its interpretation. Consistent with this flexibility, the ostensible instigating event need not be a thought at all; actions can serve as previews for future actions.

### The "Sequential Will" Study

In this study, subjects were asked to perform a series of action sequences. Importantly, each action in a sequence was performed without knowing which action would follow next. All subjects were given the same 24 initial actions (e.g., make a fist) but subsequent actions in each sequence differed across subjects. In any given sequence, the actions were either *unrelated* to each other (make fist, knock on the desk with the other hand), *disrupted* by an intervening action (make fist, tap left foot, knock on the desk with the fist), *delayed* (make fist, wait five seconds, knock on the desk with the fist), or *related* (make fist, knock on the desk with the fist). Each subject performed each of the 24 action sequences only once, and counterbalancing ensured that the sequence conditions were

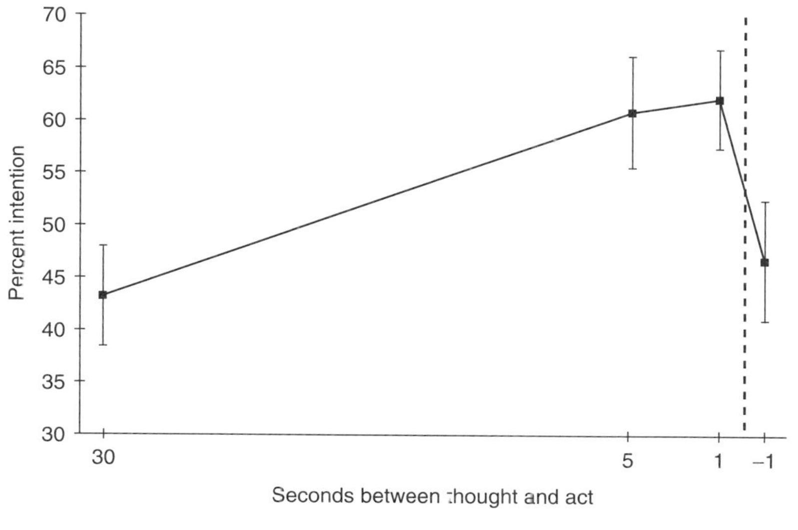


**Figure 13.1** Mean percentage of intentionality perceived for forced stops (Wegner & Wheatley, 1999). 0 ("My partner intended the stop")–100% (I intended the stop").

balanced across subjects. Immediately after each sequence was performed, subjects were asked to rate the first action, last action, or entire action sequence for how much they felt that they had performed it willfully vs. mechanically. Willfully was described as feeling "like the action was coming from you . . . like you are consciously initiating your actions, as an active participant." Mechanically was described as "operating on autopilot, responding mindlessly to what is being asked of you without being engaged or consciously involved." The empirical question was whether the first actions would be misremembered as more or less willful depending on the relatedness of the subsequent actions.

As predicted, the ratings of the first action differed significantly depending on the subsequent actions. Specifically, actions followed immediately by a related sequence were rated as having felt more willfully authored compared to actions followed by disrupted or unrelated sequences. Importantly, these first actions could not have differed at the *time* they were performed because participants did not know what the next action would be (and thus whether it would be related). The experience of will for the first action was revised by subsequent actions. Uncharacteristically, William James was incorrect when he stated that: "The willing terminates with the prevalence of the idea; and whether the act then follows or not is a matter quite immaterial" (James, 1890). In all of these experiments, illusory versions of priority, consistency, and exclusivity evoked an illusory feeling of will. The cognitive mechanism underlying this illusion is unclear, but there are at least two possibilities.

## Explaining Illusory Will

### Retrospective Inference

The most intuitive explanation of these effects is retrospective inference: participants deduced the intentionality of their actions after the fact. This explanation suggests that people are essentially outside observers of their own behavior, a conclusion that squares with many findings in social psychology. The seminal paper by Nisbett and Wilson (1977), "Telling More Than We Can Know," provides several illustrations in which people fabricated reasons for their behavior when they were ignorant of the true cause. For example, mall shoppers were asked to select the best pantyhose among four alternatives. All four pantyhose samples were identical but people overwhelming chose the right-most pair. Shoppers appeared to have no knowledge of this position effect, and instead claimed that their choices were based on more normative reasons such as the superiority of the weave. Indeed, when asked directly about whether they were influenced by position, the shoppers "denied it, usually with a worried glance at the interviewer suggesting that they felt either that they had misunderstood the question or were dealing with a madman" (Nisbett & Wilson, 1977). The shoppers observed their behavior and retrospectively inferred the most plausible, albeit incorrect, reason.

In the case of the I Spy study, retrospective inference might sound something like this: "I was the only one who heard the word 'swan,' then we stopped on the swan, . . . I suppose I must have been the one responsible for the stop." Despite presenting this reasoning as a quote, it should be noted that retrospective inference does not necessarily imply conscious awareness. This explanation simply suggests that a deduction was made retrospectively that led the participant to tag the event as willed. As the participant could not foresee the impending action in either the I Spy or Sequential Will study, it seems strange to argue that the creation of will was anything *but* retrospective. However, Patrick Haggard has suggested that a second phenomenon may be at play that is not retrospective at all (Haggard & Clark, 2003; Haggard, 2005; Moore & Haggard, 2008).

### Neural Prospection

Haggard and colleagues refer to the alternative phenomenon as neural prediction. Broadly speaking, a neural prediction is the brain's preparatory activity for a predicted action or event. In the domain of motor control, neural predictions allow the brain to evaluate the success of a motor plan by predicting the visual, motor, and proprioceptive feedback associated with an action (Blakemore, Wolpert, & Frith, 2002). Haggard posited that conscious intention may be an immediate consequence of these predictive processes. That is, the feeling of agency may arise in a feed-forward, constructive manner rather than, or perhaps as well as, via retrospective inference. Haggard et al. (2003, 2008) convincingly demonstrated that the experience of action is tied to the preparation and perceived realization of a specific motor prediction. Although this research has focused on the neural prediction of a specific motor plan, there is reason to believe that the phenomenon of neural prediction, broadly construed, is a general mechanism of brain function.

The broad view of this idea may be more consistent with the term "neural prospection" than "neural prediction." "Neural prediction" and "predictive coding" commonly refer to the mapping between a cause (motor command) and its specific sensory effect (e.g., visual or proprioceptive feedback; Kilner, Friston, & Frith, 2007). In contrast, neural *prospection* refers to mental forecasting: "the capacity to imagine, simulate, or pre-experience episodes in the future" (Schacter & Addis, 2007).

In contrast to neural prediction, neural prospection is likely to be a general mechanism across multiple sensory systems and operate at larger time-scales. Simply put, it is the sensitization of neural pathways based on recent experience. What we experience at Time 1 readies our brains to process related experiences at Time 2. Recently, there has been a shift in neuroscience to consider the brain as a predictive machine. In the (very) big picture, this conceptualization is long overdue.

## THE PROACTIVE BRAIN

Several million years of evolution honed the brain to be an incessant forecaster. Predators, weather, and social hierarchies could yield unfavorable conditions rapidly; thus an efficient predictive system was essential to not being eaten, rained on, or socially outcast. Moreover, survival prioritized the overestimation of cause-effect relationships rather than veridical accuracy: better to falsely impute the presence of a snake from the sound of rustling leaves than process the sound veridically and miss the potential implications. In short, natural selection ensured that the brain generates continuous predictions in order to selectively amplify potential biologically relevant information within streams of fleeting and ambiguous input.

The predictive nature of the brain fits a broader characterization of the brain as storyteller. A wealth of research from psychological and brain sciences has shown that the brain is not a veridical recording device but fills in gaps and even manipulates space and time to make sense of incoming sensory input (see Wheatley, 2009, for a review). To this end, even basic cognitive processes such as perception and memory are actively constructed and embellished, often without our awareness. The visual system, for example, operates by making assumptions: converging lines indicate distance, a dark line is seen as an edge, and so on. Through recurrent processing with higher order areas, these assumptions help us translate two-dimensional retinotopic input into a sensible three-dimensional model of the world. Moreover, these perceptual assumptions facilitate the prediction of later events. Representational momentum is one illustrative example.

In the first demonstration of representational momentum, Freyd and Finke (1984) presented participants with four sequential presentations of a rectangle that only varied in terms of where the rectangle appeared onscreen. The first three rectangles were presented consecutively in either a clockwise or counterclockwise direction. The participant's task was to judge whether the fourth rectangle appeared in the same position as the third. Interestingly, participants made a consistent error: they were more likely to respond "same" if the fourth rectangle was slightly beyond the location of the third, along the expected trajectory. That is, participants couldn't help but be biased by a kind of perceptual inertia. In 1996, Reed and Vinson examined whether this perceptual prediction was an impenetrable, low-level visual phenomenon or whether it could be modulated by prediction-relevant conceptual knowledge. In their study, participants were told that the rectangle (now with a pointy top) was a "rocket" or a "steeple." Participants told that the shape was a "rocket" experienced more representational momentum than participants told that the shape was a "steeple," but only when the shape ascended in a vertical trajectory, as a rocket would. This finding illustrates that top-down semantic knowledge can influence bottom-up stimulus processing to ensure that our perceptual predictions are consistent with our knowledge of the world.

The need to predict can be observed at all levels of information processing from the retina to complex social behavior. Gilbert, Pelham, and Krull (1988) showed that a cursory glance of someone's behavior floods our minds with thoughts about that person's personality, intentions, and emotional state. Being able to attribute internal states from the actions of others is invaluable. Simply observing that Alex bought the *Washington Post* has little predictive value in and of itself. Using the same observation to infer that Alex is probably a well-educated, politically aware, mid-Atlantic resident with Democratic leanings is potentially far more useful in predicting his future behavior. Clearly, the brain must generate predictions at multiple, interacting levels of analysis (Bar, 2007). How this prospection is realized in the wet matter of glia and neurons is not well understood. However, adaptation and prospective coding may be two relevant indices.

## The Neurobiology of Prospection

### Adaptation

One way to probe the processing characteristics of a particular cortical region is to observe its adaptation dynamics. If neurons adapt (fire less) to a repeated stimulus, it suggests that the first presentation of the stimulus facilitated those neurons. That is, the first presentation *potentiated* particular neural pathways through which subsequent presentations are processed more rapidly. Several researchers have suggested that this neuronal adaptation, and its hemodynamic correlate "repetition suppression," reflects the brain's ability to make predictions in order to increase efficiency (see Henson, 2003; Schacter & Buckner, 1998; Wiggs & Martin, 1998, for reviews). Part of this efficiency is the speed with which the neurons resolve "prediction error" (Grill-Spector, Henson, & Martin, 2006). Prediction error is defined as the difference between the prediction and the actual occurrence (evidence). If you expect to get a painful injection but feel nothing, the prediction error is larger than if the predicted pain occurred. Prediction error is resolved through recurrent processing and is an essential mechanism of learning. How quickly neurons adapt to a stimulus reflects the size of the prediction error. Thus, neural adaptation may be considered an index of the "goodness of fit" of a neural prediction. The more accurate the prediction, the smaller the prediction error and the more efficient the processing.

Adaptation is not limited to tracking identical visual repetitions. Instead, it appears to be a general neural mechanism. In the inferotemporal cortex, adaptation is robust to whether a stimulus (e.g., chair) changes in size and location, indicating that this region cares about semantic categories more than specific visual details (Ito, Tamura, Fujita, & Tanaka, 1995; Lueschow, Miller, & Desimone, 1994; in humans: Dehaene et al., 2004; Grill-Spector, Kushnir, Edelman, Avidan, Itzchak, & Malach, 1999). Purely conceptual information can also show adaptation effects. Reading the word "dog" produces less activity after another animal word (e.g., "horse") than after the word "cup." As the letters of words are arbitrary symbols, the reduced activity in this example can only be caused by the conceptual repetition (Wheatley, Weisberg, Beauchamp, & Martin, 2005). More recently, adaptation has been used as a tool to probe even higher order judgments, including the understanding of self and other (Jenkins, Macrae, & Mitchell, 2008). In sum, neuronal adaptation appears to be a useful index for the strength of *any* neural prediction.

Most commonly, adaptation has been used to probe the contents of particular brain areas. If seeing an apple for the second time reduces activity in brain region X, then brain region X is assumed to care about apples. The focus of research has been on neural prediction (the mapping of neural commands to their effects), not neural prospection (the prediction of future events). However, it could be used in this way.

For example, in the sequential will study, making a fist likely readied the brain for the act of knocking because the two are temporally correlated. If so, the act of knocking would have required less energy (more adaptation) than doing something unrelated to having made a fist. Perhaps one reason why adaptation has been underutilized as a prospective trace is that it requires an inference of its own—that the observed adaptation was caused by prior facilitation. A more direct index of prospection would gauge the facilitation itself. Single cell recordings with monkeys and recent multivoxel pattern analysis with humans suggest that it is now possible to measure neural codes that directly predict upcoming thoughts and actions.

### Prospective coding

Prospective coding refers to the anticipatory or predictive component of neuronal firing. Neurophysiological research has shown that neurons in the lateral prefrontal cortex of rhesus macaques predict the monkey's next action (Rainer, Rao & Miller, 1999) and the reward value of upcoming trials (Watanabe, Hikosaka, Sakagami, & Shirakawa, 2002). Of course we cannot infer from these results that the monkey is consciously thinking ahead, but part of the brain appears to be anticipating the monkey's next move. More recently, similar prospective codes have been demonstrated in humans.

Soon, Brass, Heinze, and Haynes (2008) updated the classic Libet paradigm by having subjects decide whether to press a button with their left or right hand while lying in a functional magnetic resonance imaging (fMRI) machine. Similar to Libet's "planned action" condition, subjects reported that they decided to act about a second before they pressed the button. Soon et al., were curious to find out whether these decisions could be detected earlier in the brain data. That is, could hemodynamic activity reveal subjects' decisions before they even knew it themselves? By using machine learning algorithms to detect patterns associated with upcoming decisions, Soon and colleagues found something remarkable. Two regions in the brain predicted subjects' upcoming decisions several seconds in advance, much earlier than the time at which subjects first became aware of these decisions. These two regions were located in the posterior parietal and lateral prefrontal cortices.

While subjects' decisions could be predicted by the brain data much earlier than phenomenology, the accuracy of these predictions was not 100% or even 80%. It was simply, but importantly, above chance. This suggests that Soon et al., were not tapping into a specific prospective code linked to a single motoric decision. Instead, this weak but reliable prediction several seconds in advance may best be characterized as a *biasing* of the system. As one gets closer to the actual decision, this biasing may narrow into a single, stronger prospection.

From diffuse biasing to specific action codes, prospection appears to be the modus operandi of multiple sensory and motor systems in the human and other mammalian brains. Herein lies the rub. If neural prospection is a general process across species, how could it further our understanding of a phenomenological experience presumed to be unique to human minds? The following section offers a theoretical account of how this general mechanism of neural prospection may be fundamental to the feeling of will.

## NEURAL PROSPECTION AND THE FEELING OF WILL

In all mammals, environmental unpredictability leads to poor physical and mental health. Rats given unpredictable electric shocks develop extensive stomach ulcers and give up pressing a bar for food. When the identical series of shocks are paired with a warning sound the negative outcomes are greatly reduced (Weiss, 1970). From rats to humans, predictability impinges as much or more on physical and mental health as the nature of the situation itself. In humans, unpredictable negative events can lead to posttraumatic stress disorder and panic disorders which in turn exacerbate anxiety to unpredicted threats (Grillon, Lissek, Rabin, McDowell, Dvir, & Pine, 2008). Predictability affords a level of control. Even though I cannot control the weather directly, I can grab an umbrella in response to a rainy forecast. Even if I know I will receive an electric shock, I can prepare myself psychologically. The occasional surprise party aside, knowing exactly what is coming down the pike is the preferred state of affairs. And even when we don't know what will happen next, we find comfort in believing that somewhere, Someone has a master plan. On a more micro time scale, prospective coding may offer a measure of the predictability we desire.

The kind of predictability afforded by prospective coding is very different from foretelling whom we will marry, but it may provide something nonetheless powerful: the feeling of being in command. A paradox of human behavior is that even when we have no conscious awareness of what we are about to think, say or do, our thoughts, words, and deeds rarely surprise us. Though we do not know exactly what we are about to say, the words tumble out sounding reasonable. Gestures are unplanned yet feel natural. Even when we find ourselves picking lint off our sweater it feels as if somehow, deep down, we knew we would do it.

In Wegnerian terms, realized prospective codes are fulfilled previews. Thus, prospective codes can contribute two of the three necessary ingredients of will: priority and consistency. However, these two ingredients cannot by themselves yield the full experience of will. For that, we must perceive that we are the sole and voluntary author of our actions (exclusivity).

### Authorship

Exclusivity refers to the knowledge that the action, thought, or event was initiated voluntarily by oneself without external manipulation. In the I Spy paradigm, participants did not misattribute will if they believed that the confederate heard the same preview words as themselves (Wegner & Wheatley, unpublished). Hearing the preview word and seeing the consistent stop was not enough—participants needed to think that the preview was theirs alone.

Exclusivity provides authorship; defined as "*I initiated this action.*" Recent neuroimaging evidence suggests that this perceived authorship may require activity in the ventral medial prefrontal cortex (vmPFC). This region is engaged when introspecting about oneself (Blakemore, Winston, & Frith, 2004; Mitchell, Banaji, & Macrae, 2005) and shows relevant adaptation effects: self-reflections activate this area less if prior thoughts were also self-relevant (Jenkins, Macrae, & Mitchell, 2008). Thus, thinking about oneself activates this region, which then facilitates more self-relevant processing. Together, the realization of prospective codes and the attribution of authorship fulfill the three sources of will. The following section examines how these ingredients of will may combine in different strengths to produce a variety of phenomenological experiences.

## PROSPECTION AND AUTHORSHIP

As can be seen in Figure 13.2, prospective coding and authorship may interact to produce several perceptions associated with the feeling of will (or lack thereof). The following paragraphs detail these categories, organized by the nature of the prospection.

### No Prospection

The first column in the figure is the least likely to be associated with will. Here, actions occur without any relevant, anticipatory neuronal activity. This is commonly the case when watching others act in unpredictable ways. However, this can also occur when one behaves so quickly—so reflexively—that prospective codes have no chance to develop.

#### Without Authorship

If a completely unexpected action occurs and we feel no authorship for it, it is impossible to experience the act as willed or intentional. Our predictions about what may happen in the near future are incorrect, violating the tenets of priority and consistency. Moreover, we feel that we are not the one performing the action, additionally violating the principle of exclusivity. Because these actions are unpredictable, they may seem strange and misplaced. Imagine that a colleague stands up in a meeting and starts doing jumping jacks. Nothing in the environment, or in our past knowledge about this colleague, could have facilitated such a prediction, thus there would have been no relevant prospective neural activity. No will is evoked.

| Perceived authorship | Neural prospection: None | Neural prospection: Unattended | Neural prospection: Attended |
|---|---|---|---|
| No | **No authorship, no prospection**<br>Unpredicted acts of others | **No authorship, unattended prospection**<br>Predicted, unattended acts of others post hypnotic suggestion | **No authorship, attended prospection**<br>Predicted, attended acts of others |
| Yes | **Authorship, no prospection**<br>Unpredicted acts of self e.g., reflex, instinct | **Authorship, unattended prospection**<br>Predicted, unattended acts of self e.g., gestures, gait, conversation | **Authorship, attended prospection**<br>Predicted, attended acts of self e.g., willed action |

**Figure 13.2** Interactions of Prospection and Authorship.

### With Authorship

This category contains unpredicted actions of the self. Here authorship is fulfilled—the action is deemed self-initiated—but no relevant prospective codes are in place. Such a situation may occur if an action happens so quickly that it cannot engage a predicted neuronal association (e.g., reflexive behavior). The potential lack of a prospective code may help explain why people who impulsively risk their lives to rescue others are uncomfortable with the label "hero." Recent newspapers report two such examples. In one, passer-by Michael Warburton spotted an elderly woman struggling to escape a burning building. He ran to help, grabbed a neighbor's ladder and climbed up to the roof. Later he eschewed the label: "I'm not a hero. Instinct just took over." Likewise, a cop who grabbed the loaded gun of an assailant thereby thwarting a homicide clarified: "I wasn't being brave, I was just reacting." Their discomfort with the label may be caused by the lay belief that heroic acts must be *decided in advance*, with full knowledge of the consequences. Instinctive acts may feel unwilled because they are too rapid to gain a prospective neural foothold. Our body does the acting while our mind lags behind. Five minutes before he climbed to the roof of the burning building, Michael Warburton was looking out the window of his girlfriend's car. Jumping out of the car and racing toward fire would not have felt predictable despite the undeniable fact that it was his body doing the racing. Instinctive and reflexive actions hijack our bodies regardless of whatever Bayesian neural facilitation was leading us to expect.

## Unattended Prospection

The second column of Figure 13.2 refers to prospective codes that are fulfilled but unattended. Such prospective codes are likely to occur for everyday actions that typically unfold without our attention (e.g., walking). These codes may be singular (as in the specific facilitation of putting one step in front of the other) or diffuse. Diffuse prospective codes may occur when multiple associations are facilitated with the strength of each being inversely proportional to the total number. Thus diffuse prospective codes may be inherently weaker than prospective codes for a specific event.

### Without Authorship

This category refers to the situation in which we have a vague idea of what we may see, hear, or feel but no concomitant sense of authorship. Returning to our overathletic colleague, it may seem strange to witness his jumping jacks in the middle of a meeting, but reasonable to witness the same behavior at a gym. Entering a gym primes us to detect acts of athleticism, broadly defined. Thus the processing of jumping jacks is facilitated, albeit weakly, along with other athletic acts one might expect given the setting. Clearly, vague expectations of others' actions are unlikely to feel willed. It may also seem obvious that only the acts of others would end up in this category. However, posthypnotic suggestion may be an unusual case in which a subject's own actions feel predicted but not self-initiated.

Posthypnotic suggestions are commands given during hypnosis that are intended to be obeyed once the subject is out of the hypnotic state. For example, a hypnotist might say "after you awaken from hypnosis, you will turn your head every time you hear me cough." Typically, these suggestions are combined with a suggestion of amnesia: "but you won't remember that I told you to do so" (Shor & Orne, 1962). This begs the question: how does the subject forget the instruction and remember to do it at the same time? For now this mystery remains unsolved though it suggests a stratified nature of consciousness (Schooler, 2002). Most importantly for the present discussion is how a posthypnotic suggestion *feels*. In collaboration with Dan Wegner, we ran several studies using posthypnotic suggestion and were surprised by the consistency of subject's self reports. Subjects referred to feeling a powerful urge to do the act without knowing why. One participant later described feeling as though a battle was occurring between his conscious and unconscious mind:

> It was an awkward experience. I felt like there were different parts of me speaking at the same time—different parts of me were analyzing the situation. It was like "I see this apple and this orange" and one part of me was saying "pick it up" but there was another part of me questioning why and then one part of me forces me to do it and the other part still questioning why. Almost like two sides. I didn't feel too whole to tell you the truth.

Even though the actions were self-performed and predictable once the cue was given, subjects lacked a coherent sense of authorship. This is all the more striking given the nature of the suggestions: juggling with fake fruit, rolling a ball along the floor, covering ones ears, and talking into a plastic banana as though it were a telephone. These were not rapid, reflex-like actions nor could they be mistaken for mindless gestures. These were complex behaviors that looked nothing if not self-initiated and intentional. However, the experience of the subject could not have been further from a feeling of will.

The feeling of will for a posthypnotic suggestion was examined via self-report—we simply asked subjects how intentional the action felt. Self-report is the measurement of choice for questions of phenomenology. As Libet put it: "one begins with the premise that the subjective event is only accessible introspectively to the subject himself, some kind of report of this by the subject is therefore a requirement" (Libet, 1993, p. 272). In short, if you want to learn how a person feels, you must ask them.

In order to thwart suspicion in our study, subjects were asked how a variety of actions felt rather than just the posthypnotic suggestion. To reduce the possibility of malingering, subjects were asked how these actions felt over an intercom while they were alone in a room, observed by a hidden camera. A constant stream of sounds played over their speaker allowed for the insertion of an auditory, posthypnotic cue at particular times. Subjects were left alone to play with various toys, knowing that every now and then they would be asked to report out loud what they were doing and how intentional it felt using a seven-point scale (1—not at all intentional; 7—very intentional). The most surprising finding across these studies was the sheer absence of will for the hypnotically suggested acts. The mean intentionality for all normal (nonsuggested) actions was around a 5. In contrast, the modal response for a posthypnotic suggestion was a 1. To put this in perspective, we sometimes asked participants to report on "nonactions" such as staring into space, yawning, or stretching absentmindedly. The purpose of this was simply to avoid suspicion of a hidden camera, but the results provided a useful baseline. Even though participants sheepishly admitted to not doing much of anything at these times, the modal rating was a 3 on a 7-point scale. Staring into space was a "3"! In contrast, deliberately walking over to a particular bookcase in order to use a plastic banana as a telephone was rated as a "1." Something unusual was a foot. Subjects knew what they were about to do but felt like living marionettes. Why?

One intriguing possibility is that posthypnotically suggested actions have unconscious, prospective codes that offer predictability but that these actions are not tagged with a coherent authorship signal.

### With Authorship

The bulk of our daily actions reside in the unattended, self-authored category. While the decision to walk to the post office may feel willed, the subsequent actions that get us from point A to point B are only vaguely anticipated in consciousness. The same goes for normal conversation: we may be conscious of the topic and tone but have little access to the specific words that will pop out of our mouths. Nonetheless, conversation is not the worse for wear. A colleague of ours recently commented that he had no idea how to answer a student's question but started talking anyway because he "trusted that the words would come out ok" and they did. Even though we are not actively attending to these actions, we feel a sense that they were self-initiated. To use driving as a metaphor, the experience may be akin to driving a car down a familiar route, as if on autopilot. And similar to driving, when the spotlight of attention shifts to the action at hand, our phenomenological experience becomes more agentic.

## Attended Prospection

The final column of Figure 13.2 is the most strongly associated with the feeling of will. Here, fulfilled prospective codes guarantee priority and consistency, and attention intensifies the concomitant phenomenology. Under these conditions, the addition of perceived authorship evokes the prototypical sensation of will. However, even without authorship, a "proxy" or "pseudo" will may arise.

### Without Authorship

As noted earlier, the ability to predict future events is comforting and may evoke a sense of mastery. This may help explain why strong predictions of events external to ourselves may sometimes produce a sensation similar to will. Pretend for a moment that you are playing bingo; you are very close to winning and B-13 is the only open spot left on your card. Next, you close your eyes and concentrate as hard as you can on "B-13." Suddenly it is called, and you cry out, "BINGO!" While your rational mind may remind you that this is purely chance, it *feels* as though it was your concentration that tipped the odds in your favor.

The same "proxy will" may be felt by sports fans who feel that their team's performance depends on their own attendance at the game or on what they are wearing. The presence or absence of a lucky sock, for example, may determine the predicted outcome in the fan's mind: "I am wearing my lucky sock therefore they will win." The importance of the game amplifies attention, and the fulfillment of the prediction evokes a sense of personal responsibility.

A similar scenario may apply to the phenomenon "basking in reflected glory," in which fans are more likely to use the collective pronoun after a win ("we won") than after a loss ("they lost"; Cialdini, Borden, Thorne, Walker, Freeman, & Sloan, 1976). The common explanation for this effect is that people attempt to gain social stature by associating with successful others and distancing themselves from unsuccessful others. However, prospection may also be at play, since people often expect their favorite team to do well. This "rooting on" may facilitate the experience of positive outcomes (e.g., hitting the ball). When those prospections are fulfilled (the player hits the ball), it may feel like a collective event. When those predictions are not fulfilled (the player misses), it may feel like the player was acting on his own. Of course, no sane person would admit to willing the Red Sox to victory. However, if forced to be honest with ourselves, it sometimes *feels* that way.

### With Authorship

The final category is an easy one. The strongest sense of will occurs when we attend to our own, prospected actions. We feel as though we are in the driver's seat and fully engaged. Thus, this category represents the full-blown, subjective experience of agency, regardless of whether the experience itself is causally effective vis-à-vis action.

## PROSPECTION VS. RETROSPECTIVE INFERENCE

By comparing prospection and retrospective inference as two explanations for the experience of will, we do not wish to imply mutual exclusivity. The evidence for neural prospection of will is currently outnumbered by demonstrations of retrospective inference that could not be explained in any feed-forward way (Banks & Isham, 2009; Johansson, Hall, Sikstrom, & Olsson, 2005; Kassin & Kiechel, 1996, Loftus, 1993). Most likely, the feed-forward mechanisms of prospection and authorship work in tandem with retrospective inference to create the full range of subjective experience. Also, the distinction drawn between prospection and retrospective inference is largely temporal (prospective vs. retrospective) rather than inferential (no inference vs. inference). As Wegner notes, "the inference process that yields conscious will does its job throughout the process of actual action causation, first in anticipation, then in execution, and finally in reflection" (Wegner, 2002, pp. 68–69). Thus, prospection and authorship are susceptible to inference if not inferences themselves. The difference between them and retrospective inference is that they occur earlier in time.

## SUMMARY

Prospection gives us a sense of agency, a feeling that the world is a predictable place and we are in command. This may well be illusory. We know that normal, healthy adults can be misled in matters of will, that patients can feel will for actions they can't perform (e.g., for phantom limbs) and lack will for actions they do perform (e.g., alien hand syndrome). Thus, the feeling of will can be imputed, manipulated, and taken away—all inappropriately and independent of action. Currently there is no evidence that the feeling of will is any more than an illusion.

And yet the illusion not only persists, it thrives. Regardless of whether the feeling of will does anything in a causal sense, the perception that everything happens for a reason and that our conscious selves are at the helm allows us to experience life more fully. Those who overestimate true contingencies between their actions (e.g., button press) and an outcome (flash of light) are less likely to be depressed than those who are more accurate. The depressed are "sadder but wiser" (Alloy & Abramson, 1979). The proactive nature of our brains helps keep us sane, comforted, and feeling as though we are in command of all of our actions even as we stare into space.

## REFERENCES

Alloy, L. B., & Abramson, L. Y. (1979). Judgment of contingency in depressed and nondepressed students: Sadder but wiser? *Journal of Experimental Psychology: General, 108,* 441–485.

Banks, W. P., & Isham, E. A. (2009). We infer rather than perceive the moment we decided to act. *Psychological Science, 20,* 17–21.

Bar M. (2007). The proactive brain: using analogies and associations to generate predictions. *Trends in Cognitive Science,11*, 280–289.

Bar, M. (2009). The proactive brain: Memory for predictions. *Philosophical Transactions of the Royal Society B, 364,* 1235–1243.

Blakemore, S.-J., Winston, J., & Frith, U. (2004). Social cognitive neuroscience: Where are we heading? *Trends in Cognitive Sciences, 8,* 216–222.

Blakemore, S. J., Wolpert, D. M., & Frith, C. D. (2002). Abnormalities in the awareness of action. *Trends in Cognitive Sciences, 6,* 237–242.

Choi, H., & Scholl, B. J. (2006). Blindness to swapping features in simple dynamic events. *Journal of Vision, 6,* 299.

Cialdini, R. B., Borden, R. J., Thorne, A., Walker, M. L., Freeman, S., & Sloan, L. R. (1976). Basking in reflected glory: Three (football) field studies. *Journal of Personality and Social Psychology, 57,* 626–631.

Dehaene, S., Jobert, A., Naccache, L., Ciuciu, P., Poline, J. B., Le Bihan, D., et al. (2004). Letter binding and invariant recognition of masked words: Behavioral and neuroimaging evidence. *Psychological Science, 15,* 307–313.

Freyd, J. J., & Finke, R. A. (1984) Representational momentum. *Journal of Experimental Psychology: Learning, Memory, and Cognition, 10,* 126–132.

Gilbert, D. T., Pelham, B. W., & Krull, D. S. (1988). On cognitive busyness: When person perceivers meet persons perceived. *Journal of Personality & Social Psychology, 54,* 733–740.

Grillon, C., Lissek, S., Rabin, S., McDowell, D., Dvir, S., & Pine, D. S. (2008). Increased anxiety during anticipation of unpredictable but not predictable aversive stimuli as a psychophysiologic marker of panic disorder. *American Journal of Psychiatry, 165*, 898–904.

Grill-Spector, K., Kushnir, R., Edelman, S., Avidan, G., Itzchak, Y., & Malach, R. (1999). Differential processing of objects under various viewing conditions in the human lateral occipital complex. *Neuron, 24*, 187–220.

Grill-Spector, K., Henson, R., & Martin, A. (2006). Repetition and the brain: Neural models of stimulus-specific effects. *Trends in Cognitive Sciences, 10*, 14–23.

Haggard, P. (2005). Conscious intention and motor cognition. *Trends in Cognitive Sciences, 9*, 290–295.

Haggard, P., & Clark, S. (2003). Intentional action: Conscious experience and neural prediction. *Consciousness and Cognition, 12*, 695–707.

Haggard, P. (2008). Human volition: towards a neuroscience of will. *Nature Reviews Neuroscience, 9*, 934–946.

Henson, R. N. (2003). Neuroimaging studies of priming. *Progress in Neurobiology, 70*, 53–81.

Ito, M., Tamura, H., Fujita, I., & Tanaka, K. (1995). Size and position invariance of neuronal responses in monkey inferotemporal cortex. *Journal of Neurophysiology, 73*, 218–226.

James, W. (1890). *The principles of psychology* (vol. 1). New York: Henry Holt.

Jenkins, A. C., Macrae, C. N., & Mitchell, J. P. (2008). Repetition suppression of ventromedial prefrontal activity during judgments of self and others. *Proceedings of the National Academy of Sciences, 105*, 4507–4512.

Johansson, P., Hall, L., Sikstrom, S., & Olsson, A. (2005). Failure to detect mismatches between intention and outcome in a simple decision task. *Science, 310*, 116–119.

Kassin, S., & Kiechel, K. (1996). The social psychology of false confessions: Compliance, internalization, and confabulation. *Psychological Science, 7*, 125–128.

Kilner, J. M., Friston K. J., & Frith, C. D. (2007). Predictive coding: An account of the mirror neuron system. *Cognitive Processing, 8*, 159–166.

Lau, H. C., Rogers, R. D., & Passingham, R. E. (2007). Manipulating the experienced onset of intention after action execution. *Journal of Cognitive Neuroscience, 19*, 1–10.

Libet, B. (1993). *Neurophysiology of consciousness: Selected papers and new essays by Benjamin Libet.* Boston: Birkhäuser.

Loftus, E. (1993). The reality of repressed memories. *American Psychologist, 48*, 518–537.

Lueschow, A., Miller, E. K., & Desimone, R. (1994). Inferior temporal mechanisms for invariant object recognition. *Cerebral Cortex, 5*, 523–531.

Mitchell, J. P., Banaji, M. R., & Macrae, C. N. (2005). The link between social cognition and self-referential thought in the medial prefrontal cortex. *Journal of Cognitive Neuroscience, 17*, 1306–1315.

Moore, J., & Haggard, P. (2008). Awareness of action Inference and prediction. *Consciousness and Cognition, 17*, 136–144.

Nisbett, T. D., & Wilson, R. E. (1977). Telling more than we can know: Verbal reports on mental processes. *Psychological Review, 84*, 231–257.

Rainer, G., Rao, S. C., & Miller, E. K. (1999) Prospective coding for objects in the primate prefrontal cortex. *Journal of Neuroscience, 19*, 5493–5505.

Schacter, D. L., & Addis, D. R. (2007). The cognitive neuroscience of constructive memory: Remembering the past and imagining the future. *Philosophical Transactions of the Royal Society B, 362*, 773–786.

Schacter, D. L., & Buckner, R. L. (1998). Priming and the brain. *Neuron, 20*, 185–195.

Schooler, J. (2002). Re-representing consciousness: Dissociations between experience and metaconsciousness. *Trends in Cognitive Sciences, 6*, 339–344.

Shor, R. E., & Orne, E. C. (1962). *Harvard Group Scale of Hypnotic Susceptibility: Form A.* Palo Alto, CA: Consulting Psychologists Press.

Soon, C. S., Brass, M., Heinze, H.-J., & Haynes, J. D. (2008). Unconscious determinants of free decisions in the human brain. *Nature Neuroscience, 11*, 543–545.

Watanabe, M., Hikosaka, K., Sakagami, M., & Shirakawa, S. (2002). Coding and monitoring of motivational context in the primate prefrontal cortex. *Journal of Neuroscience, 22*, 2391–2400.

Wegner, D. M. (2002). *The illusion of conscious will.* Cambridge, MA: MIT Press.

Wegner, D. M., Fuller, V. A., & Sparrow, B. (2003). Clever hands: Uncontrolled intelligence in facilitated communication. *Journal of Personality and Social Psychology, 85*, 5–19.

Wegner, D. M., Sparrow, B., & Winerman, L. (2004). Vicarious agency: Experiencing control over the movements of others. *Journal of Personality and Social Psychology, 86,* 838–848.

Wegner, D. M., & Wheatley, T. P. (1999). Apparent mental causation: Sources of the experience of will. *American Psychologist, 54,* 480–492.

Wegner, D. & Wheatley, T. The exclusivity of will. Unpublished data.

Weiss, J. M. (1970). Effects of coping behavior in different warning signal conditions on stress pathology in rats. *Journal of Comparative and Physiological Psychology, 72,* 153–160.

Wheatley, T. (2009). Everyday confabulation. In B. Hirstein (Ed.), *Confabulation: Views from neuroscience, psychiatry, psychology, and philosophy* (pp. 205–225). Oxford: Oxford University Press.

Wheatley, T., Weisberg, J., Beauchamp, M. S., & Martin, A. (2005). Automatic priming of semantically related words reduces activity in the fusiform gyrus. *Journal of Cognitive Neuroscience, 17,* 1871–1885.

Wiggs, C. L., & Martin, A. (1998). Properties and mechanisms of perceptual priming. *Current Opinion in Neurobiology, 8,* 227–233.

# CHAPTER 14

# The Phenomenology of Agency and the Libet Results

*Terry Horgan*

Benjamin Libet became justly famous for his experimental finding that the experienced moment of action-commencement, as reported by his experimental subjects, typically was later in time than the time at which a readiness potential for the action was detectable in a subject's motor cortex. Daniel Wegner and others have since reported similar results. Wegner maintains, largely on the basis of such findings, that the experience of conscious will is an illusion—i.e., that humans do not really initiate their behavior by means of consciously willing it. Do Libet-style experimental results constitute strong evidence for Wegner's contention? I am among those who maintain that the answer is No. Here I will set forth my reasons for this claim—reasons that turn largely on considerations somewhat different from those usually emphasized by skeptics about the import of the Libet data.

I will focus mainly on the phenomenal character of agentive experience—i.e., what it is like to experience oneself as the conscious author of one's behavior.[1] Experiences with this distinctive kind of "what-it's-like-ness," have *representational content*—i.e., they represent oneself, to oneself, as *willfully generating* one's actions. I maintain, and will here assume, that the representational content of agentive experience is determined by its phenomenal character.[2]

My principal argument will take this form: the representational content of act-commencement experience, as determined by the phenomenal character of such experience, is quite *compatible* with the possibility that action-triggering neural activity in the motor cortex is already occurring at a point in time prior to the onset of the experience of conscious act-commencement; hence, even if one were to grant (at least for the sake of argument) that the work of Libet and others really does establish that the acts experienced as willfully produced are causally initiated by brain-events that occur prior to the experienced onset of act-commencement, this presumptive fact would *not* show that the experience of conscious will is an illusion.

## 1. INTROSPECTION AND THE PHENOMENOLOGY OF AGENCY[3]

Direct your introspective attention to your own agentive experience. What do you find it to be like? Suppose that you deliberately perform an action (or anyway you have an experience as of doing so)—say, holding up your right hand and closing your fingers into a fist. What is your experience like? To begin with, there is of course the purely behavioral aspect of the phenomenology—the what-it's-like of being visually and kinesthetically presented with your own right hand rising and its fingers moving into clenched position. But there is more to it than that, of course, because you are experiencing this bodily motion *as your own action*.

In order to help bring into focus this specifically actional phenomenological dimension of the experience, it will be helpful to approach it in a negative/contrastive way, via some observations about what the experience is *not* like.

For example, it is certainly not like this: first experiencing an occurrent wish for your right hand to rise and your fingers to move into clenched position, and then passively experiencing your hand and fingers moving in just that way. Such phenomenal character might be called *the phenomenology of fortuitously appropriate bodily motion*. It would be very strange indeed, and very alien.

Nor is the actional phenomenological character of the experience like this: first experiencing an occurrent wish for your right hand to rise and your fingers to move into clenched position, and then having an overall causal-process experience whose etiological dimension is exclusively as-of this occurrent wish-state causing your hand to rise and your fingers to move into clenched position. Such phenomenal character might be called *the exclusively state-causal phenomenology of the mental etiology of bodily motion*.[4] People often do experience state-causal processes *as* state-causal processes, of course: the collision of a moving billiard ball with a motionless billiard ball is experienced as causing the latter ball's subsequent motion; the impact of the leading edge of an avalanche with a tree in its path is experienced as causing the tree to become uprooted; and so on. Sometimes, too, people experience state-causal processes as occurring within themselves—and, furthermore, the etiological dimension of the experience is *exclusively* as-of state-causation. This is what it is like, for instance, when one experiences one's body falling to the ground as a result of one's having just tripped over an unnoticed log. But it seems patently clear that one does not normally experience one's own actions in that way; i.e., the etiological aspect of agentive experience is not exclusively as-of the state-causal generation of bodily changes by occurrent mental states, where both cause and effect happen to be states of oneself rather than states of external objects.[5] That too would be a strange and alienating sort of experience.

How, then, should one characterize the agentive phenomenal dimension of the act of raising one's hand and clenching one's fingers, given that it is not the phenomenology of fortuitously appropriate bodily motion, and it also is not the exclusively state-causal phenomenology of the mental etiology of bodily motion? Well, it is the what-it's-like of *self as source* of the motion. You experience your arm, hand, and fingers as being moved *by you yourself*—rather than experiencing their motion either as fortuitously moving just as you want them to move, or experiencing their etiology exclusively as a matter of their being caused by your own mental states. You experience the bodily motion as generated by *yourself*.

The language of causation-by-self seems apt here too: you experience your behavior as caused by you yourself. Metaphysical libertarians about human freedom—i.e., advocates of the doctrine that free will is both real and incompatible with state-causal determinism—sometimes speak of "agent causation" (or "immanent causation"), and such terminology seems phenomenologically appropriate regardless of what one thinks about the intelligibility or credibility of metaphysical libertarianism.[6] Chisholm (1964/2004) famously argued that immanent causation (as he called it) is a distinct species of causation from event causation (or "transeunt" causation, as he called it). But he later changed his mind (Chisholm, 1995), arguing instead that agent-causal "undertakings" (as he called them) are actually a species of event-causation themselves—albeit a very different species from ordinary, nomically governed, event causation. Phenomenologically speaking, there is indeed something episodic—something temporally located, and thus "event-ish"—about experiences of self-as-source. Thus, the expression "state causation" works better than "event causation" as a way of expressing the way behaviors are not presented to oneself in agentive experience. Although agentive experience is indeed "event-ish" in the sense that one experiences oneself as undertaking to perform actions at specific moments in time, this temporally specific etiological aspect does not consist exclusively (or perhaps even partially) in experiencing one's behavior as caused by *states* of oneself—not even momentary, episodic, states. The experience as-of *me* now commencing to raise my arm and close my fist is palpably different in kind from an experience exclusively as-of the *state-causal* mental generation (perhaps by short-lived mental states, also naturally characterized as "events") of the movement of my arm and hand.[7]

The self-as-source aspect of experience is ubiquitously familiar, since it is a phenomenological dimension of virtually all ordinary agentive experience. And some features of it seem introspectively self-evident: for instance, it obviously is not the phenomenology of fortuitous bodily motion, nor the exclusively state-causal phenomenology of the mental etiology of bodily motion. These introspectively self-evident facts will be important below.

On the other hand, I maintain—and elsewhere have argued at some length—that *some* important questions about the nature of agentive phenomenology are ones whose answers are not directly and reliably available to introspection (Horgan, 2007a, 2007b, in press). One such question is this: Does agentive experience represent one's behavior as *not state-caused*? You might think that the answer to this question is indeed available to introspection, and is obviously "Yes." But I claim that this would be a mistake. Although it is indeed introspectively obvious that agentive experience, in its etiological aspect, does *not* exclusively represent one's behavior *as state-caused*, introspection alone does not reliably reveal whether or not agentive experience also represents behavior *as not state-caused*. (Maybe, for instance, agentive experience is just representationally *noncommittal* about whether or not the behaviors one experiences as one's own actions are state-caused. But even if it is representationally committal on the matter, the point is that one cannot reliably ascertain such a commitment just by introspectively attending to one's own agentive experience.)

Another pertinent introspective limitation concerns matters of temporal simultaneity. Often one does not notice any time-lag between different aspects of experience—say, a lag between one's visual experience of someone's mouth moving in pronunciation of a certain word and one's auditory experience of that very word. But can one reliably ascertain, by introspection alone, whether or not one's sensory experience literally represents the two phenomena *as simultaneous*, as opposed (say) to merely *not* representing them as *nonsimultaneous*? Arguably, no. There is no good reason to think that introspection is that powerful.[8]

So introspection is potentially important in two ways to the interpretation of the Libet results—first because of what introspection reliably reveals about agentive experience, and second because of the limits of introspection concerning certain other aspects of agentive experience and also concerning matters such as the representation of temporal sequencing.

## 2. A POTENTIAL DEFLATIONARY CONSTRUAL OF THE LIBET RESULTS

According to what I will call "the standard construal" of the data obtained in the Libet paradigm, such data shows that action-initiating motor-cortex activity occurs earlier in time than the onset of conscious act-commencement experience. My main concern in this paper is to argue that even if the standard construal is correct, this would not constitute strong evidence for Wegner's claim that humans do not really initiate their behavior by means of consciously willing it. But before proceeding to that, let me briefly describe a way of calling the standard construal into doubt: a potential deflationary construal of the Libet results that seems fairly plausible, and that differs in important respects from other kinds of deflationary construals often discussed in the literature.

The proposed interpretation goes as follows: Libet-style experiments require subjects to do some self-monitoring of their own conscious act-commencement; typically they are asked to pay attention to when they decide to undertake the relevant action (e.g., a wrist flexing)—say, by noticing the time displayed on a moving clock-face at the moment of conscious act-commencement. Perhaps the conscious registering of a conscious act-commencement is a process that itself *takes time*—so that there is a brief time lag between (a) the conscious act-commencement itself, and (b) the higher-order conscious registering of that first-order conscious act-commencement.[9] The higher-order conscious registering need not occur simultaneously with the occurrence of the first-order conscious state itself. Also, a brief time lag could occur without being consciously noticed or introspectively accessible—just as, for instance, an unnoticed time lag could occur between a visual lip-moving experience and an associated auditory word-hearing experience. If there is such an unnoticed time lag, then what the subject's report really indicates is not the moment of conscious act-commencement itself, but rather the moment of conscious *registering* of the conscious act-commencement. And in that case, it is entirely possible that the conscious act-commencement—as distinct from the conscious registering thereof—occurs temporally prior to the occurrence of the readiness potential (the RP) in the motor cortex. That is, perhaps the conscious act-commencement is a *common cause* of both the RP and the agent's conscious registering of the conscious act-commencement.[10] (On this account the RP, which certainly is causally operative in producing the act, is temporally intermediate between the conscious act-commencement and the act itself; and the RP might, or might not, be an intermediate link in the causal chain leading from the conscious act-commencement to the subsequent conscious registering of the conscious act-commencement.)

Under this construal of the data, the experience of conscious will is veridical in representing one's action, to oneself, as having been brought about by one's consciously willing it—even though subjects are systematically slightly mistaken about when the experience occurs. On one variant of the account, there is no experiential illusion at all; rather, there is just a slightly mistaken *judgment*, based on a failure to notice a subtle time lag in one's experience. On a different variant, there is indeed a slight experiential illusion: the higher-order monitoring-experience represents the first-order conscious experience as occurring slightly later than when it actually occurs. But on neither version is the first-order experience an illusion *itself*; rather, people really are conscious authors of their own actions, just as they experience themselves to be.[11]

I leave it to those with expertise in the relevant neuroscience to assess the merits of this potential deflationary construal of the Libet data, including the comparative merits of the two alternative variants of it.[12] As a philosopher, I have three principal comments about it. First, it describes a perfectly coherent-looking logical possibility. Second, this possibility is largely overlooked in the literature I am familiar with concerning the Libet results. Third, the possibility should *not* be overlooked; on the contrary, it should be explicitly assessed for neurophysiological plausibility.

Having described this potential way of giving the Libet data a deflationary construal, let me now set it aside. For the remainder of the paper I will suppose, at least for argument's sake, that the standard construal is correct—i.e., that the RP causally instigates the act that the agent experiences as being under conscious control, and that the RP starts earlier in time than the agent's own experience of consciously undertaking the act.[13] I will argue that this standard construal of the Libet data need not conflict with the phenomenologically constituted representational content of agentive experience—and, moreover, that a good case can be made for taking as the default presumption that there is no genuine conflict at all. According to such a default assumption, conscious agentive experience is not illusory.

## 3. WEGNER ON THE EXPERIENCE OF CONSCIOUS WILL

Daniel Wegner is perhaps the best-known contemporary proponent of the claim that the experience of conscious will is an illusion. He offers a range of arguments in support of this claim in his influential book *The Illusion of Conscious Will*. To my mind, the strongest of these arguments appeals to the standard construal of Libet-style experimental data, including such data obtained by Wegner himself and his collaborators. He summarizes the standard construal this way: "The conscious willing of finger movement occurred at a significant interval *after* the onset of the RP but also at a significant interval *before* the actual finger movement" (p. 53).

But when one scrutinizes carefully Wegner's argument from the standard construal to the conclusion that conscious will is an illusion, one finds that it depends heavily on a dubious phenomenological characterization of the experience of conscious will itself, which goes as follows:

> Will is experienced as a result of an interpretation of the *apparent* link between the conscious thoughts that appear in association with action and the nature of the observed action. *Will is experienced as the result of self-perceived mental causation.* (pp. 65–66)

Wegner is saying, I take it, that the experience of conscious will is entirely a matter of experiencing an apparent *state-causal* link between one's conscious thoughts and the observed action. In light of my own discussion of the phenomenology of agentive experience in section 1 above, it should be clear what the problem is. An experience of the kind Wegner describes would be quite different from an agentive ordinary experience. Rather than being an experience of the *self* as source of the action (as is actual agentive phenomenology), instead it would be what I earlier called "the exclusively state-causal phenomenology of the mental etiology of bodily motion." People do occasionally have experiences of this latter kind—for instance, when one experiences one's fear causing one's body to tremble, or one's embarassment causing one's face to feel hot with blushing. But the bodily changes involved in these cases are not experienced as one's own *actions*.

Let me be clear. I am not denying that there is something temporally specific, something "event-ish," about the experience of willfully undertaking an act. On the contrary, normally one does experience oneself as beginning to actively undertake one's action at some specific moment in time. My point is rather this: this temporally located experience is as-of *oneself* undertaking the behavior, rather than being, in its etiological aspect, the exclusively state-causal phenomenology as-of certain *mental states* of oneself triggering the behavior.

That is a difference that potentially matters enormously, concerning the question whether humans really initiate their behavior by consciously willing it. On one hand, suppose it were really true that agentive experience is exclusively as-of one's thoughts state-causally triggering one's behavior. Then the veridicality of such experience would indeed be seriously called into question by the standard construal of the Libet results: the internal states that really state-causally initiate the behavior would be occuring earlier in time than do the pertinent mental states, and this presumably would mean that these mental states themselves are just epiphenomenal vis-à-vis the onset of action. The experience of agency would represent one's acts as state-causally triggered by one's own mental states, whereas in reality they are not triggered that way at all. So, the experience of conscious will would indeed be an illusion.

On the other hand, suppose I am right that agentive experience is *not* the exclusively state-causal phenomenology of the mental etiology of bodily motion. Then the Libet results might not directly threaten the veridicality of agentive experience at all. For, the possibility now arises that the representational content of a self-as-source experience—including the temporal aspect whereby one experiences oneself as willfully commencing one's act *just now*—is compatible with the presence of act-generating state-causes that occur temporally prior to the onset of the self-as-source experience.[14] In the next two sections I will describe two respective ways in which this possibility could be realized.

## 4. STANDING INTENTIONS AND THEIR IMPLEMENTATION

An important feature of the psychological situation of subjects in Libet-style experiments is this: both before they perform the specified action (say, wrist-flexing) and when they actually do perform it, they *consciously intend* to perform that act at some time or other within a short time-interval (say, roughly one minute as indicated by a moving second-hand on a clock) after the experimental trial commences. This conscious mental state is a *standing* intention, in the sense that it persists through time rather than being fleeting and momentary. Also important is the fact that this standing intention is (as per the experimenters' instructions) *temporally nonspecific*: there is no specific upcoming moment (say, the moment when the second hand will reach a specific location on the clock-face) such that the agent's standing intention is to perform the act at *that* moment. Rather, the standing intention is to perform the act *spontaneously*, at some not-previously-selected moment within a short-term time-interval after the experimental trial commences.

This standing intention figures psychologically in the state-causal etiology of the subject's specific action, even though it does not by itself suffice to constitute a state-causal "trigger" of the action. Some additional, momentary, state of the mind/brain *implements* this standing intention, by state-causally triggering a wrist-flexing at some moment within the temporal interval associated with the intention. Perhaps the triggering-episode is an unconscious *mental* state—one that initiates a state-causal chain that includes the RP in the motor cortex as an intermediate link, and leads to the action. Or perhaps the triggering-episode is a brain-event that is not itself mental at all—maybe the RP itself, or maybe a (nonmental) brain-event that state-causes the RP (which in turn is a more proximal state-causal trigger of the behavior).

What is the state-causal etiological role of the standing intention? The specific answer to this question depends on various empirical facts about how mentality gets physically realized by brain activity. However, the following generic picture looks very plausible, regardless of how the neurophysiological details might go. The *onset* of the standing intention instigates a process P in the brain whereby a triggering-episode that generates a wrist-flexing will happen some time in roughly the next minute, provided that P evolves unimpeded. Furthermore, the *persistence* of the standing intention is a background condition for the unimpeded evolution of process P; i.e., were the intention to be no longer present, then P would thereby get truncated.[15]

As long as the standing intention plays the kind of role just described, it seems clearly correct to say that the action occurs *because of the intention*—where the operative sense of "because" is a state-causal sense. Standing conditions can perfectly well play a state-causal role of the kind just sketched, even though a triggering-episode needs to enter in at some moment too.

Suppose, then, that in the Libet paradigm, the following circumstances all obtain. First, the agent's standing intention to flex her wrist within a given one-minute interval *does* play the kind of state-causal role just described. Second, this standing intention gets implemented by a triggering-episode E that occurs at a time t, prior to the moment t+δ at which the agent begins to have the experience of undertaking the wrist-flexing. And third, once the agent does begin to have self-as-source phenomenology vis-à-vis wrist-flexing, the persistence of this phenomenology thereafter figures causally as a *sustaining condition* for the completion of the action; were the conscious-will phenomenology to be no longer present, prior to the completion of the action, this circumstance would tend to squelch the action.[16] (The third condition is closely related to Libet's own idea of a "veto response." I say that cessation of conscious-will experience vis-à-vis the action would *tend* to squelch it because in some cases the completion of the action might occur so quickly that a momentarily prior cessation of conscious-will experience, and/or a momentarily prior veto response, cannot stop it.)

Is more than this required, in order for the experience of conscious will in the Libet paradigm to count as veridical rather than illusory? In particular, does veridicality also require that the onset of agentive phenomenology is *itself* the triggering-episode that implements the agent's standing wrist-flexing intention? It is entirely possible, I submit, that the answer is No—i.e., that the etiological dimension of the experience of *commencing* an action does not involve, either wholly or in part, an experience as-of this commencing-episode *state-causally triggering* the action.

I am here using the expression "entirely possible" in an epistemological sense. The claim I mean to be making is that one here encounters yet another limitation in the powers of introspection with respect to agentive phenomenology, alongside the other kinds of limitation discussed earlier. I submit that one just cannot reliably determine, by direct introspection alone, whether or not one's experience as-of *undertaking* an action is also an experience as-of this very undertaking-episode being a *state-causal trigger* of the action.

Suppose that the undertaking-experience is not itself experientially represented as a state-causal trigger of the action. In that case, there is no particularly good reason why the undertaking-experience would need to *be* the state-causal trigger of the action, in order for one's experience of conscious will to be veridical. On the contrary, the default presumption should be that veridicality really only requires the other circumstances mentioned above: a standing intention that initiates and causally sustains a process leading to an unconscious episode that implements that very intention, together with subsequent agentive phenomenology that itself causally sustains the completion of the action. This should be the default presumption about veridicality requirements because it is theoretically more conservative, and because it better accommodates agentive phenomenology. It is theoretically more conservative because it deploys fewer hypotheses; specifically, it eschews the hypothesis that the onset of action-commencing experience is itself represented, in one's overall experience, as a state-causal trigger of one's action. And it better accommodates agentive phenomenology because it treats that phenomenology as being normally veridical, rather than as being systematically illusory.

So here is where we have gotten to, dialectically. First is a claim about the limits of introspection: one cannot reliably tell, just by means of direct introspective attention to one's phenomenology, whether or not the onset of action-commencement experience is itself experientially represented as state-causally triggering the action. Second is a claim about epistemic possibility: it is therefore entirely possible—i.e., it is a live and viable epistemic possibility—that the onset of action-commencement experience is *not* experientially represented as state-causally triggering the action. Third is a conditional claim (labeled "C" for "conditional"):

> (C) *If* the onset of action-commencement experience is not experientially represented as state-causally triggering the action, *then* even if the standard construal of the Libet data is correct, nevertheless the default presumption is that the experience of conscious will is not illusory, for subjects in the Libet-style experimental paradigm.

So the upshot, so far, is this: it is entirely possible—it is a live epistemic possibility—that the experience of conscious will is not illusory, even if the standard construal of the Libet data is correct.

This conclusion can be strengthened. There is a good case to be made in support of the following claim (labeled "N" for "negative"):

> (N) The onset of action-commencement experience is not experientially represented as state-causally triggering the action.

Even though one cannot reliably tell whether (N) is true or false just by direct introspective attention to agentive phenomenology, this certainly does not preclude the possibility of garnering other kinds of evidence for or against it. One kind of evidence is itself phenomenological: viz., other aspects of agentive phenomenology that on one hand seem to reveal themselves quite clearly in introspection, and on the other hand are evidentially relevant to (N). Let me mention some pertinent phenomenological data, and then explain why that data abductively supports (N).[17]

A ubiquitous feature of ordinary agentive phenomenology is the aspect of *freedom*—the experience of oneself as freely willing to undertake one's action, and as freely willing one's continuation of the action, and (echoes again of Libet's "veto response") as being capable of freely willing to abort it prior to its completion. On the other hand, paradigmatic experiences of state-causation seem fairly clearly to lack any such aspect of freedom; rather, the effect is experienced either (i) as being outright *necessitated* (given the circumstances) by its state-cause, or at any rate (ii) as being rendered *probable* (given the circumstances) by its state-cause in such a way that nonoccurrence of the effect-event would have been a matter of *chance* rather than an exercise of agentive freedom. (Recall my earlier examples of experiences of mental state-causation: fear causing trembling, and embarassment causing felt blushing.) This very striking phenomenological contrast between ordinary agentive experience on one hand, and paradigmatic experiences of state-causation on the other hand, is best explained by hypothesis (N): part of what it is for one's action to be experientially represented as *free* is for the action *not* to be experientially represented as *state-caused*.[18] So there is a heavy additional burden of proof on someone who would deny (N) and would claim instead that the onset of action-commencement experience *is* experientially represented as state-causally triggering the action—viz., the burden of explaining how and why this kind of alleged experiential representation as-of state-causation could deviate so far, and so dramatically, from *paradigmatic* state-cause experiences. Ceteris paribus, and in the absence of a plausible and well-motivated way of discharging that explanatory burden, inference to the best explanation favors hypothesis (N): the best explanation for this striking contrast between agentive experience and paradigmatic experiences of state-causation is that the experience of *undertaking* an action simply is not itself experientially represented as a *state-causal trigger* of the action. Self-as-source experience is suffused with the phenomenological aspect of freedom—an aspect not present in experiences of state-causation, and an aspect whose presence requires that one's overall agentive experience not represent one's action as being state-caused by the episodic experience of act-undertaking. The experience is as-of *you* bringing about the act (and doing so freely)—not as-of your act-undertaking episode being a state-causal trigger of the act.[19]

So there is strong—albeit abductive and hence nondemonstrative—evidence in support of (N). And there are also good methodological grounds, as explained above, for accepting the conditional claim (C). From (C) and (N) together, we obtain the following conclusion (by the deductive principle of inference *modus ponens*). Even if the standard construal of the Libet data is correct, nevertheless the default presumption is that the experience of conscious will is not illusory, for subjects in the Libet-style experimental paradigm.[20]

## 5. BEYOND STANDING INTENTIONS

In the Libet paradigm itself, the subject has a standing intention to perform a specific act spontaneously at some random moment in the short-term future. On a conservative version of the standard construal of the Libet data, the scope of the standard construal is confined to situations of that kind. But such data is often taken to support a much more liberal version of the standard construal, asserting that *in general* people's actions are triggered by an RP that temporally precedes the onset of the experience of consciously willing the action. What might be said about this liberal version, given that it includes actions not covered by my discussion in section 4?

The first thing to say is that Libet-style data by itself provides very little evidence for the liberal construal. Subjects in the Libet paradigm always are acting in accordance with a preformed standing intention, which means that data from the paradigm provides no good reason at all for extrapolating any conclusions about cases where such a standing intention is absent. This fact seems to be seriously underappreciated, and sometimes overlooked altogether, by those who take the Libet results to provide good evidence for the claim that the experience of conscious will is *generally*—maybe even always—an illusion.

Suppose, however, that there were to arise convincing empirical evidence for the following claim (labeled "PCC" for "pre-conscious causation"):

> (PCC) Often (or typically, or always), even in the absence of a pre-formed standing intention, an act-initiating readiness potential occurs in the brain's motor strip at a moment t that is temporally prior to the moment t+δ at which the conscious agent first has an act-undertaking experience.

Would strong empirical evidence for (PCC) constitute good evidence that the experience of conscious will is often (or typically, or always) an illusion?

No. For, there would remain a live, and prima facie quite plausible, epistemic possibility about what goes on in these cases that would be compatible with the claim that the experience of conscious will is veridical (rather than illusory). Unless and until good evidence could be provided *against* this possibility, it would count as the most credible default hypothesis (by inference to the best explanation). And this would mean that evidence for (PCC), by itself, simply would not provide strong support for the hypothesis that the experience of conscious will is illusory. Good evidence would have to be provided *against* the default hypothesis, before the evidence for (PCC) could count as providing strong support for the illusion hypothesis.

The possible scenario I have in mind, for how (PCC) might be true without the experience of conscious will being illusory, involves the following multistep etiology of an action. First is the act-initiating episode, which is the occurrence of an *unconscious* mental state—for instance, a total mental state comprising an unconscious *wish* for a certain outcome, together with an unconscious *thought* that such-and-such an act would bring about that outcome.[21] Second is the readiness potential (RP) in the motor strip; this RP is itself state-caused by the act-initiating unconscious mental state, and in turn the RP state-causes the initial portion of the bodily motion constituting the action. Third is the experience of conscious will vis-à-vis the action, which has the following features: (i) it is caused by the temporally prior unconscious mental state that triggered the action; (ii) it replicates the doxastic and conative content of the unconscious state, but now consciously (rather than unconsciously) and with the attendant phenomenal aspect of self-as-source; and (iii) the persistence of this agentive phenomenology thereafter figures causally as a *sustaining condition* for the completion of the action (so, were the conscious-will phenomenology to be no longer present, prior to the completion of the action, this circumstance would tend to squelch the action).[22]

Let the hypothesis of *unconscious psychological state-causal act-initiation* (the UPSCAI hypothesis) be the assertion that in cases that conform to (PCC), the action is produced in the manner just described. Two claims about this hypothesis both look very plausible. First, if indeed there are actions that conform to (PCC), then these actions also conform to the UPSCAI hypothesis. Second, for any action that conforms to the UPSCAI hypothesis, the agent's experience of conscious will is veridical—rather than illusory. Let me take up these claims in turn.

If everyday actions sometimes (or always) conform to (PCC), then there are some striking facts about such actions that need explaining. One such fact is that the acts are experienced by the agent not as arising "out of the blue," but rather as being in accord with the agent's ongoing sense of what she is doing and why. A second, related, fact is that "intentions in action" (as they are called in Searle, 1983) are also experienced not as arising "out of the blue," but rather as cohering well with the agent's own longer-term goals, desires, and beliefs. And a third fact is that such behavior typically makes good sense, from the perspective of external observers. Why should all this be so, for actions that conform to (PCC)? One hypothesis is that it is the product of massive, self-deceptive, confabulation: bodily motions really are triggered by motor activity in the motor cortex, but once they commence they are then consciously interpreted by the agent in a confabulational way. The real reasons for the agent's behavior are quite unrelated to the reasons that the agent *thinks* motivate the behavior. Amazingly enough, people's bodily motions happen to systematically lend themselves to such confabulatory interpretation as purposive actions, both from the perspective of the agent and from the perspective of external observers—even though the bodily motions always really are state-causally triggered in ways that have absolutely nothing to do with an agent's goals, beliefs, or other psychological states![23]

Well, if you believe *that*, then perhaps I can sell you a fine pre-owned automobile that is up on blocks in my back yard. (Don't mind that it's a bit rusty.) There is another potential explanation that is vastly more theoretically economical, and hence vastly more plausible, viz., this: if there are actions conforming to (PCC), then they also conform to the UPSCAI hypothesis. That is, the actions are state-causally initiated by unconscious *psychological* states such as occurrent wishes and occurrent thoughts. These unconscious psychological states trigger the RP in the motor cortex, which in turn triggers the onset of action. And the unconscious psychological states also state-cause conscious agentive phenomenology which itself both (i) state-causally sustains the action through to completion, and (ii) incorporates in conscious form the psychological factors that initially were unconscious when they initiated the action.[24] On this alternative explanation, there is no need to treat as a massive coincidence the fact that people's actions typically make good sense, to themselves and to others; and there is no need to posit a massive psychological "confabulation mechanism" whereby people are constantly mistaken about why they behave the way they do.

So, inference to the best explanation strongly warrants the following hypothetical claim: *if* there are actions that conform to (PCC), *then* those actions conform to the UPSCAI hypothesis. Now comes this question: given that the UPSCAI hypothesis is true of those actions that conform to (PCC), is the experience of conscious will *veridical* in the case of such actions, or is it *illusory*? At this point, my reasoning in section 4 kicks in again, mutatis mutandis, in support of veridicality. The main difference is this. In section 4, I was allowing for the possibility that the RP in the motor strip is the state-causal episode that literally *initiates* the action. Even so, a pertinent psychological factor is state-causally involved anyway, in the etiology of the action—viz., the (conscious) standing intention to perform the act at some random moment during a given short-term time interval. (According to the model in section 4, recall, that standing intention is a background condition for the onset and persistence of the process in the brain leading up to the RP that triggers the action; the conscious intention *state-causally sustains* the brain process.) In the case of actions conforming to (PCC), on the other hand, there is not a conscious standing intention in play; rather, there is an unconscious, psychological, episode that state-causally initiates the act by initiating a state-causal chain in which the RP is an intermediate link. But, with that difference duly noted, my reasoning in section 4 can be directly adapted in support of this claim: in cases that conform both to (PCC) and to the UPSCAI hypothesis, the agent's experience of conscious will is veridical, not illusory.

To summarize this section: If there are actions that conform to (PCC), then they also conform to the UPSCAI hypothesis. For actions that conform to both (PCC) and the UPSCAI hypothesis, the experience of conscious will vis-à-vis such actions is veridical. Therefore, if there are actions that conform to (PCC), then the experience of conscious will vis-à-vis such actions is veridical.

## 6. CONCLUSION

The Libet data is striking and surprising, because nothing in agentive experience suggests it, and because the character of agentive experience easily fosters the belief that one's actions do not commence until one consciously wills them. But the fact that this data is striking and surprising hardly warrants concluding that the experience of conscious will is an illusion. For one thing, the possibility remains open that the first-order experience of conscious will occurs slightly earlier than does the higher-order conscious registering of that experience, and moreover that the first-order experience occurs prior to the occurrence of the RP in the motor strip. This possibility would need to get excluded by empirical investigation, before the standard construal of the Libet data could be considered secure. (And the numerous other challenges to the standard construal also would need to be satisfactorily answered, of course.) But even if the standard construal is correct, the experience of conscious will is very probably veridical anyway, rather than being an illusion. This is the lesson that emerges from abductive reasoning that assigns due and appropriate evidential significance to introspectively accessible facts about the phenomenology of agency, while at the same time also acknowledging and respecting the apparent limits of introspection.

## ACKNOWLEDGMENTS

For valuable feedback and discussion I thank audiences and discussion groups at "Toward a Science of Consciousness 2008" in Tucson (at the pre-conference workshop on Benjamin Libet), the Australian National University, and the University of Sydney. I also thank Dianne Horgan, Uriah Kriegel, Shaun Nichols, Adina Roskies, Jonathan Schaffer, Declan Smithies, Mark Timmons, and especially Walter Sinnott-Armstrong.

## NOTES

1. I will assume throughout that all behavior that one experiences as one's purposive action counts as exhibiting what Wegner calls "the experience of conscious will"—even if the action is spontaneous or routine. Wegner (2002) seems to me most plausibly interpreted this way. In any event, I think that my overall argument in this paper would still remain in force relative to a narrower interpretation of what Wegner means by "the experience of conscious will."
2. For some recent philosophical argumentation in support of the claim that *sensory* phenomenology is richly representational, see for instance Siegel (2005, 2006a, 2006b), and chapter 7 of Siewert (1998). For some recent argumentation specifically in support of the claim that *agentive* phenomenology is richly representational, see for instance Graham, Horgan, and Tienson (2007), Horgan (2007a, 2007b, in press), Horgan, Tienson, and Graham (2003, 2004), and Horgan and Tienson (2005).
3. In this section I draw freely on papers in note 2 of which I am author or coauthor.
4. This is a mouthful, but I am trying to be as accurate as I can in describing the kind of phenomenology I have in mind. Here and throughout I speak of "state-causation" rather than "event-causation." More presently on my reasons for this choice of terminology. States as here understood can be short-lived and episodic, and often when they are they also fall naturally under the rubric "event."
5. This leaves open the question whether or not the etiological aspect of agentive experience is *partly*—albeit not exclusively—as-of the mental state-causal generation of bodily behavior. Maybe it is, or maybe not. More below on this question.
6. Some readers might think that the metaphysical issue is the more important one, and indeed is the one to which the Libet data is mainly relevant—and hence that my present emphasis on the *phenomenology* of agentive experience is just misplaced. To my mind, such a thought would be confused—in at least two ways. First, if the fundamental question one is focusing upon is whether or not human actions are free in the metaphysical-libertarian way, then there is already an enormous body of scientific evidence suggesting that the answer is "No"—evidence to the effect that everything physical that happens in the brain and the body is the product of purely physical causes. The Libet data is a minor sideshow, compared to all that other evidence. Second, I submit that a principal reason one might be inclined to think that genuinely free action must conform to the heavyweight-libertarian conception is that one thinks—perhaps without putting it to oneself in just this way—that the phenomenology of agentive experience represents one's actions, to oneself, as generated in the metaphysical-libertarian way.
7. Some readers might think that I am really cheating here by using the term "state" rather than the term "event," despite what I say about short-lived states being naturally describable as "events." Why does it seem natural (such a reader might ask) to say, "I did it because I chose to do it"? Isn't such a choice an *event*, and isn't it being cited as *cause*? Well, to my ear such a response seems more vapid than natural: a natural response would be one that cites my *reason* for doing it, rather than citing some *event* that caused the behavior. And in any case, the fact that my choosing to do it occurred at some specific moment does not alter the fact that the behavior was experienced etiologically as being generated (at that moment) *by me myself*, rather than being exclusively experienced, etiologically, as being generated by some event *within* me.
8. Note well: I am not saying that there is no good reason to think that experience represents the two phenomena as simultaneous. Maybe it does, or maybe not. Rather, I am saying that there is no good reason to think that one's introspective capacities are so powerful that one can reliably ascertain, just by introspectively attending to one's experience, whether or not it represents the phenomena as simultaneous.
9. Relevant to this hypothesis is the question whether there are such time lags in the

conscious registering of other kinds of conscious experiences, such as sensations. If not, then that would be evidence against the hypothesis. On the other hand, there might be specific reasons, perhaps somehow associated with features of decision making that are not present in the passive registering of conscious sensory experience, why it would take longer to consciously register an experience of act-commencement than to consciously register a sensation.

10. Some readers might think that it makes no sense to construe a mental occurrence that has not yet been consciously registered or noticed as already being part of one's current phenomenal consciousness—i.e., part of the overall "what-it-is-like" of one's current experience. In my view, that thought is seriously mistaken. One's overall visual phenomenology, for example, can include features that are *present* in one's current visual conscious experience without being *noticed*. Take, for example, the phenomenon of "change blindness." One well-known visual display that typically induces change blindness consists of a repeating sequence of two alternating photos of a parked jet airliner, with passengers climbing steps and boarding it. Subjects typically stare at the sequence for a long while without noticing any difference between the two successive displays, even though in the center of one image there is an enormous engine attached to the jet's wing, whereas in the center of the other image there is no engine there. Although subjects typically do not initially notice this difference, I submit that it is just *wildly* implausible to claim that their visual phenomenology is the same when viewing each image. On the contrary, one visual experience is phenomenologically as-of a parked jet with an engine attached to its wing, whereas the other experience is phenomenologically as-of a parked jet without an engine attached to its wing, *even though this experiential difference is not initially noticed.*
11. It would be a methodologically subtle business to determine which variant is better. A key question here, not readily answerable by introspection alone, is whether one's overall, self-monitoring-infused, agentive phenomenology represents the first-order experience *as simultaneous* with the higher-order experience, as opposed to merely *not* representing these as *nonsimultaneous.* Recall my earlier remarks about the limitations of introspection about such matters.
12. See, in particular, the contribution by Adina Roskies to the present volume (Chapter 2).
13. Also, in section 3, I will follow the common practice in the literature of not distinguishing between two versions of the standard construal: a conservative version, which restricts itself to behavior performed under the relatively specific conditions of the Libet paradigm, and a liberal version, which takes the data to support the claim that actions in general are initiated by an RP that occurs prior to the onset of the experience of conscious will. In sections 4 and 5, however, the differences between these two versions of the standard construal will become salient and important.
14. A reader might object as follows: even if the agentive *experience* is not illusory, the Libet results would still undermine the widely held *belief* that people's conscious choices cause their actions—a belief that arguably is commonly held, and that arguably is essential to the law. I myself suspect, however, that this objection misstates what is commonly believed and what is essential to the law. The common belief—and the one that is really essential to the law—is that *persons* often bring about their own actions, via willful choice.
15. On an alternative potential variant of the picture I am sketching, process P could proceed ahead even if the standing intention has meanwhile faded, as long as no *contrary* intention has replaced it. That standing intention would still be implicated in the etiology of the action.
16. Conscious-will phenomenology could remain present, however, without remaining *salient*—e.g., because the agent becomes distracted while still (willfully) completing the action.
17. It should be noted that thesis (N) constitutes a negative answer to the question posed in note 5 above.
18. I hasten to reiterate a point I made earlier: *not* experientially representing an action *as state-caused* is different from, and weaker than, representing the action *as not state-caused.* It is obvious introspectively that agentive experience does not represent actions as *passively* state-caused—i.e., as state-caused by states of oneself other than the episode of one's own act-undertaking itself. But introspection alone cannot directly ascertain whether or not agentive

experience represents actions as *not* state-caused. And I have just been maintaining that introspection is evidently limited in another way too: introspection alone cannot reliably ascertain whether or not experiential episodes of act-undertaking are themselves represented in experience as state-causes of one's behavior. I am presently arguing for (N) not by claiming that its truth is directly manifest to introspection, but rather abductively, by inference to the best explanation. (N) explains why there is such a stark phenomenological contrast between agentive experience and paradigmatic experiences of state causation; more specifically, (N) best explains the aspect of freedom in agentive experience, an aspect which has no counterpart in paradigmatic experiences of state causation.

19. An issue now looming is whether the aspect of freedom is itself an illusion—and whether, if it is, then this is already enough to render the experience of conscious will illusory too (quite apart from the standard construal of the Libet data). Let me make just two brief remarks about this here. First, even if the freedom aspect is indeed illusory, this would not undermine my contention that hypothesis (N) better accommodates this feature of agentive experience than does the hypothesis that act-undertakings are experientially represented as state-causal triggers of one's behavior. Second, I have argued elsewhere that the aspect of freedom in agentive experience is not illusory (Horgan, 2007a, 2007b, in press).
20. I wasn't born yesterday. I fully expect that fans of the claim that conscious will is an illusion are apt to regard the argument in the present section as mere sophistry. Let me say that I, in turn, regard those fans as having a skewed epistemological sensibility that underwrites a tendency to leap much too quickly, and without sufficient evidence, to very radical conclusions. One person's mere sophistry is another person's reliance on epistemologically sound principles about how to reason from empirical evidence to theoretical hypotheses.
21. What justification could there be for positing these kinds of unconscious states, one might ask? The justification comes from the explanatory benefits of doing so—as explained presently.
22. Most real-life actions take time, and are physically constituted by complex temporal sequences of bodily activity. The RP could be a sufficient cause for the initial portion of such bodily activity, even if the phenomenology is a necessary condition for the completion of the whole sequence.
23. I do not mean to suggest that this hypothesis is explicitly, or even implicitly, advocated by any fans of the liberal version of the standard construal of the Libet data. I do mean to be underscoring, however, the explanatory burden they face—and how challenging it is to meet that burden plausibly.
24. The remarks in note 22 are again applicable here, concerning the idea that typically, agentive phenomenology state-causally sustains the act through to completion.

## REFERENCES


Chisholm, R. (1995). Agents, causes, and events: The problem of free will. In T. O'Connor (Ed.), *Agents, causes, and events: Essays on indeterminism and free will.* Oxford: Oxford University Press.

Chisholm, R. (2004). Human freedom and the self [Langley Lecture (University of Kansas), 1964]. Reprinted in J. Feinberg and R. Shafer-Langua (Eds.), *Reason and responsibility: Readings in some basic problems of philosophy* (12th ed., pp. 452–459). East Windsor, CT: Wadsworth Press.

Graham, G., Horgan, T., & Tienson, J. (2007). Consciousness and intentionality. In M. Velmans & S. Schneider (Eds.), *The Blackwell companion to consciousness* (pp. 468–484). Oxford: Blackwell.

Horgan, T. (2007a). Agentive phenomenal intentionality and the limits of introspection. *Psyche, 13*(2), 1–29.

Horgan, T. (2007b). Mental causation and the agent-exclusion problem. *Erkenntnis, 67,* 183–200.

Horgan, T. (in press). Causal compatibilism about agentive phenomenology. In T. Horgan, M. Sabatos & D. Sosa (Eds.), *Essays in honor of Jaegwon Kim.* Cambridge, MA: MIT Press.

Horgan, T., & Tienson, J. (2005). The phenomenology of embodied agency. In M. Saagua and F. de Ferro (Eds.), *A Explicacao da Interpretacao Humana: The explanation of human interpretation; Proceedings of the Conference Mind and Action III—May 2001* (pp. 415–423). Lisbon: Edicoes Colibri.

Horgan, T., Tienson, J., & Graham, G. (2003). The phenomenology of first-person agency. In S. Walter and H. D. Heckmann (Eds.), *Physicalism and mental causation: The metaphysics of mind and action* (pp. 323–340). Exeter, UK: Imprint Academic.

Horgan, T., Tienson, J., & Graham, G. (2004). Phenomenal intentionality and the brain in a vat. In R. Schantz (Ed.), *The externalist challenge* (pp. 297–317). Berlin: Walter de Gruyter.

Searle, J. (1983). *Intentionality: An essay in the philosophy of mind*. Cambridge, UK: Cambridge University Press.

Siegel, S. (2005). The contents of perception. *Stanford Encyclopedia of Philosophy*. http://plato.stanford.edu/entries/perception-contents/ Published Fri Mar 18, 2005

Siegel, S. (2006a). Which properties are represented in perception? In T. Gendler Szabo & J. Hawthorne (Eds.), *Perceptual experience*. Oxford: Oxford University Press.

Siegel, S. (2006b). Subject and object in the contents of visual experience. *Philosophical Review, 115*, 355–388.

Siewert, C. (1998). *The significance of consciousness*. Princeton, NJ: Princeton University Press.

Wegner, D. (2002). *The illusion of conscious will*. Cambridge, MA: MIT Press.

# CHAPTER 15

## The Threat of Shrinking Agency and Free Will Disillusionism

*Thomas Nadelhoffer*

> *The death of free will, or its exposure as a convenient illusion, some worry, could wreak havoc on our sense of moral and legal responsibility. According to those who believe that free will and determinism are incompatible . . . it would mean that people are no more responsible for their actions than asteroids or planets. Anything would go.*
>
> —Dennis Overbye, *The New York Times* (2007)

> *This is the excellent foppery of the world, that when we are sick in fortune, often the surfeits of our own behavior, we make guilty of our disasters the sun, the moon, and stars; as if we were villains on necessity; fools by heavenly compulsion; knaves, thieves, and treachers by spherical predominance; drunkards, liars, and adulterers by an enforced obedience of planetary influence; and all that we are evil in, by a divine thrusting on—an admirable evasion of whoremaster man, to lay his goatish disposition on the charge of a star.*
>
> —William Shakespeare, *King Lear* (1610/2005)

## INTRODUCTION

During the past few years the popular press has become increasingly interested in free will, agency, and responsibility, with stories appearing in mainstream media outlets such as *The New York Times*, *The Economist*, *Forbes Magazine*, *Wired*, and *FOX News*. As psychologists continue to demystify the mind by uncovering the mechanisms that undergird human behavior, what was once an issue that fell mostly under the purview of philosophers and theologians has started to pique the curiosity of the public more generally. This interest is quite understandable. If free will provides the foundation for our traditional moral beliefs and practices, and its existence is incompatible with the gathering data from the so-called "sciences of the mind," then free will isn't just a topic fit for philosophers—it is a psychological, sociological, cultural, and policy issue as well. To the extent that scientific advancements undermine or threaten our traditional views about human agency, we ought to carefully consider what impact this might have on our moral and legal practices.

In an attempt to address this issue, philosophers have recently begun thinking about what we ought to do in light of the gathering threats to human agency and responsibility. From Saul Smilansky's illusionism (2000, 2002) and Derk Pereboom's hard incompatibilism (2001) to Shaun Nichols's antirevolutionism (2007), one finds several novel attempts to wrestle with what we should to in the face of the possible "death of free will"—to borrow a phrase recently used in *The New York Times* by Dennis Overbye.[1] Given the timeliness, gravity, and complexity of the issues at stake, these philosophers are to be applauded for their efforts. However, I also believe that their respective views share one shortcoming—namely, each focuses primarily (if not exclusively) on the threat of determinism.

In this respect, I share Eddy Nahmias's view that the focus on determinism that is often the hallmark of the free will debate can lead us to overlook more pressing threats to agency coming from psychology that are orthogonal to worries about the fundamental laws of the universe, the general nature of causality, and other related issues (Nahmias, in press).

Whereas the traditional free will debate focused on the *free* part of "free will"—with an emphasis on alternative possibilities and the ability to do otherwise—many of the new threats from psychology pose potential problems for the *will* part as well. My primary goal in this paper is to shed some light on the nature of these potential psychological threats. In doing so, I first set the stage by explaining and clarifying some key terms and exploring some of the key issues from the free will debate (§1). Then, I examine several potential threats to free will that I am going to collectively call the *Threat of Shrinking Agency* (§2). In piecing this general threat together, I discuss the work of several prominent psychologists including Jonathan Bargh, Benjamin Libet, Daniel Wegner, and others. My goal is not to argue that these threats actually do undermine free will and responsibility. Trying to accomplish this admittedly difficult task is beyond the scope of the present essay. Instead, my aim is simply to trace the boundaries of the potential threats that I examine and to show that they are not dependent on other potential threats such as determinism, mechanism, reductionism, and the like. Having canvassed some of the salient research from psychology, I will then end by briefly lobbying for philosophers to take a more active role in the paradigm shift that I believe is already under foot. On my view, rather than marshaling our forces together to stem the spread of skepticism as some philosophers have suggested (e.g., Smilansky, 2000, 2002; Nichols, 2007), I believe that we should instead be active agents of disillusionment and change when it comes to traditional views about human agency (§3).

## 1. SETTING THE STAGE

The dominant issue in the free will debate has traditionally been whether free will and responsibility are compatible with determinism—i.e., the thesis that given the fixity of the past and the laws of nature, there is always only one possible future (Van Inwagen, 1983). The attempt to address the compatibility question has spawned a litany of positions.[2] Incompatibilists, for instance, run the gamut from pro–free will libertarians who suggest that we are unmoved movers (e.g., Chisholm, 1982) to free will skeptics who claim that we can't be free and responsible regardless of the truth of determinism (e.g., Strawson, 1986). A number of incompatibilists lie on a continuum between these two extremes. The two broadest pro–free will incompatibilist views are event-causal libertarianism (e.g., Ekstrom, 2000; Kane, 1996) and agent-causal libertarianism (e.g., Clarke, 1996, 2003; O'Connor, 1993, 2000)—each of which maintains that determinism is false and that human beings are (sometimes) free and morally responsible. Nonrealism about free will and moral responsibility, on the other hand, comes in several stripes as well (e.g., Double, 1991; Honderich, 1998; Smilansky, 2000, 2002; Pereboom, 2001; Sommers, 2007; Strawson, 1986)—some of which are driven by worries about determinism and some of which are not.

Predictably, there are just as many varieties of compatibilism. Compatibilists known as soft determinists, for instance, claim that free will and responsibility actually *require* determinism (e.g., Ayer, 1982; Stace, 1960). Most compatibilists, however, are merely committed to the weaker conditional view that we could be free even if determinism were true.[3] Of course, even this is an issue about which compatibilists disagree. Semicompatibilists, for instance, think that while determinism may very well preclude free will, it is does not undermine moral responsibility (e.g., Fischer 1994, 2007; Fischer & Ravizza, 1998). On this view, the latter does not require us to have alternative possibilities. Instead, moral responsibility merely requires us to have the capacity for understanding and acting (or not) upon moral reasons. If this were correct, free will would not be a necessary condition for responsibility—which is something most compatibilists would deny. But despite their differences, semicompatibilists and compatibilists agree that we could be morally responsible even if determinism is true.

Given that the free will literature is a vast and tangled web, a few more clarifications are in order before we examine the data from psychology.[4] First, when talking about the kind of free will that is at stake between the fighting factions *within* the incompatibilist camp, I will use either the term *libertarian free will* or simply *free will*. Libertarians claim that we have it. Free will skeptics claim that we don't. Second, when talking about the kind of free will that is usually in the offing by the compatibilist camp, I will use a cluster of related terms such as *compatibilist control*, *self-regulation*, and *practical deliberation*. However, since I believe calling this kind of control "free will" unnecessarily muddies the dialectical waters, I will break with both compatibilists and revisionists and refrain from doing so here. On my view, if we do not have *libertarian* free will, we do not have free will at all.

My main reason for limiting the application of the term "free will" to the kind of metaphysically spooky stuff that immaterial souls are made of is that I do not believe that the kinds of cognitive capacities that compatibilists try to reconcile with determinism adequately capture the full spectrum of folk intuitions about free will. But that is an admittedly messy empirical question that has recently received a fair amount of attention.[5] As it stands, however, the verdict is still out. So, for now, I am simply going to assume for the sake of argument that the commonsense notion of free will is loosely libertarian and that we don't have it. Adequately defending either of these assumptions is beyond the scope of this essay. For present purposes, the important point is that even though I do not believe that we have free will in the traditional sense, I still believe that we could have the capacity for self-control and practical reason even if determinism were true. Moreover, I believe that these kinds of cognitive capacities are enough to ground some pared down kind of responsibility—which brings us to our next important distinction.

When talking about responsibility in this paper, I will always try to make it clear whether I am talking about desert-based responsibility or consequentialist-based responsibility. Moreover, I will focus primarily on the kind of responsibility that underpins punishment since it helps illuminate the key difference between saying that someone is *answerable* in some minimal way for violating a norm and saying someone *morally deserves* to suffer for violating a norm. On my view, to say that an agent is desert-based responsible for breaking some moral or legal norm *x* is to say that she deserves to suffer for *x-ing*, even if the suffering produces no other tangible benefits.[6] To say that an agent is consequentialist-based responsible for *x-ing*, on the other hand, is to say that she ought to suffer only if the suffering would decrease the likelihood that she (and others) will *x* in the future. The main difference between the two is that whereas the former maintains that making agents suffer for knowingly violating moral and legal norms is intrinsically valuable, the latter places merely instrumental value on the suffering. So, for instance, if there were two *equally effective* penalties available for a particular norm violation in terms of deterrence—one of which involves suffering and the other of which does not—the proponent of a desert-based approach must opt for the former while the proponent of a consequentialist approach must opt for the latter.

By my lights, when examining what's at stake in the free will debate, we must resist the temptation to conflate these two kinds of responsibility. After all, one could be an *incompatibilist* about determinism and moral desert but a *compatibilist* with respect to determinism and consequentialist-based responsibility—which is essentially the kind of view that I hold. Unfortunately, people are not always sufficiently careful when it comes to maintaining a clear line between these twin faces of responsibility. Keep in mind that one of the key issues in the debate between libertarians and free will skeptics is *moral desert*. Are human beings the kinds of creatures that deserve to suffer for their wrongdoings even if the suffering is otherwise noncompensatory? Libertarians and skeptics both agree that if humans are to be morally responsible in the robust desert-based sense, we would need to have libertarian free will. The two camps simply disagree about whether we actually have it.

Compatibilists, on the other hand, are not always clear on this point. One can find them sliding back and forth between desert-based and prevention-based responsibility—a move that is facilitated by the fact that we can use the same general term to refer to both. Consider, for instance, the following pair of remarks by Daniel Dennett:

1. Is she [i.e., the free will skeptic] going to jettison our system of law and punishment? Is she going to abandon the social leverage by which we encourage people to take responsibility for their actions? Is she prepared to dismiss the distinction between honesty and cheating as just another myth fostered by the traditional concept of free will? (2008, p. 255)
2. We ought to admit, up front, that one of our strongest unspoken motivations for upholding something close to the traditional concept of free will is our desire to see the world's villains get what they deserve. And surely they do deserve our condemnation, our criticism, and—when we have a sound system of laws in place—punishment. (2008, p. 258)

The way Dennett frames the debate here between the realists and nonrealists about free will is misleading, since he makes it seem as if skeptics are denying that we should have systems of social and legal norms. But the skeptic does not need to reject the importance of norms any more than she needs to reject the distinction between honesty and deceit. Instead, she merely denies that people who lie deserve to suffer for doing so. This is not to suggest that we don't need sanctions in place to deter people from lying—it's just to say that the point of the sanctions is forward rather than backward looking.

Perhaps Dennett presents free will skeptics in an unduly implausible light because he has conflated the rejection of moral desert with the rejection of any mechanisms of accountability whatsoever. If so, this is a mistake. For even though I happen to believe that determinism precludes both free will and moral desert, I am nevertheless able to consistently maintain that social stability requires a system of social and legal norms, that practical deliberation and self-control are two key elements of responsible agency, and that these two cognitive capacities are compatible with determinism. Given that one can be both a compatibilist (of sorts) and an incompatibilist (of sorts) in this way, we must maintain a bright line between the different kinds of responsibility when arguing about free will.

Another undesirable side effect of failing to adequately distinguish desert-based from consequentialist-based responsibility is that it misleadingly makes it look like there is a deep rift between compatibilists and free will skeptics when in many cases I would argue that the disagreement between the two camps is mainly terminological. After all, both camps typically agree about several key issues. First, each camp believes that we do not have libertarian free will. Second, each camp nevertheless believes that we have a bounded capacity for self-regulation and rational deliberation. Finally, compatibilists and free will skeptics also agree that there are important practical considerations that necessitate that we have a formalized system for holding people accountable for breaking social and legal norms. Given these similarities, the two main issues that distinguish compatibilists from free will skeptics are (a) whether we should call compatibilist control "free will," and (b) whether compatibilist control is enough to ground moral desert. Resolving this last issue is only possible if we avoid conflating desert-based and consequentialist-based responsibility.

The most obvious solution would be to limit the term "moral" to desert-based responsibility. We could then call the other kind of responsibility something else—e.g., answerability, accountability, etc.[7] This move is in line with my earlier insistence that we limit our application of the term "free will" to instances of libertarian free will. My goal in each of these cases is not to be unduly contrarian. Nor am I engaging in mere semantic quibbling. Rather, I think that what we call things matters. And I also think the terms "free will" and "moral responsibility" carry an awful lot of both metaphysical and historical baggage. From the story about free will's role in our purported fall from grace in the Garden of Eden to the Cartesian dualism that aimed to make room for free will in an otherwise mechanistic universe, in the Western tradition the notion of free will has often been aligned with that which is supernatural within us—that ephemeral ghost that so curiously haunts our lowly bodily machine. Moreover, it has historically been conceptualized as that part of us that separates us from "the beasts," makes us morally responsible for our behavior, and determines whether we end up with eternal damnation (or salvation). Given this web of historical associations I do not think that we should revise the terms "free will" and "moral responsibility." If we don't have the kind of agency and responsibility that people have traditionally thought we had, we invite confusion by continuing to use the old terms to talk about what we actually do have—especially when we could simply use other terms which are less loaded.

Another frustration that has always lurked in the background of the free will debate is that it is unclear what kind of evidence could possibly establish whether universal determinism is true. As it stands, the scientific consensus is that causality is indeterministic at the quantum level. Whether this quantum indeterminacy "bubbles up" in a way that would help libertarians such as Robert Kane (1996) is entirely unclear. Consequently, a number of incompatibilists will continue to remain hostage to future developments in quantum physics. Compatibilists, on the other hand, often reject this kind of waiting game outright. John Martin Fischer, for instance, recently claimed that, "our most fundamental views of ourselves as free and responsible should not, as it were, 'hang on a thread'—should not depend on subtle and arcane deliverances of theoretical physicists" (Fischer, 2007, p. 71). Regardless of whether one shares Fischer's deflationary attitude toward the threat of determinism, it is clear that philosophers will remain at an argumentative impasse until we know more about the fabric of the universe.

In the meantime, I think philosophers and psychologists should focus on other threats that are both more pressing and more challenging than the specter of determinism. The issue is not whether the mind is deterministic or mechanistic—the scientific consensus seems to be that it is both (see, e.g., Walter, 2001, p. 162)—but rather whether the conscious mind plays the central etiological role that we have traditionally assumed. For instance, if our conscious mental states are merely epiphenomena as some psychologists have suggested (e.g., Wegner, 2003), then regardless of the truth of determinism it wouldn't make sense to say that we are free. At the end of the day, *indeterministic* epiphenomenalism is no less worrisome than *deterministic* epiphenomenalism. Either way, there wouldn't be room for libertarian free will because there wouldn't be room for conscious will at all. Only the buzzing and whirling of the unconscious would have any real etiological role to play.

In light of this kind of worry, Nahmias has recently identified himself as a "neurotic compatibilist" (in press)—i.e., someone who thinks free will and responsibility are compatible with determinism but who nevertheless worries that developments in psychology could pose an independent threat. There are at least two important components to his view. First, he is worried that future developments in psychology could be incompatible with *both* libertarian free will *and* compatibilist control (hence, the neurotic part). Second, Nahmias nevertheless believes that determinism per se is compatible with free will and moral desert (hence, the compatibilist part). So, while he is confident that determinism does not pose a threat, he is nervous that perhaps future developments in psychology could. I, on the other hand, am outright skeptical about the existence of free will and moral desert on both fronts.

First, when it comes to the traditional compatibilism debate, I believe that libertarian free will is what is needed to undergird moral desert, and that libertarian free will is incompatible with the truth of determinism. That makes me an incompatibilist in the traditional sense. At the same time, I also believe that self-control and practical reason are compatible with determinism, and these capacities are enough for consequentialist-based responsibility even if they are not enough for moral desert. In this respect, I am also a compatibilist of sorts. However, regardless of whether these self-regulative capacities are compatible with determinism, they could be incompatible with a number of other things (e.g., manipulation, mental illness, automaticity, epiphenomenalism, etc.). These "other things" are the ultimate source of Nahmias's aforementioned unease—and for good reason.

On my view, the gathering data from psychology that we will examine in the following section are inconsistent with our traditional view of ourselves as fully free and autonomous moral agents. So, on this front, I am actually pessimistic when it comes to the fate of free will rather than merely anxious or neurotic. However, while Nahmias and I admittedly disagree when it comes to how concerned we presently ought to be, we nevertheless share a common methodological starting point. On both of our views, the old compatibility question is less interesting and less pressing than the potential threats posed by the literature on the automaticity of the mind, situationism, introspection, and epiphenomenalism. As such, we both advocate that philosophers focus more of their attention on what could helpfully be called the *New Compatibility Problem*—a problem that has often been obscured by orthogonal worries about determinism, mechanism, physicalism, and reductionism. That being said, it is finally time to turn our attention to the collective threat from psychology that is the focus of the present paper.

## 2. THE THREAT OF SHRINKING AGENCY

The first thing worth pointing out about what I am calling the threat of shrinking agency is that it is driven by developments in several different areas of psychology. While it is doubtful that any particular data set or research program could sound the death knell of free will and desert-based responsibility, I nevertheless think that the literature examined in the following pages collectively shifts the burden to those who maintain that our traditional conceptions of human agency are compatible with the picture of the mind that is being pieced together by psychologists. But I am getting ahead of myself. There will be time for shifting burdens down the road. For now, one more preliminary distinction needs to be made.

As we will see in the following pages, there is an important difference between partial agential threats and global agential threats. A partial agential threat is one that merely constrains or shrinks the domain of our conscious agency and control. A global agential threat, on the other hand, is one that does not leave any room for conscious volition at all. Examples of the former can be found in the literature on automaticity (e.g., Bargh) while examples of the latter can be found in the literature on epiphenomenalism (e.g., Wegner). It is also worth pointing out that the partial and global agential threats we are going to examine have nothing to do with whether (a) the laws of the universe are deterministic, (b) the conscious mind can be reduced to underlying mechanisms in the brain, (c) all mental events are caused by prior physical events, or (d) all mental events supervene on physical events. Instead, the agential threats that we will be examining here are ultimately fueled by the fact that the conscious mind exercises less control over our behavior than we have traditionally assumed. It is this deflationary view of conscious volition that is potentially agency undermining. After all, the less conscious *willing* we are able to do, the less free *will* we are able to have—which is true independently of traditional threats to free will such as determinism.[8]

Consider, for instance, the fascinating work by Bargh on the role of the unconscious mind. On his view, the data on automaticity indicate that "most of our day-to-day actions, motivations, judgments, and emotions are not the products of conscious choice and guidance, but must be driven instead by mental processes put into operation directly by environmental features and events" (Bargh & Chartrand, 1999, p. 465). According to Bargh, it's not that conscious mental states don't have any volitional role to play. Rather, it's just that this role is markedly more circumscribed than we previously thought. In light of the gathering evidence, Bargh predicts that:

> [T]he more we know about the situational causes of psychological phenomena, the less need we have for postulating internal conscious mediating process to explain these phenomena.... [I]t is hard to escape the forecast that as knowledge progresses regarding psychological phenomena,

> there will be less of a role played by free will or conscious choice in accounting for them. . . . That trend has already begun . . . and it can do nothing but continue. (Bargh, 1997, p. 1)

In attempting to understand Bargh's pessimistic stance toward the fate of free will, it would be instructive for us to examine some of what I take to be the more interesting and important priming studies. The first involved exposing participants to words that were related either to being polite (e.g., considerate, respect, polite) or to being rude (e.g., impolite, obnoxious, rude) (Bargh & Chartrand, 1999). In each condition, the primed terms were interspersed with a number of other random words for the purposes of the experiment. The participants were told that once they were done reading through the list, they were to ask the experimenter for directions for the second step of the experiment. At this point, they would each find the experimenter speaking with a confederate in the hall. This set up the crux of the study which was to determine whether those who were primed with polite words would be more patient and polite than those primed instead with rude words. Whereas the majority of the participants in the "rude" condition interrupted (67%), far fewer participants interrupted in the other two conditions (38% in the control condition and 16% in the "polite" condition).

In another one of Bargh's studies, participants were primed (or not) with an achievement goal (Bargh & Chartrand, 1999). They were then asked to identify and write down as many words as they could, based on a set of seven Scrabble letter tiles. A few minutes later, they were told over an intercom to stop. Hidden video cameras recorded the participants' behavior throughout to see how many of them continued to search for and write down words after they were told to stop doing so. Whereas only 21% of the participants in the control condition cheated, more than half of the participants in the "achievement" condition (55%) ignored the instructions to stop.

Finally, in a similar study run by Guido Hertel and Norbert Kerr (2000), participants were exposed either to terms such as fair, impartial, prejudiced, and favoritism (in the equality condition) or to terms such as trustworthy, betrayal, and disloyal (in the loyalty condition). Having been individually exposed to one of these two sets of words, participants were then brought together to take part in a minimal group paradigm experiment. Hertel and Kerr found at least two interesting and important results. First, participants in the "loyalty" condition showed greater in-group favoritism with respect to resource allocation and they exhibited a stronger identification with their in-group than the participants in the "equality" condition. Second, participants in the "loyalty" condition also experienced higher self-esteem the more group favoritism they showed. Participants in the "equality" condition, on the other hand, experienced lower self-esteem the more favoritism they showed.

By my lights, the existing data on priming and automaticity collectively establish that morally insignificant situational cues and stimuli both can and do have a significant effect on our moral behavior.[9] Moreover, it appears that our conscious minds are often blind to the forces that drive our behavior—even when these forces are ones that we would neither endorse nor identify with if asked to do so. For instance, other studies have shown that our moral behavior is sensitive to contextual variables such as the level of ambient noise in our immediate environment (Mathews & Cannon, 1975), (b) how many people happen to be standing around at the time (Latane & Darley, 1970), (c) whether the person telling us to do something morally suspect happens to be wearing a lab coat (Milgram, 1974), (d) whether or not we find a dime on a public telephone (Isen & Levin, 1972), (e) whether or not we are in a hurry (Darley & Batson, 1973), and (f) whether or not we have recently been primed to think about a ghost (Bering, McLeod, & Shackelford, 2005).[10] In each case, one finds morally extraneous situational variables having a stark effect on people's moral behavior without their awareness—an effect they often understandably deny when pressed.

If nothing else, the literature on automaticity puts pressure on what Bargh aptly calls the assumption of "conscious primacy"—i.e., the view according to which most of our overt behavior is ultimately driven by high level conscious mental states. Indeed, Bargh suggests that the only reason we find the literature on automaticity and situationism so surprising is that we view it against the backdrop of the assumption of conscious primacy. Yet, as intuitive as this assumption happens to be, Bargh claims that it flies in the face of the gathering data. On his view, the unconscious mind is "the rule in nature, not the exception" (2008, p. 149). So, while it is true that our subjective phenomenology "has given us the strong sense, difficult to overcome, that our ethereal free will is the source of our behaviors, judgments, and goal pursuits" (2008, p. 146–147), we no longer need to appeal to the conscious will to explain even some of our most complex actions.

One obvious response to the automaticity literature is to optimistically fall back on introspection in an effort to stave off the situationist threats to our moral agency. Unfortunately, as tempting as this response might appear at first blush, introspection isn't likely up to the task. For instance, in a series of papers in the late 1970s, Richard Nisbett and Timothy Wilson provided evidence that "there may be little to no direct introspective access to higher order cognitive processes" (1977, p. 231). On their view:

> Subjects are sometimes (a) unaware of the existence of a stimulus that importantly influenced the response, (b) unaware of the existence of the response, and (c) unaware that the stimulus has affected the response. It is proposed that when people attempt to report on their cognitive processes, that is, on the processes mediating the effects of a stimulus on a response, they do not do so on the basis of any true introspection. Instead, their reports are based on a priori, implicit theories or judgments about the extent to which a particular stimulus is a plausible cause of a given response. (Nisbett & Wilson, 1977, p. 231)

Given these limitations, introspection is unlikely to enable us to fully escape the clutches of automaticity and situationism. The less conscious access we have to the root causes of our behavior, the less conscious control we have over how our lives unfold—which will be a recurring theme in the pages ahead.

At this point, we can draw two conclusions. First, our moral behavior can be *both* initiated *and* driven by processes that lie beneath the veil of consciousness (e.g., Bargh). Second, introspection is unlikely to give us reliable access to the ultimate causes of our own complex behavior (e.g., Nisbett & Wilson). In short, our conscious minds play a less prominent role in how our lives unfold than we previously assumed. Moreover, the role they do play seems to be quite fragile. For present purposes, I am going to call this collective threat to autonomy the *Rarity Thesis*. And while this view admittedly leaves room for conscious agency, it does not leave nearly as much as most libertarians and compatibilists would presumably prefer. Minimally, I think the rarity thesis can be used to motivate a deflationary view of agency and moral responsibility. Fleshing out what this pared down view might look like would take us too far afield. For now, I want to turn our attention instead to two more radical threats to free will that are already lurking in our midst—the first of which is based upon the groundbreaking work of Benjamin Libet.

In Libet (1999), for instance, participants were trained to focus their attention on the "first awareness of a wish or urge to act" (Libet, 1999, p. 49).[11] Once they had grown accustomed to identifying the onset of their conscious urges, they were asked to perform a simple flick of the wrist whenever they felt the urge to do so (in 30-second increments). Information about the participants' respective readiness potentials—i.e., the slow electrical charges that have been shown to precede "self-paced" voluntary actions—were recorded via readings of their scalps. As Libet correctly points out, "in the traditional view of conscious will and free will, one would expect conscious will to appear before, or at the onset, of the RP, and thus command the brain to perform the intended act" (Libet, 1999, p. 49). However, this is not what appeared to happen at all. According to Libet's interpretation of the data, the brain processes that prepared the participants for their voluntary actions preceded conscious awareness by 400 ms (Libet, 1999, p. 51). In short, Libet claims that his participants' brains were forming *decisions* or *intentions* prior to conscious awareness.[12]

A series of recent studies by John-Dylan Haynes and colleagues produced similarly surprising results. In one study, participants could freely choose to press a button with either their left hand or their right hand (Soon, Brass, Heinze, & Haynes, 2008). Their task was to remember the precise time at which they consciously settled on a choice. The researchers were able to use brain signals from the participants to predict their choice up to seven seconds before they consciously made their decision. Using highly sophisticated computer programs and advanced imaging techniques, Haynes and colleagues used micropatterns of activity in participants' frontopolar cortexes to predict their choices up to *seven seconds* before they became consciously aware of which button they were going to push.

In light of these results, it might be tempting to conclude that conscious mental states don't have any etiological role to play at all. But, as Libet is quick to point out, even in his own studies conscious awareness appears approximately 150 ms before muscle activation. So, even though conscious awareness appears after the onset of RP, it could nevertheless affect the output of volitional processes. In light of this possibility, Libet claims that our conscious will may have a kind of veto-power over the actions that our bodies antecedently prepare us to perform. On this view—which I am going to call the *Gatekeeper Thesis*—the "conscious will might block or veto the process, so that no act occurs" (Libet, 1999, p. 52).[13] As Libet claims:

> The role of conscious free will would be, then, not to initiate voluntary action, but rather to control whether the act takes place. We may view the unconscious initiatives for voluntary actions as "bubbling up" in the brain. The conscious will then selects which of these initiatives may go forward to an action or which ones to veto and abort, with no act of appearing. (1999, p. 52)

But if the conscious mind merely serves as a sentinel—allowing some unconscious action plans to come to fruition while blocking others—then it is unclear to me how we could have free *will*. At best, it appears that Libet provides us with what others have called free *won't* (Ohbi & Haggard, 2004).

For now, I want to set aside the question of whether the gatekeeper thesis is true. Instead, I simply want to emphasize that the potential threat that Libet's veto power poses to our traditional conception of agency is entirely independent of the issue of determinism—which is something Libet himself seemingly fails to realize. Consider, for instance, his claim that the view that we are "genuinely free in the non-determined sense," is "at least as good, if not better, scientific option than is its denial by determinist theory" (1999, p. 56). These remarks suggest that Libet has misunderstood the novel threat posed by his studies. The worry isn't (a) whether the laws of nature are deterministic, (b) whether our minds are mechanistic, or (c) whether our conscious mental states are determined by prior unconscious mental states. After all, the gatekeeper thesis—like the aforementioned rarity thesis—is neutral with respect to these traditional threats to free will.

The real worry raised by Libet's data is that our conscious mental states do not appear to play the etiological role we have traditionally assumed. Moreover, when our capacity for inhibition and practical deliberation is as flimsy as Roy Baumeister's work on ego-depletion suggests, we have all the more reason to be concerned (see, e.g., Baumeister, 2008). For not only is my conscious self not the volitional source of my behavior, but my limited capacity to control my unconsciously initiated urges, intentions, and plans is sensitive to many factors about which I am unaware and over which I do not have control. By my lights, the more circumscribed our conscious minds become, the less room there will be for libertarian free will and desert-based responsibility. That being said, it is worth pointing out that the gatekeeper thesis is nevertheless consistent with some deflationary notions of conscious agency. For while it may turn out that the conscious mind is regulative rather than volitional, it could still play an important role in how our lives unfold.

If, on the other hand, we don't at least have the kind of minimal control that one finds in Libet's veto power, then epiphenomenalism would be the only remaining possibility. According to Libet, if this were the case, it would undermine our moral agency altogether:

> In such a view, the individual would not consciously control his actions; he would only become aware of an unconsciously initiated choice. He would have no direct conscious control over the nature of the preceding unconscious processes. But a free will process implies one could be held consciously responsible for one's choice to act or not to act. We do not hold people responsible for actions performed unconsciously, without the possibility of conscious control. (Libet, 1999, p. 52).

Given the deep entrenchment of our moral reactive attitudes and our belief in the causal efficacy of the conscious mind, Libet thinks the burden is on those who would deny the existence of conscious agency.

Daniel Wegner is one psychologist who takes up the challenge.[14] On his view, the traditional picture of the conscious will is not easily reconciled with the complex picture of the mind that is slowly being pieced together by psychologists. As he says:

> The mechanisms underlying the experience of will are themselves a fundamental topic of scientific study. We should be able to examine and understand what creates the experience of will and what makes it go away. This means, though, that conscious will is an illusion. It is an illusion in the sense that the experience of consciously willing something is not a direct indication that the conscious thought has caused an action. Conscious will, viewed in this way, may be an extraordinary illusion indeed. (Wegner, 2003, pp. 2–3)

According to Wegner, while it is important to better understand why we *think* the conscious mind is volitional, at the end of the day our self-conception on this front is illusory. Unfortunately, Wegner's account of the illusory nature of our views about mental causation is a bit vague. While he sometimes appears to be arguing for the kind of epiphenomenalism one finds in the literature on the philosophy of mind—i.e., the view that conscious mental states are entirely causally inert—at other times it seems as if he has something else in mind. If conscious mental states were *wholly* causally inefficacious, then it wouldn't make sense to say that they do anything positive for us or that they help us in any way. However, Wegner suggests that these conscious states do play a role in how our lives unfold, just not the role we previously thought.[15]

Nahmias has suggested that perhaps the best way to interpret Wegner on this front is to assume that he is developing *modular epiphenomenalism*. On this view, "it is not that conscious mental states in general are epiphenomenal but that specifically those thoughts and intentions we experience just before actions as the cause of those actions do not in fact cause our actions" (Nahmias, 2002, p. 530). This interpretation fits quite nicely with several things Wegner says when explicating his view. Consider, for instance, the following two comments:

1. Still the automatisms and illusions of control that lie off this diagonal remind us that action and the feeling of doing are not locked together inevitably. They come apart often enough to make us wonder whether they may be produced by separate systems in the mind. The processes of mind that produce the experience of will may be quite distinct from the processes of the mind that produce the action itself. As soon as we accept the idea that the will should be understood as an experience of the person who acts, we realize that conscious will is not inherent in action—there are actions that have it and actions that don't. (Wegner, 2003, p. 11)
2. Perceiving mind and causal agency [via intentions, beliefs, desires, and plans] is a significant human ability. It is possible that this achievement is accomplished by a fairly narrow mental module, a special skill unit of mind that does not only this, and that in different individuals this module can thus be particularly healthy, damaged, or even nonfunctional. (Wegner, 2003, p. 24)

In supporting his view, Wegner appeals to studies that show that participants' experience of control over an action can be severed from their actual performance (or nonperformance) of the action. On the one hand, we sometimes find what appears to be otherwise purposive behavior which participants nevertheless perceive to be foreign to or outside their conscious control (e.g., hypnosis and alien hand syndrome). On the other hand, we find agents who think they are exercising control when they are not (e.g., positive illusions of control). According to Wegner, these kinds of studies highlight the fact that our experience of conscious will cannot, in and of itself, be taken as evidence that our conscious will is the ultimate source of our actions. After all, if feelings of will (or lack thereof) can be entirely decoupled from purposive behavior, then we can't assume that just because we experience the former that we are the ultimate cause of the latter. In short, while we often consciously experience an "internal oomph" when performing actions that we take to be voluntary and intentional, there is no guarantee that this experience is veridical.

According to Wegner, while the experience of will misleads us into believing in the "magic of our own causal agency," the actual causal springs of our behavior dwell below the veil of consciousness (2003, p. 28). On this view:

> The mind is a system that produces appearance for its owner. . . . The mind creates this continuous illusion; it really doesn't know what causes its own actions. Whatever empirical will there is rumbling along in the engine room—an actual relation between thought and action—might in fact be totally inscrutable to the driver of the machine (the mind). The mind has a self-explanation mechanism that produces a roughly continuous sense that what is in consciousness is the cause of action—the phenomenal will—whereas in fact the mind can't ever know itself well enough to be able to say what the causes of its actions are. (Wegner, 2003, p. 28)

If Wegner were right that our conscious minds don't have access to the actual causes of our behavior, it is unclear how we could be said to behave freely and responsibly. As we saw earlier when we examined the gatekeeper thesis, free will and desert-based responsibility require that our conscious mental states are volitional. In this respect, both Libet's veto power and Wegner's illusion of conscious will threaten our traditional conception of human agency. However, Wegner's view is potentially much more corrosive.

Keep in mind that while Libet's veto power may not be enough for libertarian free will and desert-based responsibility, it is nevertheless enough for compatibilist control, self-regulation, etc. Wegner's view, on the other hand, does not appear to leave room for our conscious mental states to play any real etiological role at all. So, whereas Libet's view merely shrinks the domain over which we exercise control, Wegner seemingly leaves the conscious mind out of the causal loop altogether. After all, if the unconscious mind is the captain of our proverbial ship—with conscious mental states merely serving the lowly role of compass as Wegner suggests—then the unfolding of our lives ultimately depends on the former and not the latter. For it is the captain, not the compass who decides where the ship is going in the first place.

As such, Wegner's view—which I am going to call the *Bypassing Thesis*—represents a global and not merely partial agential threat. By my lights, if the bypassing thesis were correct, then our conscious minds would simply be along for the ride, etiologically speaking. This would have far reaching implications as far as free will is concerned. Not only would we not have libertarian free will, but we wouldn't even have the kind of conscious control that compatibilists have tried to use to ground moral desert. In the face of the bypassing thesis, what's left of moral responsibility—if anything is left at all—is little more than moral luck. By leaving "us" out of the story about agency and action, it removes us from the sphere of moral desert altogether. Only my body and brain—neither of which I can directly control—are left to "blame" for our behavior. And if you, like me, don't think it makes sense to say that people deserve blame (or praise) for things over which they have no ultimate control, then epiphenomenalism represents the greatest threat of all to free will and desert-based responsibility. At the end of the day, Wegner's bypassing thesis threatens to leave us adrift on a sea of unconscious forces that we are powerless to change. So, while I am presently unpersuaded by Wegner's attempts to empirically motivate some form of epiphenomenalism, I nevertheless appreciate the fact that in light of the research on apparent mental causation, it is an open possibility that one day soon we may have to radically alter how we view human cognition and agency.

## 3. TAKING STOCK

My primary goal in this paper was to explore the unique problems and issues that arise when trying to rectify our traditional views about human agency and responsibility with the gathering data from the sciences of the mind. Fully plumbing the depths of these threats is a task for another day. For present purposes, I simply wanted to sketch the boundaries of the threats that I believe are already under foot and to show that they are independent of the issues that have traditionally been the focus of the free will debate. In this respect, I disagree with researchers who do not think advancements in psychology pose any new threats to free will above and beyond antecedently existing threats such as determinism, mechanism, reductionism, and the like (see, e.g., Roskies, 2006). On my view, the new picture of human agency (or lack thereof) that is being pieced together by psychologists has the potential to radically transform the way we view ourselves both in relation to one another and to the world around us. Moreover, I believe that to the extent that these developments turn out to undermine our traditional views about free will, philosophers and psychologists ought to take an active roll in disabusing the public of their mistaken views on this front. By my lights, if our beliefs are inconsistent with the best available scientific data, these beliefs ought to be discarded just like the myriad other views that litter the ideological dustbins of human history.

In this respect, I break with philosophers such as Smilansky and Nichols, who both point to the alleged benefits of believing in libertarian free will and moral desert as grounds for leaving these beliefs in place. Whereas Smilansky suggests that we ought to keep quiet about the nonexistence of free will (2000, 2002)—since our illusory beliefs on this front undergird our community of moral responsibility—Nichols similarly suggests that to the extent that nihilism about free will threatens to undermine social cooperation, we should either "relinquish or ignore" incompatibilism even if we otherwise find it to be intuitive (2007). In this sense, both philosophers may accurately be identified with what Nichols calls a "counter-revolutionary agenda." On each of their respective views, the potential costs of a revolution about free will and responsibility outweigh whatever benefits we might derive from it.

I, on the other hand, would prefer to throw my lot with the revolutionaries in the event that the potential threat of shrinking agency discussed in this paper is further borne out by future research. At the end of the day, I advocate what might helpfully be called *free will disillusinonism*—i.e., the view that to the extent that folk intuitions and beliefs about the nature of human cognition and moral responsibility are mistaken, philosophers and psychologists ought to do their part to educate the public—especially when their mistaken beliefs arguably fuel a number of unhealthy emotions and attitudes such as revenge, hatred, intolerance, lack of empathy, etc. By my lights, humanity must get beyond this maladaptive suite of emotions if we are to survive. To the extent that future developments in the sciences of the mind can bring us one step closer to that goal—by giving us a newfound appreciation for the limits of human cognition and agency—I welcome them with open arms.

Of course, not everyone will be so sanguine in the face of the potential death of free will. Indeed, they will likely share the worry captured by the following remarks from Wegner:

> Many of the most strident arguments for free will hinge on the idea that a scientific understanding of human behavior could potentially ruin everything. The magic will be undone, the glorious human spirit will be cheapened, demystified, and rendered grotesque. We will uncover the trolls operating the machinery in the dungeon, and we will never again be able to appreciate the sparkling radiance of the Magic Kingdom of the self. Or, more realistically, we will uncover the genetic codes that produce neural structures that allow incoming sensations by social and situational factors to contribute to the cognitive computations that incline our motor output processes to lead us to behave—and then we lose the magic. (Wegner, 2008, p. 235)

Wegner believes that this worry is overstated. On his view, the illusion of self—much like an optical illusion—will survive the onslaught at the hands of psychologists. As he says, "the magic is here to stay" (Wegner, 2008, p. 243). Unlike Wegner, however, I have no time for magical powers and fairy tale endings—especially when they often do more harm than good. Indeed, not only do I think that developments in psychology will radically alter our conception of human agency, but I also happen to think that these potential changes represent a step in the right direction. As such, I am a disillusionist about free will and responsibility both descriptively and normatively. Figuring out which of us is right about the proper fate of free will is a thorny issue that will require philosophers and psychologists to continue to reach across disciplinary boundaries. But that, too, is a story for another day.

## ACKNOWLEDGMENTS

I would first like to thank the students in my seminar on free will and science at Dickinson College for their helpful feedback on the ideas contained in this paper. It was a pleasure to explore these issues with such eager minds. I also owe a special thanks to Eddy Nahmias—whose approach to the free will debate has had a formative effect on my own. So, even though we may disagree concerning the fate of free will, we nevertheless agree when it comes to the future direction the debate ought to take.

## NOTES

1. A copy of the article can be found at: http://www.nytimes.com/2007/01/02/science/02free.html
2. For a very helpful introduction to the major views in the free will debate, see Fischer, Kane, Pereboom, and Vargas (2007).
3. For recent overviews of the several faces of contemporary compatibilism, see Berofsky (2002); Haji (2002); Mele (2006); and Russell (2002).
4. There are several other major views in the free will literature that do not fit into either the incompatibilist or the compatibilist camps but that I will not have time to discuss here. Examples include Saul Smilansky's fundamental dualism (2000, 2002), Al Mele's agnostic autonomism (2001), and Manuel Vargas's revisionism (2005, 2007)—to name just a few.
5. See, e.g., Nadelhoffer and Feltz (2007); Nahmias, Morris, Nadelhoffer, and Turner, (2005); (2006); Nahmias (2006); Nichols and Knobe (2007); and Woolfolk, Doris, and Darley (2006).
6. For ease of exposition, I will focus on bad actions and blameworthy agents in this paper, but the same notion of moral desert applies to good acts and praiseworthy agents as well.
7. Gary Watson helpfully distinguishes between what he calls accountability and attributability (2004, pp. 260–283).
8. This is not to say that these other things don't pose a threat—it's just to say that to the extent they pose a threat, they do so independently of the psychological threats that are the topic of the present paper.
9. For criticisms of the automaticity literature, see Kihlstrom (2008); Logan (1997); and Pashler (1998).
10. Both John Doris (1998, 2002) and Gilbert Harman (1999, 2000) have relied upon the data on automaticity and situationism to criticize the empirical credibility of virtue ethics. On their view, virtue ethics does not comport with what researchers are discovering about the nature of moral cognition and social behavior. For responses on the part of virtue ethics, see Kamtekar (2004); Miller (2003); Sabini and Silver (2005); and Solomon (2003).
11. See, also, Libet (1985, 2001, 2004); and Libet, Gleason, Wright, and Pearl (1983).
12. Libet has been widely, and I believe correctly, criticized on this point. One particularly exacting criticism has been developed by Al Mele (see, e.g., Mele 2004 2006, 2008a, 2008b). On his view, a rival interpretation of the data that he calls the "urge hypothesis" not only does a better job of explaining Libet's results, but it also leaves room for the traditional view of conscious agency. For other critical responses to Libet's work see Bayne (2006); Gallagher (2006); Pacherie (2006); Pockett, Banks, and Gallagher (2006); Ross (2006); and Zhu (2003).
13. Baumeister (2008) develops a similar nonvolitional notion of conscious control.
14. For other work on apparent mental-causation, see Brown (1989); Claxton (1999); Michotte

(1963); Spence (1996); and Thompson, Armstrong, and Thomas, (1998).

15. Wegner draws a curious analogy between the role played by our conscious mental states and the role played by a compass. Just as the latter guides us without causing us to go one way or the other, so the conscious self purportedly shapes our behavior by helping us distinguish the things we do from the things we don't do. See, e.g., Wegner (2003, ch. 9).

## REFERENCES

Ayer, A. J. (1982). *Freedom and necessity*. In G. Watson (Ed.), *Free will* (pp. 15–23). New York: Oxford University Press.

Bargh, J. (1997). The automaticity of everyday life. In R. S. Wyer & T. K. Srull (Eds.), *Advances in social cognition* (Vol. 10, pp. 1–61). Mahwah, NJ: Erlbaum.

Bargh, J. (2008). Free will is unnatural. In J. Baer, J. Kaufman, & R. Baumeister (Eds.), *Are we free? Psychology and free will* (pp. 128–154). New York: Oxford University Press.

Bargh, J. A., & Chartrand, T. L. (1999). The unbearable automaticity of being. *American Psychologist, 57*(7), 462–479.

Baumeister, R. (2008). Free will, consciousness, and cultural animals. In J. Baer, J. Kaufman, and R. Baumeister (Eds.), *Are we free? Psychology and free will* (pp. 65–85). New York: Oxford University Press.

Bayne, T. (2006). Phenomenology and the feeling of doing. In S. Pockett, W. Banks, & S. Gallagher (Eds.), *Does consciousness cause behavior? An investigation of the nature of volition* (pp. 169–186). Cambridge, MA: MIT Press.

Bering, J. M., McLeod, K., & Shackelford, T. K. (2005). Reasoning about dead agents reveals possible adaptive trends. *Human Nature, 16,* 360–381.

Berofsky, B. (2002). Ifs, cans, and free will: The issues. In R. Kane (Ed.), *The Oxford handbook of free will* (pp. 181–201). New York: Oxford University Press.

Brown, J. W. (1989). The nature of voluntary action. *Brain and Cognition, 10,* 105–120.

Chisholm, R. (1982). Human freedom and the self. In G. Watson (Ed.), *Free will* (pp. 24–35). New York: Oxford University Press.

Clarke, R. (1996). Agent causation and event causation in the production of free action. *Philosophical Topics, 24*(Fall), 19–48.

Clarke, R. (2003). *Libertarian accounts of free will*. Oxford: Oxford University Press.

Claxton, G. (1999). Whodunnit? Unpicking the "seems" of free will. *Journal of Consciousness Studies, 6,* 99–113.

Darley, J. M., & Batson, C. D. (1973). From Jerusalem to Jericho: A study of situational and dispositional variables in helping behavior. *Journal of Personality and Social Psychology, 27,* 100–108.

Dennett, D. (2008). Some observations on the psychology of thinking about free will. In J. Baer, J. Kaufman, & R. Baumeister (Eds.), *Are we free? Psychology and free will* (pp. 248–259). New York: Oxford University Press.

Double, R. (1991). *The non-reality of free will*. New York: Oxford University Press.

Doris, J. M. (1998). Persons, situations, and virtue ethics. *Noûs, 32,* 504–530.

Doris, J. M. (2002). *Lack of character: Personality and moral behavior*. New York: Cambridge University Press.

Ekstrom, L. (2000). *Free will: A philosophical study*. Boulder, CO: Westview Press.

Fischer, J. M. (1994). *The metaphysics of free will*. Oxford: Blackwell Publishers.

Fischer, J. M. (2007). Compatibilism. In J. Fischer, R. Kane, D. Pereboom, & M. Vargas (Eds.), *Four views on free will* (pp. 44–84). Oxford: Blackwell Publishing.

Fischer, J., Kane, R., Pereboom, D., & Vargas, M. (Eds.). (2007). *Four views on free will*. Oxford: Blackwell Publishing.

Fischer, J. M., & Ravizza, M. (1998). *Responsibility and control: An essay on moral responsibility*. Cambridge, UK: Cambridge University Press.

Frankfurt, H. (1988). *The importance of what we care about*. Cambridge, UK: Cambridge University Press.

Gallagher, S. (2006). Where's the action? Epiphenomenalism and the problem of free will. In S. Pockett, W. Banks, & S. Gallagher (Eds.), *Does consciousness cause behavior? An investigation of the nature of volition* (pp. 109–124). Cambridge, MA: MIT Press.

Haji, I. (2002). Compatibilist views of freedom and responsibility. In R. Kane (Ed.), *The Oxford handbook of free will* (pp. 202–228). New York: Oxford University Press.

Harman, G. (1999). Moral philosophy meets social psychology: Virtue ethics and the fundamental attribution error. *Proceedings of the Aristotelian Society, 99,* 315–331.

Harman, G. (2000). The non-existence of character traits. *Proceedings of the Aristotelian Society, 100,* 223–226.

Hertel, G., & Kerr, N. L. (2000). Priming in-group favoritism: The impact of normative scripts in the minimal group paradigm. *Journal of Experimental Social Psychology, 37*(4), 316–324.

Honderich, T. (1988). *A theory of determinism.* Oxford: Oxford University Press.

Isen, A. M., & Levin, P. F. (1972). Effect of feeling good on helping: Cookies and kindness. *Journal of Personality and Social Psychology, 21,* 384–388.

Kamtekar, R. (2004). Situationism and virtue ethics on the content of our character. *Ethics, 114,* 458–491.

Kane, R. (1996). *The significance of free will.* New York: Oxford University Press.

Kane, R. (Ed.). (2002). *The Oxford handbook of free will.* Oxford and New York: Oxford University Press.

Kihlstrom, J. F. (2008). The automaticity juggernaut—or, Are we automatons after all? In J. Baer, J. Kaufman, & R. Baumeister (Eds.), *Are we free? Psychology and free will* (pp. 155–180). New York: Oxford University Press.

Latane, B., & Darley, J. (1970). *The unresponsive bystander: Why doesn't he help?* New York: Appleton-Century Crofts.

Libet, B. (1985). Unconscious cerebral initiative and the role of conscious will in voluntary action. *Behavioral and Brain Sciences, 8,* 529–566.

Libet, B. (1999). Do we have free will? *Journal of Consciousness Studies, 6*(8–9), 47–57.

Libet, B. (2001). Consciousness, free action, and the brain. *Journal of Consciousness Studies, 8,* 59–65.

Libet, B. (2004). *Mind time.* Cambridge, MA: Harvard University Press.

Libet, B., Gleason, C.,Wright, E., & Pearl, D. (1983). Time of unconscious intention to act in relation to onset of cerebral activity (readiness potential). *Brain, 106,* 623–642.

Logan, G. D. (1997). The automaticity of academic life: Unconscious applications of an implicit theory. In R. S. Wyer & T. K. Srull (Eds.), *Advances in social cognition* (pp. 157–179). Mahwah, NJ: Erlbaum.

Mathews, K. E., & Cannon, L. K. (1975). Environmental noise level as a determinant of helping behavior. *Journal of Personality and Social Psychology, 32,* 571–577.

Mele, A. (2001). *Autonomous agents: From self-control to autonomy.* New York: Oxford University Press.

Mele, A. (2004). The illusion of conscious will and the causation of intentional action. *Philosophical Topics, 32,* 193–213.

Mele, A. (2006). *Free will and luck.* New York: Oxford University Press.

Mele, A. (2008a). Recent work on free will and science. *American Philosophical Quarterly, 45*(2), 107–130.

Mele, A. (2008b). Psychology and free will: A commentary. In J. Baer, J. Kaufman, & R. Baumeister (Eds.), *Are we free? Psychology and free will* (pp. 325–346). New York: Oxford University Press.

Michotte, A. (1963). The perception of causality (T. R. Miles & E. Miles, Trans.). New York: Basic Books.

Milgram, S. (1974). *Obedience to authority.* New York: Harper and Row.

Miller, C. (2003). Social psychology and virtue ethics. *The Journal of Ethics, 7,* 365–392.

Nadelhoffer, T., & Feltz, A. (2007). Folk intuitions, slippery slopes, and necessary fictions: An essay on Smilansky's free will illusionism. *Midwest Studies in Philosophy, 13*(1), 202–213.

Nahmias, E. (2002). When consciousness matters: A critical review of Daniel Wegner's *The illusion of conscious will. Philosophical Psychology, 15*(4), 527–541.

Nahmias, E. (2006). Folk fears about freedom and responsibility: Determinism vs. reductionism. *Journal of Cognition and Culture, 6*(1–2), 215–237.

Nahmias, E. (in press). The psychology of free will. In J. Prinz (Ed.), *The Oxford handbook on the philosophy of psychology.* New York: Oxford University Press.

Nahmias, E., Morris, S., Nadelhoffer, T., & Turner, J. (2005). Surveying free will: Folk intuitions about free will and moral responsibility. *Philosophical Psychology, 18*(5), 561–584.

Nahmias, E., Morris, S., Nadelhoffer, T., & Turner, J. (2006). Is incompatibilism intuitive? *Philosophy and Phenomenological Research, 73,* 28–53.

Nichols, S. (2007). After incompatibilism: A naturalistic defense of the reactive attitudes. *Philosophical Perspectives, 21,* 405–428.

Nichols, S., & Knobe, J. (2007). Moral responsibility and determinism: The cognitive science of folk intuition. *Nous, 41,* 663–685.

Nisbett, R., & Wilson, T. (1977). Telling more than we can know: Verbal reports on mental processes. *Psychological Review, 84,* 231–259.

O'Connor, T. (1993). Indeterminism and free agency: Three recent views. *Philosophy and Phenomenological Research, 53,* 499–526.

O'Connor, T. (2000). *Persons and causes: The metaphysics of free will.* New York: Oxford University Press.

Ohbi, S. S., & Haggard, P. (2004). Free will and free won't. *American Scientist, 92,* 358–365.

Overbye, D. (2007, January 2). Free will: Now you have it, now you don't. *The New York Times.*

Pacherie, E. (2006). Toward a dynamic theory of intentions. In S. Pockett, W. Banks, & S. Gallagher (Eds.), *Does consciousness cause behavior? An investigation of the nature of volition* (pp. 146–168). Cambridge, MA: MIT Press.

Pashler, H. E. (1998). *The psychology of attention.* Cambridge, MA: MIT Press.

Pereboom, D. (2001). *Living without free will.* Cambridge, UK: Cambridge University Press.

Pockett, S., Banks, W., & Gallagher, S. (2006). Does consciousness cause behavior? An investigation of the nature of volition. Cambridge, MA: MIT Press.

Roskies, A. (2006). Neuroscientific challenges to free will and responsibility. *Trends in Cognitive Science, 10*(9), 419–423.

Ross, P. (2006). Empirical constraints on the problem of free will. In S. Pockett, W. Banks, & S. Gallagher (Eds.), *Does consciousness cause behavior? An investigation of the nature of volition* (pp. 105–144). Cambridge, MA: MIT Press.

Russell, P. (2002). Pessimists, pollyannas, and the new compatibilism. In R. Kane (Ed.), *The Oxford handbook of free will* (pp. 229–256). New York: Oxford University Press.

Sabini, J., & Silver, M. (2005). Lack of character? Situationism critiqued. *Ethics, 115,* 535–562.

Shakespeare, W. (2005). *King Lear.* In S. Wells, G. Taylor, J. Jowett, & W. Montgomery (Eds.), *The Oxford Shakespeare: The complete works* (2nd ed., pp. 1153–1184). New York: Oxford University Press. (Original work 1610).

Smilansky, S. (2000). *Free will and illusion.* New York: Oxford University Press.

Smilansky, S. (2002). Free will, fundamental dualism, and the centrality of illusion. In R. Kane (Ed.), *The Oxford handbook of free will* (pp. 489–505). New York: Oxford University Press.

Solomon, R. (2003). Victims of circumstances? A defense of virtue ethics in business. *Business Ethics Quarterly, 13,* 43–62.

Sommers, T. (2007). The objective attitude. *The Philosophical Quarterly, 57,* 321–342.

Soon, C. S., Brass, M., Heinze, H. J., & Haynes, J. D. (2008). Unconscious determinants of free decisions in the human brain. *Nature Neuroscience, 11,* 543–545.

Spence, S. A. (1996). Free will in the light of neuropsychiatry. *Philosophy, Psychiatry, and Psychology, 3,* 75–90.

Stace, W. (1960). *Religion and the modern mind.* Philadelphia: Keystone Books.

Strawson, G. (1986). *Freedom and belief.* Oxford: Clarendon Press.

Thompson, S. C., Armstrong, W., & Thomas, C. (1998). Illusions of control, underestimations, and accuracy: A control heuristic explanation. *Psychological Bulletin, 123,* 143–161.

Van Inwagen, P. (1983). *An essay on free will.* Oxford: Oxford University Press.

Vargas, M. (2005). The revisionist's guide to responsibility. *Philosophical Studies, 125*(3), 399–429.

Vargas, M. (2007). Revisionism. In J. Fischer, R. Kane, D. Pereboom, & M. Vargas (Eds.), *Four views on free will* (pp. 126–165). Oxford: Blackwell Publishing.

Walter, H. (2001). Neurophilosophy of free will: From libertarianism illusions to a concept of natural autonomy. Cambridge, MA: MIT Press.

Watson, G. (Ed.). (1982). *Free will.* New York: Oxford University Press.

Watson, G. (2004). *Agency and answerability.* New York: Oxford University Press.

Wegner, D. (2003). *The illusion of conscious will.* Cambridge, MA: MIT Press.

Wegner, D. (2008). Self is magic. In J. Baer, J. Kaufman, & R. Baumeister (Eds.), *Are we free? Psychology and free will* (pp. 226–247). New York: Oxford University Press.

Woolfolk, R. L, Doris, J. M., & Darley, J. M. (2006). Identification, situational constraint, and social cognition: Studies in the attribution of moral responsibility. *Cognition, 100,* 283–301.

Zhu, J. (2003). Reclaiming volition. *Consciousness and Cognition, 10,* 61–77.

# CHAPTER 16

## Libet and the Criminal Law's Voluntary Act Requirement

*Gideon Yaffe*

### INTRODUCTION

Imagine someone who says, "Thanks to the pioneering work of Benjamin Libet it is well-established that there is a surge of brain activity, registering on the EEG as 'the readiness potential,' prior to the moment that agents take themselves to make a decision. People say they decided at a particular moment, but their EEGs tell us that their brains were very active some moments earlier. From this we learn that although people think they act voluntarily, they never do in fact. Since it is unjustifiable to hold people criminally liable when they did nothing voluntarily, nobody is justifiably held criminally liable. Thus, our prisons are filled with people we are unjustified in imprisoning. Our courts are clogged with cases that ought to be decided immediately for the defense on the basis merely of a proper appreciation of Libet's discovery."

This imagined person reaches a lot of big conclusions in a few short sentences. My focus here is on the concept of the voluntary that figures in this train of reasoning. For the startling conclusions about the law to follow in the way proposed from the facts that Libet uncovered, it must be the case that the property, labeled "voluntariness," that Libet's discoveries are said to show our acts to lack is in fact required for justified criminal liability.[1] In thinking about this, it is important not to be misled by our language. There might be perfectly good usages of the term "voluntary" under which Libet has indeed shown our acts not to be voluntary; and there are, of course, perfectly good usages of the term under which an act must be voluntary if a person is to be criminally punished for it. Our question is whether these two perfectly good usages of the term are close enough in meaning to warrant important conclusions about criminal liability. Are the terms more than just homophones?

We'll start on the legal side. What is meant by the term "voluntary" in the law? What little can be gleaned in answer to this question from contemporary legal materials is discussed in section 1. As we'll see in section 2, we can make some further headway on that question not just by looking at today's law, but also by looking at the theory of voluntary action popular in seventeenth- and eighteenth-century Britain during the period in which the criminal law's voluntary act requirement became what it is today, a theory disseminated in part at least through the works of John Locke. Then in section 3 we'll turn to Libet: Has Libet shown our acts not to be voluntary in the sense that is of relevance to the law? The answer to this last question is, given some plausible empirical assumptions, probably no. However, in the end I describe schematically a type of experiment that might help us to decide the question with more certainty.[2]

### 1. THE LAW'S SCHEMATIC CONCEPTION OF VOLUNTARY ACTION

As every law student learns in the 1L course in criminal law, a defendant is never guilty of a crime, in our system, unless he is shown beyond a reasonable doubt to have performed some voluntary act.[3,4] A voluntary act, the law tells us, is a bodily movement that is appropriately guided by the mental state of volition. The theory of voluntary action embedded in the law does not, by itself, rule out the possibility that *mental* events can themselves be voluntary acts; my *thinking* about my upcoming Paris trip can, itself, be an activity guided by volition, as when I put aside some time to give it some thought. But the law's voluntary act requirement cannot be met through showing that the defendant did something mental voluntarily; what must be shown is that the defendant engaged in some relevant bodily motion that was guided by volition. The thought is that even though there can be voluntary mental acts, there are no crimes of pure thought; crime requires bodily motion.

1Ls are also taught that every crime has two parts: the actus reus and the mens rea. Defendants must be shown, that is, both to have done something and to have had certain mental states. If a statute specifies a penalty for, say "intentionally damaging public property," a defendant charged with that crime must be shown beyond a reasonable doubt to have damaged public property (the actus reus of the crime) and to have intended to (the mens rea of the crime). The voluntary act required for liability is part of the actus reus, not the mens rea. This can be confusing, since the law tells us that what makes a bodily movement a voluntary action is that it is appropriately guided by a mental state, namely a volition. So it can seem as though finding that a defendant has acted voluntarily requires first finding out that he's met at least some of the mens rea requirements of the crime. But this is only an appearance. Volition is a special mental state, distinct from those included in the mens rea. Volition is best thought of as an executory mental state: it performs the role of realizing in bodily motion the plans and purposes set out by other mental states like intention. One can intend to damage a public memorial, for instance, but one cannot have a volition in favor of that. Putting aside mental acts, one can have a volition in favor *only* of moving one's body in a particular way and more is required than bodily motion for the damage of a public memorial. The idea is that a person who intends to damage a memorial executes that intention through the formation of further mental states, volitions, that control and guide the intricate bodily motions needed to, for instance, carve one's name in the stone. But the mental states guiding those bodily movements, volitions, are not representations of the intended damage to the memorial; they are representations only of the bodily motions that they guide. The mens rea of the crime, then, includes only mental states like intention and belief, while the actus reus of the crime—involving, as it must, a voluntary act—includes something mental only in so far as it includes the executory mental state of volition. The decision to put volition under the heading of actus reus rather than mens rea is not arbitrary. The idea is that mens rea is reserved for what the Latin term actually says: the mind of the guilty. Volitions, the thought is, don't contribute to what makes your mental state into an objectionable one. What's bad is not moving your hand in a certain way; what's bad is *damaging public property*. But in so far as volitions only represent and guide bodily motions as such, independently of their legally important results, they are morally neutral.

The crucial ingredient in the legal concept of voluntary action for our purposes, then, is volition. However, the idea that the bodily motion is *appropriately guided* is important too, as one can see from simple examples: I fall from a bridge. The movement of my body is not a voluntary act since the motion is not guided by my mental activity. There's mental activity at the time alright—I'm thinking, "Good God! I'm falling off a bridge!"—but the motion of my body is not guided at all by this mental activity. Nor would the motion of my body be a voluntary action if, as I fell, I tried desperately to stop falling.

Postponing, for a moment, further reflection on the nature of volition, it is important to see that one way to argue that Libet's experiments show us never to act voluntarily is to argue that they show that even if there is relevant mental activity taking place in the moments before bodily motion, that mental activity does not appropriately guide our bodily motions. The picture is of the mental activity that we call "choice" or "decision" or "volition" as causally irrelevant to the generation of the bodily movements that we take it to cause and guide. To assess this line of thought one needs to know what is meant by "appropriate guidance" and one needs a good argument for thinking that Libet's experiments show this to be absent in our bodily motions. Although I won't make good on this claim here, I think this line of thought is very unlikely to succeed, although there are deep questions here about what any facts about the brain can tell us about the causal properties of our mental states. In any event, I am going to be assuming in what follows, controversially I know, that Libet's discoveries are at least consistent with the view that some kind of mental activity does indeed guide bodily motion.

But there is still room for the view that Libet has shown us not to act voluntarily in the sense required by the law, for even if a bodily movement is responsive to and guided by a mental state, it still might fail to be voluntary in the legal sense if the mental state is not of the right sort. And it is possible that Libet's experiments show the guiding mental activity to be of the wrong sort. I yank my hand back from the handle of the burning hot pot. The motion of my hand is responsive to brain events that underlie mental states; when my hand touched the handle this caused brain activity which in turn caused my hand to yank back. Further the brain activity in question underlies mental states—pains, and probably other states, too, such as beliefs about the heat of the handle. But the yanking of my hand is not a voluntary act. If in yanking it back I broke something of yours, I would not on those grounds be a candidate for a charge of destruction of property; there might be other bodily motions of mine that could serve to put me on the hook for that crime, but the yanking of my hand would not. What then is the law's conception of the distinctive feature of the mental states that guide bodily motions that are voluntary acts? How do they differ from mental activities such as those involved in the hot pot example?

In answering this question, we need to know how the law distinguishes between volitions and other mental activities that cause and guide bodily motions. We learn something about this by looking at the acts which fail to go over the legal hurdle that an act must go over to count as voluntary. There are so few actual criminal cases in which this is so, and in which courts explain the basis of their judgment that it is so, that theorists who have written about the voluntary act requirement tend to cite the same few examples: Huey Newton was shot in the abdomen and moments later fired a gun at and hit the police officer who shot him. He testifies to having no memory of drawing or firing his gun and expert medical testimony confirms that people suffering from such severe physical trauma often engage in complex bodily movements of which they have no memory. Was Newton conscious when he shot the police officer? In some senses of "conscious" he was, and in others he was not. He wasn't asleep, but he was clearly diminished in consciousness in comparison to people who have not just been shot in the abdomen. Newton is acquitted on the grounds that the bodily movements on which his criminal liability would have to be predicated—namely those involved in his drawing and firing his gun—are not voluntary acts because not accompanied by consciousness.[5] There's almost no question that his bodily movements are guided by mental activity—his gun is drawn and aimed at his attacker; it didn't just accidentally fire in the policeman's direction. But, the court holds, this mental activity is not conscious and so fails to be a volition. In reaching this conclusion, the court takes the position that in the meaning of the term "conscious" that is of relevance to the law, a mental state like Newton's is not conscious.

Another oft-cited example: Mrs. Cogdon has a vivid dream in which her daughter is being attacked by an enemy soldier. When she awakes she finds that while asleep she fetched an axe from the woodpile and cleaved her daughter's head in two apparently while dreaming herself to be attacking the soldier in defense of her daughter. She is acquitted on the grounds that the bodily movements that putatively constitute the act portion of her crime—her going to the woodpile, retrieving the axe and swinging it—are not voluntary because the mental activity that guided these movements is unaccompanied by consciousness.[6] Dreams involve a kind of consciousness greater than we find, for instance, in sticks and stones; but, as in *Newton*, in Cogdon's case the court reaches the conclusion that in all of the senses that matter to the law, even if not in all of the senses that are sometimes attached to the term "conscious," Cogdon's relevant mental states are not conscious.

In both Newton's and Cogdon's cases, there is no question that brain activity bearing some kind of resemblance (although how much resemblance is unclear) to that involved in ordinary action is crucially involved in the production of the relevant bodily movements. But control by such complex brain activity is not enough for criminal liability, according to the courts in those cases, for there is a crucial *psychological* difference between the mental states, if any, that Cogdon's and Newton's brain activity underlies, and those involved in ordinary voluntary action: Newton's and Cogdon's mental states are not conscious. So, the hurdle that an act must go over to count as voluntary in the legal sense is at least this high: the mental activity that guides it must be conscious. Or, put in slightly different terms, at least one necessary condition that mental activity must meet to count as volition is a condition of consciousness.

It is important to note that the requirement of consciousness is not a *causal* requirement. Say that a person's volition guides his bodily movement, but it would have guided it in just the same way even if it had not been accompanied by consciousness. In such a case, there is guidance of the bodily movement by a mental state that is conscious, and which counts as a volition in part thanks to the fact that it is conscious, but there is good reason to think that the consciousness which accompanied the mental state was not causally efficacious: conscious or not, the mental state would have the same effects. Was the bodily movement voluntary in the legal sense? Yes. The problem with Newton and Cogdon is not that consciousness was causally irrelevant. The problem is that they weren't conscious. Had they been conscious, they would have engaged in voluntary action, in the legal sense, even if it were also true that the same bodily movements would have followed even absent consciousness. The mental state has to cause bodily movement for the bodily movement to count as voluntary. It must also be accompanied by consciousness. But the mental state needn't cause the bodily movement *in virtue of the fact* that it is accompanied by consciousness. What this implies is that in considering what, if anything, Libet's experiments show us about the criminal law, we needn't concern ourselves with the question of whether or not the experiments show consciousness to be causally irrelevant to bodily movement. The question we should care about, instead, is whether they show consciousness to be absent.

The question with which we began—is voluntariness of the sort Libet has shown our acts to lack required for justifiable criminal liability?—has led us to another: is the sense of "consciousness" in which Libet has shown the mental states underlain by the brain activity registering as the readiness potential to be unaccompanied by consciousness the same sense as that in which justifiable criminal liability requires consciousness to accompany action? At this point, the 1L student discovers that the law supplies no positive description of the kind of consciousness in question, but merely provides, instead, a list of different circumstances in which the relevant sort of consciousness is absent: reflexes, and cases of hypnosis and somnambulism.[7] It also supplies some rules of evidence: the fact that a person *cannot* remember doing something does not imply, as a matter of law, that she was unconscious when she did it, although it does supply some evidence for that. And the fact that a person *can* remember doing something provides powerful, although defeasible evidence that she was conscious when she did it.

The law hasn't supplied us with much to go on. For one thing, it gives us no guidance about exactly what a person needs to be aware *of* in order to be "conscious" in the sense that Newton and Cogdon are not. The subjects in Libet's experiments, for instance, remember the mental events that take place milliseconds after the brain events that register as the readiness potential. They are aware also of the bodily movement that follows moments after that. What, exactly, must a person be aware of in order for his act to be accompanied by consciousness in the sense that matters for the law? Certainly not everything that's involved in action. I am not aware in any way that I can recall of the motion of my pinky when I pull the trigger with my index finger, even though, as biophysics discovers, the motion of the pinky against the barrel turns out to be crucial to leveraging enough force to pull the trigger. The explicit legal opinions in cases like Newton and Cogdon give us no guidance on the issue of what we need to be aware of.

In addition, and more importantly for our purposes, the legal opinions give us almost no guidance about what the awareness itself must involve; they don't tell us when an act of awareness is an instance of the kind of awareness that's required for the mental states in question to be volitions and when it is not. There is certainly some sense in which Cogdon is aware while killing her daughter; she can tell us later about the dream she was having at the time, and dreaming seems to be a form of awareness. Further, the kind of awareness she had is not insufficient for voluntariness simply because it is nonveridical. If she had dreamed that she was killing her daughter, while she was killing her daughter, she would still not have been conscious in the way required for liability. In fact, some of what she was aware of was veridical; she must have been aware of the location of the woodpile, and of the axe's location on the woodpile, when she retrieved it. It is rather that dreamlike awareness is not *consciousness* in the sense that the law has in mind. It's a different kind of awareness from the sort that we take to accompany voluntary action, independently of what it is awareness of. But this still doesn't tell us how that form of awareness differs from the kind that's necessary for criminal liability under the voluntary act requirement.

## 2. LOCKE AND THE EMERGENCE OF THE CONSCIOUSNESS REQUIREMENT

At this point, I want to change the subject and ask a different question, the answer to which will turn out to help us in clarifying both what one needs to be aware of, for legal purposes, for the mental activity guiding one's bodily movement to be a volition, and what the nature of that awareness is, how it differs from other sorts. Here's the new question: When did it come to pass that those who had a powerful influence over the formation of our criminal law determined that there must be some kind of consciousness accompanying the mental states guiding action for that action to be voluntary? In asking this question, I am not asking when those who influenced the development of the criminal law came to believe that criminal liability required a voluntary act. I am interested, instead, in the historical moment when it came to be held that volitions are distinguished from other mental states by consciousness. Oddly enough, given some plausible historical assumptions, it is possible to date this with some precision by looking at John Locke's *Essay Concerning Human Understanding*.

We now tend to think of Locke as a political philosopher because of the well-known influence of his political philosophy on the American and French Revolutions. And, to be sure, Locke was a political philosopher of the first importance; Jefferson quite clearly had Locke's *Second Treatise of Government* to hand as he wrote the *Declaration of Independence*. But in the late seventeenth and eighteenth centuries in Britain, when much of modern common law criminal law doctrine was explicitly formulated and codified, Locke was at least as well known for his views in epistemology, metaphysics, and philosophy of mind as he was for his political philosophy. The *Essay Concerning Human Understanding*, in which Locke presents his views on those topics, was in the library of every learned person in Britain, including every magistrate entrusted with the power to decide criminal cases. The book went through five editions in Locke's lifetime, and a sixth was published shortly after his death. It is plausible to think, then, that what Locke had to say about action had an effect on the criminal law of his time, and, in turn, on ours. Magistrates trying to decide whether or not a defendant's bodily motion was a voluntary act may very well have turned, for instance, to book 2, chapter 21 of Locke's *Essay* and looked carefully at section 28, a section entitled "Volition what."

Even if the influence was not as direct as this, there are other ways in which the law comes to reflect the going views on topics, and the going view of the nature of voluntary action in Britain in the late seventeenth century, and for much of the eighteenth- and nineteenth-, was Locke's. In fact, Locke's conception of action was not significantly challenged by Anglophone philosophers until the mid-twentieth century, when Gilbert Ryle and others of that period, under the influence of Wittgenstein and also behaviorism, began to question volitional theories of action. The primary concern from that quarter was with the very idea of executory mental states guiding bodily motions aimed by grander mental states like intentions. Why should we think there are any executory mental states of that sort? Donald Davidson's response to this sort of concern was to develop a theory of voluntary action under which all of the guidance of bodily motion was done by the mental states like intentions without the help of the special executory mental states the law calls "volitions." But while some of the criticisms of volitional theories have made their way into legal academic circles, and most philosophers of action now think that a theory of action like Davidson's, that grants no role to volition, is more likely to be true than a volitional theory, these lines of thought have had no influence on the law. The law in this area simply has not been revised in any significant way for a very long time.[8]

Now Locke's views on the nature of action changed significantly between the first and second editions of the *Essay*. Throughout all editions of the *Essay* Locke holds a volitional theory of voluntary action. In accord with the criminal law of today, he holds, that is, that, for instance, what makes the movement of my finger a voluntary act on my part, different from a spasmodic movement, is that the movement of the finger is guided by a mental state of volition. There may be mental causes of the spasmodic movement also, but those mental causes are not (in the ordinary case) volitions, and volition, Locke thinks, is what is special to voluntary action. So the Locke interpreter must ask the same question that we ask of the criminal law today: what is volition and how does it differ from other forms of mental activity?

To appreciate Locke's conception of volition, it is important to keep in mind a distinction that Locke makes between two kinds of awareness that one might have of a thing, or of one's own mental states (cf. *Essay* II.i.7, II.ix.1). For Locke, and, really, for all of the philosophers of mind who had an influence on the development of the common law conception of the criminal mind, every mental state was attended with some kind of awareness; that was thought to be a distinctive feature of the mental that distinguished it from bare physical states, such as the states of the bodily organs like the heart or the liver. Locke sometimes, although not always, used the term "consciousness" to refer to this kind of awareness; his more favored term, which has vastly different connotations now, was "perception."[9] In this sense of "consciousness," if we were to say that there is mental activity taking place during the readiness potential, we would also be saying that that mental activity involves consciousness. In this sense of consciousness, that is, it is a contradiction in terms to imagine mental activity that is not conscious. But nobody, much less Locke, took the fact that awareness attends every mental state to imply that those mental states were all things we could know about. The fact that a person is in a mental state implies that she is in some state of awareness, but it does not imply that she knows, can report, can remember, or in any practical way access the mental state she is in. Consider, for instance, your awareness of nonmoving objects in the periphery of your visual field while you focus intently on something in the center of the visual field. You are aware of those objects. But you can't later report on what is there, or remember what is there, or claim even at the moment, much less later, to know what is there. The kind of awareness that was thought to attend all mental states is very thin.

But this very thin kind of awareness that accompanies all mental activity is not the only kind of awareness that Locke thought us to be capable of. Locke, and, again, this was standard in the period, held that for anything of which you were aware to be something that you could know anything about, or remember later, or access in any really meaningful way, you had to *attend* to it. Awareness is one thing; awareness plus attention something much more robust. Locke uses a variety of rather elevated terms to indicate that he is talking about this kind of awareness when he is. He describes people in such a state of attentive awareness to be "contemplating" something or "knowingly" aware of it, or engaged in an act of "attentive reflection." For ease of exposition, let's call the kind of awareness that Locke took to accompany all mental activity "thin consciousness" and call the kind that he took to involve attention, and to allow for knowledge, memory, and perhaps other forms of access of what one is aware of, "thick consciousness." In these terms, there is logical space for thinking that Libet has shown that we are not thickly conscious of the mental activity taking place during the readiness potential. If there is mental activity taking place at that time, it is at most thinly conscious, but it is not thickly conscious.

Now, what does Locke take a volition to be? Locke gives an importantly different answer in the first edition of the *Essay* than he does in the second and later editions of the book. Here's one of the things he writes in the first edition of the *Essay*:

> (1) *Volition*,'tis plain, is nothing but the actual choosing or preferring the forbearance to the doing, or doing to the forbearance, of any particular Action in our power, that we think on. (*Essay*, II.xxi.15, first edition)

The term "preferring" is an umbrella term for Locke; to say that someone is "preferring" something is merely to say that he has a pro-attitude of some variety in favor of it. So, in the first edition, any thought in favor of a particular action—a desire, a preference, a wish, a whim—is a volition to perform that action. Since, under this definition, volitions are mental states, they are accompanied by thin consciousness. But nothing in Locke's definition here intimates that they are necessarily accompanied by thick consciousness. It would be possible, under this definition, to be having a volition while attending solely to something unrelated to the volition—to be attending neither to the act one's volition favors nor to the volition itself—or not to be attending to anything at all. What follows is that it is possible, under this definition of volition, to have a volition that is not thickly conscious. And if it is possible for there to be volitions that are not thickly conscious, it is possible for there to be voluntary actions the mental causes of which are unattended by thick consciousness. What we learn from Libet's experiments is, at worst, that if there is mental activity underlain by the physical events registered as the readiness potential, we are not aware of that mental activity in any way that we can access or turn into knowledge. But this shows only that we are not thickly conscious of that mental activity. That fact is pertinent here *only if* it shows that the mental activity in question is not of the sort that can qualify the resulting bodily movement as voluntary action. But it only shows *that* if it shows the relevant mental activity to be importantly different from volition. But that is not shown if Locke's first edition account of volition is the law's. So, if Locke's first edition account of volition were in line with the law's conception of voluntary action then we could quickly reach an answer to the question that concerns us here: Libet's discoveries, we would conclude, are of no relevance whatsoever to the law's voluntary act requirement.

But this would be too hasty for at least two reasons. First, Locke's first edition account of volition is philosophically indefensible. Here's a counterexample: say that A is B's marionette—B controls how A's body moves, and A knows it—but A is a thinking creature with strong desires about how his body should move. Further, B is very attuned to those desires and aims to please: B moves A's body in exactly the ways that A wants his body to move. Are A's bodily motions voluntary? Clearly not. But they are guided by A's wants. It must be that A's desires don't rise to the level of volition. But they count as volitions under Locke's first edition account of volition. So there must be something wrong with that account. That's one problem, but there is another which is more important for our purposes: there is really no reason to think that Locke's first edition account of volition is the same as today's criminal law's conception. After all, under Locke's first edition account of volition, Newton's bodily movements are voluntary: Newton's bodily movements were guided by mental activities and there is every reason to believe that Newton wanted to engage in them; he wanted to shoot the cop who shot him. So, when the law requires that Newton's mental activity be conscious to be volition, it must be requiring more than what is required by Locke in the first edition of the *Essay*.

Now notice what happens in the later editions of the *Essay*. In the second and later editions, Locke cuts passage (1) and replaces it with the following:

> (2) *Volition*,'tis plain, is an Act of the Mind knowingly exerting that Dominion it takes itself to have over any part of the man, by imploying it in, or withholding it from, any particular Action. (*Essay* II.xxi.15)

For our purposes, the crucial word here is "knowingly." Locke is telling us that it is definitive of volition that it is accompanied by *thick* consciousness; thin consciousness of the sort involved in every mental activity is not enough. To be engaging in the kind of mental activity capable of qualifying resulting bodily movement as voluntary, one must be in a position to know something about that activity. And given that knowledge about X can only derive from awareness of X when that awareness is accompanied with attention, it follows that one must be aware of something in the thick sense in order to be engaging in volition. Voluntary action involves knowing not just that your body is moving, but also something about the mental causes of that bodily movement. Locke's point here is the one that we find expressed in today's criminal law. Cogdon's and Newton's mental states are not accompanied by the kind of thick conscious awareness that is distinctive of volition, no matter what term we use to pick out that special property.

In fact, Locke's changes from the first to the second edition of the *Essay* are systematic in this regard. Every definition of volition, and virtually every remark about volition, is replaced with one that intimates that volitions involve some kind of heightened awareness. Further, and importantly, the second edition of the *Essay* includes Locke's groundbreaking discussion of personal identity in which he argues that the definitive feature of a person, what constitutes personal identity over time, in fact, is self-awareness. That now familiar idea had its birth alongside Locke's account of volition as involving thick consciousness.[10]

I conjecture, then, that the criminal law's requirement of consciousness for voluntary action and thus for criminal liability is born with Locke's rewriting of the *Essay Concerning Human Understanding* between 1689 and 1694. In 1689, Locke thinks that although volitions are accompanied by thin consciousness, they needn't be accompanied by thick. But thin consciousness does not distinguish volitions from any other kind of mental activity, and so does not help us to characterize the difference between, for instance, Cogdon's mental activity and that of a waking person who engaged in the same bodily movements. But five years later, in 1694, Locke has come to believe something very close to what today's criminal law accepts: one of the distinguishing features of volition is its accompaniment by some heightened form of awareness that goes beyond that involved in dreaming, or in the kind of complex reflexive behavior in which Huey Newton engaged.

Why does this matter to the question of the relevance of Libet's experiments to the voluntary act requirement? The reason it matters is that it suggests that if we want to understand what the law is requiring in making consciousness a necessary condition of criminal liability, we might do well to look at what, exactly, Locke was requiring. After all, if the voluntary act requirement comes to involve a requirement of consciousness because Locke took consciousness to be a necessary condition for volition, then the voluntary act requirement, originally anyway, imported Locke's conception of thick consciousness. Of course, the law may have changed. But there's reason to think it hasn't. The primary engines of change to the criminal law are statutes and judicial decisions. Legislators pass statutes that supplement, revise or overrule common law doctrines, or settle common law ambiguities. And judges make decisions that do the same things. But of all the elements of the common criminal law, it is probably no exaggeration to say that the voluntary act requirement is closer to being unsullied by legislative and judicial machinations than any other; it is simply taken as a basic axiom of the criminal law and all but untouchable.

## 3. LOCKEAN VOLUNTARY ACTION AND THE LIBET EXPERIMENTS

Recall that to make progress on the question of the relevance of Libet's discoveries to the criminal law we need to know more both about what we are thickly conscious of when we are engaging in a volition, and what the nature of thick consciousness is. When we know these things we will be in a better position to determine whether the subjects in Libet's experiments have been shown to lack thick consciousness in a way that is of relevance to criminal liability. Moving forward under the assumption that the criminal law's theory of voluntary action is Locke's, we can ask then both what Locke thinks we are thickly conscious of when engaging in volition, and what Locke takes the nature of thick consciousness to be. Reflection on both questions is aided by consideration of the following passage from Locke, a passage added to the second edition of the *Essay*:

> (3) *Volition* . . . is an act of the Mind directing its thought to the production of any Action, and thereby exerting its power to produce it. (*Essay* II.xxi.28)

As I mentioned, for Locke, and so quite possibly for the criminal law, thick consciousness involves attention in a way that thin consciousness does not. Locke's talk here of "directing [one's] thought" to something is one of his ways of making explicit the role of attentive awareness, or thick consciousness, in volition.

In this passage Locke is clear that what a person who has a volition is thickly conscious *of* is "the production of [the] [a]ction." But it is far from clear how we should understand this phrase. What, exactly, is "the production of the action"? It is easier to say what this is not than it is to say what it is. It is not to be equated with volition; being aware of a mental state does not amount to being aware of the production of anything, including those bodily movements that are caused by that mental state. Nor is the production of the action to be equated with the bodily movement that one brings about through volition. To be aware of an event is not to be aware, ipso facto, of its being produced. A person, like a professional high diver, for instance, who engages in attentive "previsualization" of a bodily movement—the twist of his shoulders, say, moments after reaching the apex of his jump from the board—does not thereby engage in a volition in favor of that bodily movement. In previsualization, he is attending to the bodily movement, not to the bringing it about, or the production of the action.[11]

In any event, however we are to understand "the production of the action," it seems clear that the object of attention here is not exactly what Libet's subjects are shown to be poor at timing. His subjects are asked to time *their volition*, a mental state, and that is not precisely what Locke thinks we are attentively aware of in volition. So, even if we grant that being bad at timing a mental state is strong evidence that one was not thickly conscious of it—an assumption that should not go unquestioned—we cannot say, from looking at Libet's experiments, whether his subjects failed to be thickly conscious of the production of the action. Whatever the production of the action is, it does not take place solely during the period of the readiness potential since that precedes the muscle contraction that in turn causes—*produces*—the bodily movement. Or, to put the point differently, Libet's subjects are thickly conscious of something that takes place after the readiness potential and before the muscle contraction; since that is precisely the period in which the action is being produced, Libet's results are consistent with thick consciousness of just the thing that Locke thinks one must be thickly conscious of in order to be engaging in a volition. So, so far anyway, there's no reason to think that Libet's experiments show the mental state taking place during the readiness potential to be unaccompanied by the kind of awareness needed for it to count as a volition. To put the point yet another way, Libet's results are consistent with the possibility that subjects are thinking attentively during the readiness potential of events that take place a few milliseconds later. When they report the time of their volition, then, they report the time of the events to which they were attending during the readiness potential, and so they report the time of their volition as a few milliseconds after the readiness potential. But since it seems plausible enough that "the production of the action" takes place a few milliseconds after the readiness potential, it seems plausible that the subjects are attending to precisely what they need to attend to for their mental states to count as volitions. If so, then the experiments are consistent with the claim that the subjects are acting voluntarily.

Still, we should not be hasty here. Perhaps a *necessary condition* of attentive awareness of "the production of action" is attentive awareness of the volition that causes the relevant bodily movement. Maybe "the production of the action" is a complex event that includes the volition plus more. If so, then a subject who was attentively aware of the production of action would also be attentively aware of his volition. Someone who attends to the play at first attends to the runner's advance to the base since, after all, the runner's advance to the base is part of the event that is the play at first. Is the volition part of the complex event that is the production of the action? It might be. But even if it is, we would need to know more about the way in which subjects assign times to events that take place over the course of a few milliseconds to know if Libet's subjects were not aware of the production of the action.

Say, for instance, that when asked to time an event that takes place over the course of the interval from zero to 100 milliseconds, subjects tend to identify the time of the event as 50 milliseconds. The fact that the event begins 50 milliseconds prior to the moment that they identify does not show that they are not aware of *the event*, or that they are not aware of it during its first 50 milliseconds. They are timing *an event*, not the instant that the event begins.[12] Say that the play at first begins at time 0, as the runner gets very close to the base, continues as the ball hits the first baseman's glove at time 50, and ends at time 100, as the runner moves up the line. A subject asked to say when the play at first took place very well might identify the moment that the ball hit the first baseman's glove, time 50, even though he was aware of the event as the runner advanced to the base at time 0. If that were so, then even if the volition is part of a complex event that continues for some time after the volition itself strikes (which we are assuming is during the readiness potential), a subject asked to report when the thing of which he was attentively aware took place very well might identify a moment some milliseconds after *the first part of that event* (namely the volition) took place.

It's plausible to think that we time complex events based on the time of their most salient parts. In the case of the play at first, the most salient part might be thought to be the moment when the ball hits the first baseman's glove. In the case of "the production of the action," the most salient part might be some milliseconds after the readiness potential. But we cannot conclude from the fact that the subject identifies the time that the ball hits the glove as the time of the play at first *that* the subject is not aware of the runner's approach to the base. And similarly, we cannot conclude from the fact that Libet's subjects identify times some moments after the readiness potential as the time of their volition that they are not aware of their volition. A subject asked when he first became aware of his volition very well might interpret the question to be asking when he first became aware of *that which he is ordinarily aware of when he acts voluntarily.* This, if Locke is right, is "the production of the action." If the subject then times that event as taking place some milliseconds after the readiness potential, he is just like the spectator to the play at first: we can conclude nothing from his answer about whether or not he was aware of the volition. I conclude, then, that even on the assumption that the volition itself is part of "the production of the action," Libet's results are consistent with attentive awareness during the readiness potential of just the sort that Locke took to be needed for the mental event taking place at the time to be a volition.

We are still not done, however. There remains a question as to whether Libet's results show us to lack a kind of awareness of the mental state taking place during the readiness potential (if there is one) that we have not yet discussed and that may be needed for voluntariness, under Locke's account. To see this, return for a moment to passage (3). Locke does not seem to hold that there are two events taking place in the mind during volition: a volition and, separately, an act of attentive awareness of the production of the action. Rather, he seems to hold that the act of attentive awareness of the production of the action <u>is</u> the volition. Volitions are a species of acts of attention. His idea is that all you do in your head when you have a volition, when you exercise executory control over your body, is to turn your attention in a particular way to the production of bodily movement. Elsewhere he says that we move our bodies "barely by a thought" (*Essay* II.xxi.4). His idea is that having an attentive mental representation of something—"the production of an action"—is all that the mind contributes to voluntary motion. But are we thickly conscious of our acts of attention? If I am attentively aware of X, am I also attentively aware of the fact that I am engaging in an act of attentive awareness?

It is very easy to get confused about this because it is easy to mix up the sense in which we are aware of the *object* to which we attend with the sense in which we are aware of the *act* of attention itself. Say that I ask you to stare at the tip of your index finger and to attend to it as closely as you can. What are you aware of when you do this? Well, you are certainly aware of more than just your index finger. You are aware, for instance, also of your middle finger (assuming it is not blocked from view), as well as everything else in your visual field. But you are somehow more vividly aware of the index finger. Now imagine that a few minutes later you are asked some questions about what you were aware of while focusing intently on your index finger. You are going to be far better at reporting the features of your index finger than at reporting the features of anything else in your visual field. It was your index finger, after all, to which you were attending. So, you were thickly conscious *of your index finger*. But what about the mental state you were in when attending to the index finger? In what sense were you aware of that mental state? In what sense were you aware of your act of attending? Are you thinly conscious of it, or thickly conscious of it? Are you in a position to report, after the fact, on any of its distinctive features? For instance, are you in a position to say when you started to attend to your index finger? For how long you attended? We're good at saying what we attended *to*; we were, after all, attending to it, and so should be good at using that awareness to generate knowledge about that to which we attended. But how good are we at saying anything about the act of attention itself, considered independently of its object? These are empirical questions, and the answers to them are not immediately obvious.

Although I don't say it with complete confidence, it seems to me plausible that Locke takes us to be only thinly conscious of the act of attention itself, except in rare cases in which we make it, itself, an object of a distinct act of attending. If this is right, then the sense in which volition, for Locke, involves thick consciousness is exhausted by the assertion that in volition we are attentively aware of the production of action, a form of attentive awareness that Libet has not shown us to lack. However, I am not entirely confident about this even as a matter of Locke scholarship; Locke just never, to my knowledge, discusses the question of whether we are thickly or thinly conscious of our acts of attention. Further, his silence on the matter suggests that in so far as the criminal law incorporates an answer to this question, it's unlikely to have come from Locke. And, of course, it is quite likely that there is no settled view about this to be found in the criminal law.

It seems to me, however, that there is little reason to think that people are more than thinly conscious of their acts of attention. They are thickly conscious of *the objects* of their acts of attending. But in so far as thick consciousness of X requires attending to X, it seems unlikely that people are thickly aware of their acts of attending since they only rarely attend to them. It is notoriously difficult to attend to more than one very different thing at the same moment. It seems extremely hard to attend, at once, to, say, the future movement of one's finger, and also to one's act of attending to that future movement. Add having, at the same time, to attend to a small dot moving around a clock, one might find that the thing that simply cannot hold one's attention is one's act of attending. Still, it would be hasty to think that the question of whether we are thinly or thickly conscious of our acts of attention can be solved from the armchair. Let me end by sketching the outline of an experiment that would help us to answer the question in a way that would help us to determine whether our acts are voluntary in the legal sense.

Libet emphasizes that subjects asked to identify the moment they were unexpectedly pricked with a pin identify a time that is closer to the moment that the brain activity underlying the pain takes place than do subjects asked to identify the moment at which they decided to do something.[13,14] But if volitions are acts of attention, if that is the sense in which they involve thick consciousness, then the relevant comparison is not with pain, but with other acts of attention. How close to the moment at which our attention is actually turned do we judge our attention to have been turned?[15] In the same way that Libet asked subjects to move their fingers spontaneously, and to note the time at which they decided to do so, the experimenter would devise for subjects' attention to be diverted and ask them to identify the moment at which this occurs. Notice that if Locke is right, volitions are acts of turning attention to something, namely the production of an action, that does not exist until after one's attention is turned to it; it is, after all, the turning of attention to it that brings it about. So, similarly, whatever it is that subjects have their attention turned to in the experiment, call it "X," must be something that is not present at the moment that attention is turned to it but appears moments later. What is needed, then, is something that is going to lead subjects to think of X instants before X appears before them and they are to be asked when they thought of that thing attentively for the first time. Ideally, the gap between the subjects' first thought of X and X's appearance should be the same as the gap between the beginning of the readiness potential and the contraction of the muscle in Libet's experiments.

Let me give an example of the kind of thing I have in mind.[16] Subjects are seated before a computer screen divided into 100 squares in a ten-by-ten grid with a clock at the top and they are monitored by EEG or by fMRI. At any given moment, each square in the grid contains a colored dot and the colors are constantly changing. For a period of time, a "priming" period, subjects are asked to say when a blue dot appears somewhere on the screen. They are not told that prior to the appearance of a blue dot a red dot appears elsewhere on the screen, signaling to them that the blue dot is about to appear. The red dot and the blue dot always appear in the same relative positions so that a subject who spotted the pattern could say where the blue dot will appear given the location of the red. (If the red appears in square (x, y), then the blue appears in (x+3, y-2), for instance.) The priming period ends when there is an EEG or fMRI event occurring in response to the appearance of the red dot that indicates that the subjects are now anticipating the appearance of the blue dot. (Ideally, they will not have explicitly figured out the pattern, but will be responding in conditioned anticipation of the appearance of the blue dot.) At the completion of the priming period, a new period starts in which subjects are asked to identify not the moment the blue dot appears, but the moment that they find themselves starting to *anticipate* its appearance; they are asked, that is, to say when they start to think that the blue dot is about to appear. The experimenter then looks to see how these reports correspond to the timing of the EEG or fMRI event that seems to indicate the turn of attention. The idea is that the EEG or fMRI event is registering the brain activity that underlies the turn of attention toward the blue dot, and the subject is being asked to say when this event occurs. If the gap between the moment that the subject takes his attention to have turned and the brain event is close to the gap in the timing of volition in Libet's experiments, then it would appear that subjects are aware of their volitions in something like the same way as they are aware of acts of turning attention. But if not, if subjects are better at timing their acts of turning attention than they are at timing the events registered as the readiness potential in Libet's experiments, then that too would be of interest since it would provide evidence suggesting that there is an important difference in our awareness of the relevant events in the one case than in the other.

## CONCLUSION

Libet himself was famously impatient with philosophers. In fact, he used the term in a clearly pejorative sense. My impression is that he was primarily impatient with the generation of hypotheses explaining his data that he took to be either intrinsically implausible, or unsupported by independent empirical results, or both. Fair enough. But plausible or not, there is a view to be found in the law about what happens when the criminal acts. Unless we're going to radically reform the law—and maybe we should—we can only compare the defendant to the picture we find in the law of the criminal and see whether the two are close enough to warrant labeling the defendant as such. What I've tried to do here is, first, to suggest that in many ways, even incorporating Libet's discoveries, there is no reason to think that defendants generally fail to match the picture we find in the law, and, second, to suggest how further empirical work can help us to develop clarity on the question.

## ACKNOWLEDGMENTS

Thanks are owed to Michael Bratman, Alfred Mele, and especially Walter Sinnott-Armstrong for comments on earlier drafts.

## APPENDIX: MOORE'S REVERSE ENGINEERING OF LOCKE

Michael Moore has developed a detailed account of the nature of voluntary action, and he has made a powerful case for thinking that the account he offers is very close to the view implicitly accepted in the criminal law.[xvii] Moore's method is to determine what questions need to be answered about voluntary action in order to resolve the sorts of cases that appear in criminal courts (cases like *Newton* or *Cogdon*) and then to determine which possible answers to those questions are most philosophically defensible. As I will indicate in this appendix, the view Moore develops through following this method is startlingly similar to Locke's position. If I am right, however, that Locke's view of voluntary action was taken up by the criminal law, this is no surprise. If that is right, then whether we start by looking at Locke's view, as I have, or by looking, instead, at the criminal law's position, as Moore has, we should end up in the same place. The fact that we do end up in the same place provides some further evidence for thinking that it is Locke's conception of voluntary action that has been accepted by the criminal law.

There is no disputing that in the criminal law, for Locke and for Moore, the crucial element in voluntary action is volition. Moore identifies nine questions that can be asked about volition, each of which can be answered in a variety of different ways. Accounts of the nature of volition can be classified, then, with respect to their answers to these nine questions. Moore and Locke give the same answers to seven of these nine questions. One of the remaining two questions is addressed only partially by Locke. That question concerns the classification of volition as desire, belief, intention, or something distinct from all of these that some have labeled "willing" or "choosing." Locke, like Moore, is clear that volition is not to be equated either with desire or belief, but he does not draw a distinction between intention and willing, and so it is hard to know how he would classify volition in this last respect. The remaining question concerns the classification of volition as a functional state, or as some other kind of state. Locke simply doesn't address this issue, although the answer that Moore gives (functional state) is not inconsistent with anything that Locke says. The similarities between Locke's position and Moore's are detailed in the table 16.1 indicating passages from Locke's *Essay* that provide evidence for thinking that he gives the same answer as Moore.

A thoroughgoing argument to the effect that each of these passages does indeed support the attribution of the position to Locke that coincides with Moore's will not be undertaken here.[xviii] But if those attributions are correct, we have further, albeit indirect evidence to suggest that the criminal law's voluntary act requirement was inherited from Locke.

**Table 16.1 Textual evidence in support of the claim that Locke's and Morre's conceptions of volition are the same.**

| Question | Answer | Passage |
|---|---|---|
| Are volitions events or agents? | Events | II.xxi.5, II.xxi.19 |
| Are volitions mere happenings or actions? | Mere happenings | II.xxi.8, II.xxi.25, II.xxi.72 |
| Are volitions desires, beliefs, intentions, or willings? | Intentions | Not desire: II.xxi.30<br>Not belief: II.xxi.15 |
| Do volitions have objects? | Yes | II.xxi.30 |
| Is a volition's object a thing or a representation of a thing, like a proposition? | Representation | IV.i.1 |
| Is the content of a volition the proposition that an action occurs or that a mere happening occurs? | Mere happening | II.xxi.30 |
| Is the propositional content of a volition an internal bodily event, a remote consequence, or a bodily movement? | A bodily movement | II.xxi.30 |
| Are volitions functional states, physical states, behavioral states, or irreducibly mental states? | Functional states | ———— |
| Are volitions states of the whole person, or of a subpersonal homunculus? | The whole person | II.xxi.16–19 |

## NOTES

1. Other reasons might be offered for thinking that Libet's discoveries undermine justifiable criminal liability. One might think, for instance, that they show that we never form criminal intent. This is a distinct line of thought from the one that I discuss here.
2. Since my concern here is with the concept of voluntariness employed by the law and the relevance of Libet's experiments to it, I will be assuming that the law in this area is justified. I will be assuming, that is, that acts labeled as voluntary by the law possess the property that is required for justifiable punishment. This assumption can, of course, be questioned. But I will not question it here.
3. Even apparent counterexamples—such as crimes of possession or crimes of omission—- turn out, on reflection, to be *merely* apparent. To be guilty of a crime of possession of an illegal drug, for instance, the defendant must have performed a voluntary act resulting in the acquisition of the possessed drug, or voluntarily performed an act through which he came to continue to hold on to the drug that he possessed. If you slip some pot into my glove compartment without my knowledge, I'm guilty of possession only if I perform a voluntary act through which I come to leave it there. The relevant section of the *Model Penal Code* allows for criminal liability for possession "if the possessor knowingly procured or received the thing possessed or was aware of his control thereof for a sufficient period to have been able to terminate his possession" (§2.01(4)).
4. It is important to see that there are senses of the ordinary term "voluntary" that are simply not at issue in the law's voluntary act requirement. For instance, imagine that I am walking toward the U.S. border from Mexico when someone puts a gun to my head and explains that if I don't carry a package for him across the border, he'll kill me. Fearing for my life, I stuff the package in my pocket and try to cross the border, where I am stopped and searched and the drugs the package contains are found. Am I guilty of attempting to smuggle drugs into the United States? No, but not because of the absence of an appropriate voluntary act in the legal sense. I voluntarily, in the legal sense if not in some ordinary senses of the term, hid the package in my pocket; I voluntarily handed my passport to the agent; I voluntarily said that I had nothing to declare, etc. I am absolved of criminal responsibility for this crime because I performed the relevant voluntary acts *under duress*. Duress undermines liability, but not because it undermines the voluntariness, in the legal sense, of the defendant's acts.
5. *People v. Newton*, 8 Cal. App. 3d 359, 87 Cal. Rptr. 394 (1970).

6. This case was unreported but has been widely discussed. The most cited discussion is Norval Morris, "Somnambulistic Suicide: Ghosts, Spiders and North Koreans," *Res Judicata* 29 (1951): 5.
7. See, for instance, *Model Penal Code* §2.01(2).
8. It is also important to note that were the law to incorporate views of voluntary action that give no place to volition, then Libet's experiments would clearly fail to imply that our acts are not voluntary in the sense that matters. The reason is that at most Libet's experiments show that we are not aware of executory mental states through which our intentions to engage in future conduct—such as the intention to comply with the experimenter's instructions—are executed. But if nothing about those executory mental states contributes to making resulting bodily movement voluntary, as on the Davidsonian theory of voluntary action, then Libet's discoveries simply aren't relevant to voluntariness. Libet's experiments, in short, would have less relevance to a criminal law that reflected post-Davidsonian thinking about the nature of action than it has for the actual criminal law, which does not.
9. At *Essay* II.xxvii.9, Locke uses both the terms "consciousness" and "perception" in the same sentence to refer to the kind of awareness that attends all mental states.
10. The systematic changes to Locke's account of volition were discovered independently by myself and Stephen Darwall in the 1990s. Their importance has been discussed by both us in print, and by others. See Stephen Darwall, *The British Moralists and the Internal 'Ought'* (Cambridge: Cambridge University Press, 1995), 149–175; Tito Magri, "Locke, Suspension of Desire, and the Remote Good," *British Journal for the History of Philosophy* 8, no. 1 (March 2000): 55–70; Gideon Yaffe, *Liberty Worth the Name: Locke on Free Agency* (Princeton, NJ: Princeton University Press, 2000).
11. There are difficult type-token questions to ask here. Is the previsualizer aware of *the type* of bodily movement that he will engage in when he jumps, or is he aware of a token of that type? For our purposes, it should not matter for whatever we wish to say about what he is aware of, we can say the same thing of the person who is in the same mental state while engaging in the dive. So however we are to understand the object of the previsualizer's awareness, it is clear that it cannot amount to a volition.
12. Could the subjects be interpreted to be timing not their volition, but *the beginning* of a distinct event, namely *their awareness* of their volition? Possibly. I suspect that most people would interpret the question, "When did you become aware of the play at first?" to be asking "When did the play at first take place?" When the event of which we are aware takes place over a very short period of time, we don't normally distinguish the time of our awareness of the event and the time of the event. Some subjects, however, might interpret the two questions differently.
13. See Benjamin Libet, "Unconscious Cerebral Initiative and the Role of Conscious Will in Voluntary Action" in *Brain and Behavioral Sciences* 3 (1985): §2.4.1, p. 534.
14. Pains are, for Locke, the quintessential example of a mental state of which we are thickly conscious. When you are in pain he thinks that your attention is inexorably drawn to that mental state and away from other things. See, for instance, *Essay* II.xxi.12.
15. An attentive reader will notice that the following two questions are distinct: (1) Are we thickly conscious of our acts of attention? (2) How accurately are we capable of timing our acts of attention? It is possible that the answer to (2) is 'not very" even though the answer to (1) is "yes." However, notice that we find the same problem in Libet's experiments. Libet, that is, takes the fact that we are poor at timing our volitions to show that we are not conscious of them It is possible that this inference is flawed. If it is, then that is a flaw in both Libet's experiments and the experiment proposed here. Still, if the answer to (2) is "not very," then that at least supplies evidence in favor of thinking that the answer to (1) is "no." The evidence is defeasible, but it is evidence nonetheless.
16. Thanks to Walter Sinnott-Armstrong for helping me to turn my sketchy thoughts about this into a concrete experiment.
17. Michael Moore, *Act and Crime* (Oxford: Clarendon Press, 1993), 113–133. The questions and answers that appear in the table below are also to be found here.
18. Many of these passages are discussed at some length in Gideon Yaffe, *Liberty Worth the Name: Locke on Free Agency* (Princeton, NJ: Princeton University Press, 2000), 75–117.

# CHAPTER 17

## Criminal and Moral Responsibility and the Libet Experiments

*Larry Alexander*

The basic unit for evaluation by the criminal law—and by the moral notions that underlie it—is the so-called voluntary act. (I shall leave to the side those few omissions that the law criminalizes and the somewhat greater number that common morality condemns. What I shall say about the Libet experiments and how they bear on criminal and moral responsibility for acts will apply, I believe, equally to illegal and immoral omissions, although in a somewhat more complicated way.) The voluntary act that is the principal focus of criminal law and morality can be characterized as a "willed bodily movement." And in case one believes there are unconscious "willings," the voluntary act can be characterized as a "consciously willed bodily movement." The culpability of such voluntary acts or consciously willed bodily movements will be determined by what the actor believes about the circumstances in which the acts take place, by what the actor believes the consequences of the acts will or might be, and by the reasons for which the actor has taken the acts. (For some, culpability is, in addition, determined by what the circumstances and consequences actually are. And for some, culpability is, in addition, determined by what the actor should have believed about the circumstances and consequences.)

If a consciously willed bodily movement is the principal unit of criminal and moral assessment, then criminal law and morality do not evaluate the following bodily movements, even if they produce harm: tics, reflexes, spasms, and other bodily movements that are not subject to the conscious will, as when one is pushed or falls.[1] (The consciously willed bodily movements that preceded and set the stage for such involuntary bodily movements may, of course, be evaluated and in some cases be deemed culpable.)

More controversial are bodily movements that are "willed" in states of "altered consciousness." These include acts undertaken while in a hypnotic trance, acts committed while sleepwalking, and acts committed in a state of automatism. The actor on such occasions is conscious to some degree: his acts appear to be goal-directed and responsive to the environment. Nonetheless, unlike one who undertakes fully conscious acts, the actor cannot recall acts committed in those altered states of consciousness.

The criminal law deems acts committed in altered states of consciousness not to be voluntary and therefore not culpable because they are not fully conscious;[2] and I suspect the criminal law is mirroring morality here as well. Interestingly, the criminal law and morality *do* treat acts committed out of habit as voluntary and potentially culpable, even though one could argue that acts committed out of habit are committed with such a low level of conscious awareness that they too are beyond recollection and thus should not be distinguished from acts committed in altered states of consciousness.[3] Perhaps it is thought that habitual acts, even if they occur in a somewhat altered state of consciousness, are nonetheless monitorable by the fully conscious mind in a way that acts affected by hypnosis, somnambulism, and automatism cannot be.

All of this is by way of setting the stage for an analysis of how Libet's experiments bear on criminal and moral responsibility. More specifically, has Libet demonstrated that the consciously willed bodily movement, the centerpiece of our notions of criminal and moral responsibility, is an illusion?

Libet's experiments purport to show that about half a second before a subject is consciously aware of a decision to act, there is an increase in brain activity. In the experiments, the subject is not deliberating about whether to act much less about what act to take. The only decision the subject makes is *when* to act. And the experiments purport to show that when the subject thinks "now" and acts, his brain had begun increasing its activity about a half second before.

Libet reached the following conclusion as a result of these experiments: "The process leading to a voluntary act is initiated by the brain unconsciously, well before the conscious will to act appears. That implies that free will, if it exists, would not initiate a voluntary act."[4]

There are, I believe, three possible interpretations of the Libet experiment. The first, and perhaps most dramatic, is that implied by Libet himself in what was just quoted, namely, that decisions to act are not initiated by the conscious will but by the nonconscious brain. The sense that we have that we are consciously willing our bodily movements is illusory or epiphenomenal.

There are two other ways to interpret the experiments, however. I will assume that the experiments demonstrate what they purport to, so my alternatives do not deny Libet's results, only his interpretation of those results. One alternative is that the decisions the actors reached were not unconscious but rather conscious, though in an altered state, beyond the subject's recall. The subjects misidentified the time they became conscious of their decision to act as the time they became robustly or fully conscious of it. They were conscious of it before that time, but not fully conscious of it.

If this interpretation of the results is correct, however, it still has major implications for criminal and moral responsibility. For as I said previously, the law and probably common morality do not regard those who act in altered states of consciousness to have acted voluntarily. They therefore cannot be deemed culpable for what they do in such states. If we are always deciding to act in altered states of consciousness and only become fully conscious of our decisions to act after we have made them, then criminal and moral responsibility is threatened every bit as much as it is on Libet's interpretation of his results. Or at least that is so if we do not change our views about acts in hypnotic, somnambulant, and similar states of altered consciousness.

The third possible interpretation of Libet's results is that they have nothing to do with the voluntariness of our acts. Rather, the brain activity that precedes our fully conscious willings is not an unconscious willing or an altered conscious willing but is instead an indicator of something else—perhaps the anxiety or tension that precedes the moment of conscious choice. Notice that in the experiments, there was no deliberation about what to do. Indeed, there was really no deliberation about when to do it, as nothing hung in the balance regarding when the act occurred. When the subject decided to move his body in the prescribed way, that was all that was up for decision. In a sense, everything had already been decided other than the precise moment of the act. It is surely conceivable that in those circumstances, when the subject was about to choose "now," some readiness activity was already welling up in his brain.

Libet points out that his experiments remove deliberation from the scene. Indeed, even the choice of when to act is not a focus of deliberation, given that absolutely nothing hangs on it.

Moreover, Libet himself, almost immediately after the quotation I gave above, backs off quite a way from being deflationary regarding conscious willings. Consider these quotations that appear only a few pages from the quote I gave:

"[Conscious free will] can control the actual outcome or performance of the act. It could permit the action to proceed, or it can veto it, so that no action occurs."[5]

"We may view voluntary acts as beginning with unconscious initiatives being 'burbled up' by the brain. The conscious will would then select which of these initiatives may go forward to an action."[6]

"On the other hand, it is possible the conscious will, when it appears, acts as a trigger to enable the unconsciously prepared initiative to proceed further to production of the act."[7]

The conception of the conscious will Libet portrays in these quotes is as a gatekeeper regarding which "unconscious initiatives" will proceed to action. That is a more pivotal role than that described in the first two interpretations. It preserves the central importance of the fully consciously willed bodily movement. It is also consistent with the experimental evidence. And it does not necessitate any revision of our pre-Libet notions of moral and criminal responsibility.

It would be interesting to know what kind of brain activity would precede a moment of choice if, unlike in Libet's experiment, the time for the choice were not at issue but were prescribed, and the subject were told either to act or refrain from acting at that time. My hunch is that brain activity would arise as the moment for choice approached whether or not the subject chose to act or to refrain. That result would be consistent with the brain's activity indicating not a prior unconscious willing but rather a prewilling state of anticipatory tension.

One should also note that professional baseball players must make a swing or no swing decision in a time period that is shorter than that described in Libet's experiments. A ninety mile per hour pitch delivered from less than sixty feet away when released must be assessed and reacted to in less than half a second. On the other hand, I suspect one would find an increase in the batter's brain activity shortly before the pitch is released.

Given the simple notion of the choice presented to Libet's subjects—again, they had no need to deliberate over how to act or whether to act; they were to act in a prescribed way, and the only question for them was when—and given Libet's own interpretation of the role of the conscious will, I see nothing in his experimental results to warrant revising the standard picture of morally and legally responsible acting or revising the standard view of the frequency with which it occurs.

## NOTES

1. *See* Model Penal Code, § 2.01(2)(a), (d).
2. *See* Model Penal Code, § 2.01(b), (c).
3. *See* Model Penal Code, § 2.01(d).
4. Benjamin Libet, *Mind time* (Cambridge, MA: Harvard University Press, 2004), 136.
5. *Id.* at 139.
6. *Id.*
7. *Id.* at 145.

# CHAPTER 18

# Libet's Challenge(s) to Responsible Agency

*Michael S. Moore*

## 1. THE ROLE OF INTENTION IN ASSESSING RESPONSIBILITY IN LAW AND MORALS

The concept of an intention lies at the heart of the attribution of both moral responsibility and legal liability in the law of torts and of crimes. It does so in two ways. The first is as a marker (arguably *the* marker) of serious culpability in the doing of wrongful actions. As the law both of crimes and of torts recognizes, doing some wrongful action because one intended to do it merits greater blame and more severe sanctions than does doing that same wrongful action recklessly or negligently. This implication of intention for responsibility is learned early on by children, who frame serious accusations of others in terms of their doing things "on purpose." As Justice Holmes famously put it, "even a dog knows the difference between being stumbled over and being kicked."[1] Criminal law shares with dogs and children this emphasis on intention as essential to serious blame. As the U.S. Supreme Court once put it, "The contention that an injury can amount to a crime only when inflicted by intention is no provincial or transient notion. It is . . . universal and persistent in mature systems of law . . . [and] is almost as instinctive as the child's familiar exculpatory, 'But I didn't mean to.'"[2]

The second way in which intention figures into attributions of responsibility has to do with wrongdoing rather than culpability. To do wrong is to *act* in a way that morality or the law prohibits, and intentions are at the root of action and agency. The very possibility of persons doing *actions* depends on persons having intentions. The old way of putting this was to say that "every action must be intentional under some description of it." A more modern rendition is to say that every action begins with an intention, in the sense that intentions must be the immediate cause of those bodily movements through which persons act, for those movements to be actions at all.[3]

At the most general level the two legal and moral uses of intention to ascribe responsibility presuppose a realism about intentions. As one common law court put it, the law supposes that "the state of a man's mind is as much a fact as the state of his digestion."[4] We suppose this in law and in ethics because any naturalist view of legal and moral qualities is committed to there being some natural property on which moral and legal properties supervene.[5] There have to be intentions for responsibility to depend on intentionality in the way that it does.

Less generally, our assessment of responsibility also supposes that the folk psychology of intention is at least roughly correct. Intention, in other words, not only exists as a distinct kind of mental state, but it is the kind of mental state the folk psychology posits it to be. One sees this supposition plainly in the way that the voluntary act and the mens rea doctrines of the criminal law are built entirely on the back of that folk psychology.

The folk psychology in question is that relating to practical rationality. On this psychology there are three sorts of representational states that cause the behavior of rational agents: there are states of desire, where we represent the world as we want it to be; states of belief, where we represent the world as we believe it is; and there are states of intention, where we represent the world as we intend to make it.[6] For rational action, these states need to be related in their contents according to the following schema:

1. Δ Desires some state of affairs S. (Motivational premise)
2. Δ Believes if he does action A, then S will obtain. (Cognitive premise)
3. Δ Intends to do A. (Conational premise)
4. Δ Believes that if he wills bodily movement BM, this will result in action A being done. (Second cognitive premise)
5. Δ Intends (or wills) BM. (Second conational premise)
6. Δ Does bodily movement BM. ("Conclusion")

The *actus reus* and *mens rea* requirements of the criminal law are built entirely on the back of this folk psychology. With regard to mens rea, the criminal law grades culpability entirely in terms of the representational states of the folk psychology. With regard to the consequences of one's action, for example, the criminal law lumps motivational states of desire with conational states of intention, finding either sufficient for "specific intent" or "purpose" (the states of most serious culpability under the common law and the Model Penal Code, respectively). The third representational state, belief, is used to mark out the states of lesser culpability: knowledge (or "general intention"), recklessness, and negligence.

Notice that the mens rea doctrines of the criminal law do not take a position in the thirty-year-old debate between those who think intention is a species of desire and those who think it is not.[7] By allowing either motivating ends or intended means to suffice for "specific intent" or "purpose," the law can accept either answer in this debate within the philosophy of mind. Whereas the criminal law does stake out a position in the equally long-running debate about whether intentions are just a kind of predictive belief,[8] the law supposing that the mental state of intention is psychologically distinct from cognitive states of belief.

With regard to the actus reus requirement that there be a voluntary action, the criminal law adopts without change the folk psychological view that intentions can be either general (as schematized in premise 3 above) or specific (premise 5), temporally distal (premise 3 above) or immediate (premise 5). As Bratman charts in detail,[9] we execute our motivations by plans consisting of a hierarchically ordered set of intentions. If defendant wants Jones's money and believes that killing Jones will get him the money, he may decide to kill Jones. Yet the general, distal intention formed by such a decision will require a hierarchy of less general, less temporally removed intentions to execute it, culminating in the most specific, most immediate intention of all, such as an intention (or willing) to move his trigger finger now.

There are a number of other suppositions (about intentions) that responsibility assessments are commonly thought to make, in addition to supposing the existence and distinctiveness of the belief/desire/intention triad. I shall consider three of them. The first is that intentions are causally efficacious. More specifically, the idea is that intentions (both distal and immediate) often cause the acts that are their object. When I go downtown *because* I intended to go downtown, the "because" is meant causally.

It is often urged that something more than causation is required here. This is thought to be shown by "deviant causal chains" kinds of cases.[10] Suppose I intend to run you down with my car; yet this intention causes such excitement in me, such conflict, etc., that I tremble, my foot slips off the brakes, hits the accelerator, and my car does indeed run you down. You are run down *because* of my intention, but my running you down was still an accident. So we must amend the supposition here: the intention must cause the bodily movement "in the right way,"[11] or better, the action must be done in execution of the intention. In any case, however this is put, *at least* the hierarchy of intentions must cause the action for one to be regarded as seriously culpable because one *intended* the wrong done.

The second additional supposition that responsibility assessments are said to make has to do with the causes of intentions rather than what intentions can cause. The supposition is that intentions are free in some sense of the word. The idea is that intentions are a species of choice, decision, and willing, and that all of these processes must be free, else they would not be what they are. This is of course nothing less than the supposition of free will, in some sense of the words.

The third additional supposition has to do with consciousness. Many think that one can have an intention only if one is conscious of what the content of that intention is.[12] Alternatively, one might think that although one can have unconscious intentions, the only intentions *that affect one's culpability* are conscious intentions.[13] As we shall see shortly, each of these three additional suppositions about intentions in our responsibility assessments generates a challenge to those assessments by neuroscience.

## 2. THE CHALLENGING FINDINGS OF THE LIBET EXPERIMENTS

The neuroscientific challenge(s) I wish to examine stem from the kind of experiments begun in the early 1980s by the late Benjamin Libet and his associates.[14] In Libet's early experiments his subjects were told to flex their right wrists or the fingers of their right hands whenever they wished. EEG readings were taken from the subject's scalps over the relevant portions of their brain, the supplementary motor area. Such readings detected a negative shift, what Libet termed a "readiness potential" (RP), beginning about 550 milliseconds prior to the time at which their muscles began to move so as to flex their wrists or move their fingers. These subjects were also told to watch a spot revolving on a spatial clock and to register when their initial awareness of intending to move their wrist/fingers began. They reported the beginnings of awareness of their decision to move their finger or wrist on average 350 milliseconds after the shift in readiness potential began. Such beginning of awareness preceded the beginning of actual movement by 200 milliseconds.

We can represent these results along a simple schema that I will use throughout the remainder of this article. Let "$t_1$" be the time of the onset of the shift in readiness potential; "$t_2$" the time of initial awareness of an intention to move, and "$t_3$" the time of the beginning of the bodily movement in question. The basic schema is represented in Figure 18.1:

| $t_1$ | $t_2$ | $t_3$ |
|---|---|---|
| (onset of RP) | (onset of awareness of intention to move) | (onset of bodily movement) |

**Figure 18.1**

The total time from $t_1$ to $t_3$ is 550 milliseconds, $t_2$ being located 350 milliseconds after $t_1$ and 200 milliseconds before $t_3$. Libet added two more times of some interest here. One is Libet's corrected time of the onset of awareness; finding from other studies an error of about 50 milliseconds in subjects' estimation of the onset of awareness of sensations generally, Libet corrected the temporal location of $t_2$ to be 50 milliseconds closer to $t_3$, and 50 milliseconds further from $t_1$, than the subjects reported. Secondly, Libet notes that (what I shall call) the "Rubicon Point"—the point beyond which the subject cannot stop the movement already decided upon—occurs 50 milliseconds prior to actual muscle movement initiation ($t_3$) and 100 milliseconds after the corrected time for onset of awareness of the decision to move ($t_2$).

The values above for $t_1$, $t_2$, and $t_3$ are given for what Libet called "type II RPs." These are readiness potentials and awareness onsets measured when subjects both were instructed to move whenever they wished and when they reported (in postmovement debriefings) no experience of any advanced preplanning to move within the next few seconds. Shifts in readiness potential measured when there was such experience of preplanning, or where subjects were not free to move spontaneously (i.e., where they moved in response to a preset signal), Libet termed "type I RPs." Type I RPs had considerably earlier onsets than did type II RPs (about 1050 milliseconds prior to movement).

In what follows I shall focus on type II RPs, as did Libet. For Libet thought "that the RP component that starts at about—550 ms, the one that predominates in type II RPs, . . . is the one uniquely associated with an exclusively endogenous volitional process."[15] It is this data that thus forms the core of the neuroscientific challenge(s) to the presuppositions about intentions made by the law and morality in their responsibility assessments.

## 3. THE CHALLENGE(S) TO THE FOLK PSYCHOLOGY FROM THE LIBET AND POST-LIBET EXPERIMENTS

Patrick Haggard has touted Libet's initial article, describing the readiness potential experiment there reported, as "one of the most philosophically challenging papers in modern scientific psychology."[16] I on the contrary think Libet's work to be philosophically challenged, not challenging. To see who is right here requires that we parse up the challenge(s) better than is usually done.

Start with one of Libet's own characterizations of his challenge(s) to the folk psychology: "If the 'act now' process is initiated unconsciously, then conscious free will is not doing it."[17] Notice the three things run together in the phrase, "conscious free will:" (1) maybe a conscious will is initiating action, but it isn't a *free* will doing the work; (2) maybe there is consciousness and freedom at the time of action initiation, but there is no *will* doing any action initiation; and (3) maybe there is a free will operating to initiate actions, but there is no *consciousness* of that will or its operations at the time it is initiating actions. I now want to show that Libet has elided three distinct challenges together.

### A. Persons Have No Free Will Because Their Willings are Caused by Unwilled Brain Events

By far the most heralded of Libet's challenges is taken to be a challenge to the possibility of there being free will. A free will is thought to be a will whose exercise of its powers would be uncaused by any other prior events, brain events included. Such a will is thought to cause the bodily movements that lie at the heart of many actions; but its activities would not themselves be the effects of earlier causes.

Libet shares with much of popular literature the thought that having a free will in this sense is essential to being morally responsible and blameworthy. Libet's thought is that if brain states precede and cause one's choices, then such choices cannot ground a true responsibility. For such choices to give one *control* (and thus responsibility), they have to be undetermined by any brain events that are outside the control of the chooser. If there are such unchosen brain events causing us to will what we do, "the individual would not consciously control his actions; he would only become aware of an unconsciously initiated choice. He would have no direct conscious control over the nature of any preceding unconscious processes. . . . We do not hold people responsible for actions performed unconsciously, without the possibility of conscious control."[18]

True enough, Libet himself draws back from consigning our blaming practices to the dustheap. Yet he does this only by positing a veto function that the will can possess.[19] According to Libet, the will does not initiate actions, it being the mere puppet of the brain events that cause it; yet the will has about a 100 millisecond window (the difference between corrected awareness time and the Rubicon Point) in which to exercise a veto over the already initiated movement. By exercising such a veto, the will can prevent a movement already initiated. Remarkably, Libet holds such preventative choices to be uncaused.[20] Unlike the *initiation* of movements, *blocking* the movements is an effort of pure will. Here, for Libet, is where free will resides (or as some wags put it, where "free won't" resides). Needless to say, many neuroscientists otherwise admiring of Libet's work do not follow him here. For them, the exercise or nonexercise of a veto function is as caused by earlier brain events that precede awareness as is the exercise of the function that initiates motor movements. For them, thus, the implication of Libet's work is that there is no free will and thus, no responsibility or blameworthiness.

### B. Persons Have No Causally Efficacious Wills Because Willings Are Always Epiphenomenal to the Actions They Putatively Cause

Quite distinct from the denial that wills are *free* of being caused is the denial that wills are themselves causes. This skeptical claim thus proceeds from what wills are thought to cause in the folk psychology, not from what willings are caused by. The epiphenomenal claim is thus quite distinct from the lack of freedom claim.

One can picture the difference in the two skeptical claims this way. The free will skeptic pictures the relation between brain states, willings, and bodily movements as a simple causal chain:

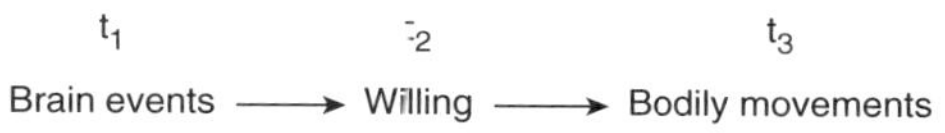


**Figure 18.2**

On this picture, willings do cause the bodily movements that are their objects. But the willings are themselves caused by certain brain events, and it is this etiological feature that the free will skeptic says robs willings of the freedom allegedly needed for responsibility. Contrast this with a second picture:

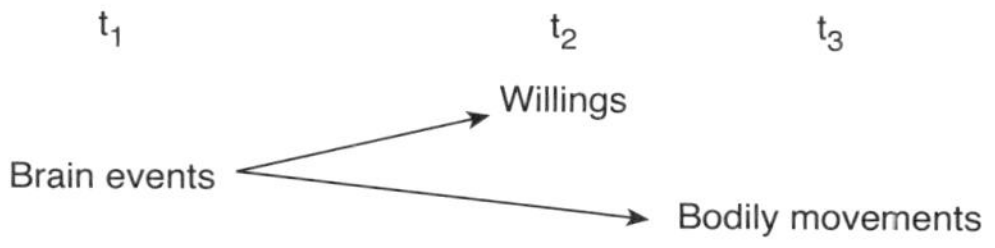


**Figure 18.3**

Willings are caused on this picture too, but what here grounds the skepticism about responsibility is not the existence of this causal relation but rather, the nonexistence of a causal connection between willings and bodily movements. Willings and bodily movements are conceived here as being epiphenomenal of each other, co-effects of a common cause, which is why they look like but are not in a causal relationship with one another.

The epiphenomenal skepticism needs fleshing out a bit. Just because brain events both cause bodily movements and precede willings does not rule out the possibility that such brain events cause bodily movements *through* such willings. The possibility is that the right picture is that depicted in Figure 18.2, where willings are causative of bodily movements even if themselves caused by earlier brain events. The epiphenomenal skeptic thus needs to say more than that the mental events of willing are preceded by brain events that cause bodily movements. Such a skeptic may have one of two additional thoughts here.

First, he might think that the brain events at $t_1$ are the last events needed for the bodily movements in question. This is the idea that not only are the brain events sufficient to produce the bodily movements, but that these early brain events do not operate through any other, subsequent brain events. Once the early brain events have occurred at $t_1$, in other words, the bodily movements at $t_3$ are going to happen without need of any other events occurring, willings included. (For a complete causal chain to exist from $t_1$ to $t_3$, there must be *states* existing, but these are not the *changes of state* we think of as events.)[21]

Alternatively, he might think that the brain events at $t_1$ cause the bodily movements at $t_3$ via a series of other brain events. For ease of exposition, assume just one other set of brain events occurring at $t_2$, call them BE'. Then the picture is that depicted in Figure 18.4:

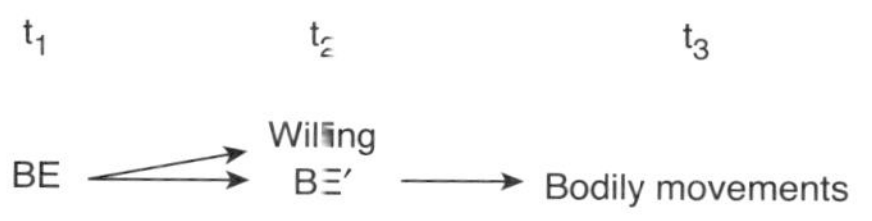


**Figure 18.4**

Willing on this picture is still epiphenomenal because BE' at $t_2$ is sufficient for the bodily movements at $t_3$, and at no point in time is there room or need for some other event, such as a "willing," to do any causing of bodily movements.

One's choice between these two pictures (Figs. 18.3 and 18.4) will not be settled by armchair philosophy. The issue is an empirical one, to be settled by the best neuroscience available. I nonetheless separate the two versions of this skepticism because how one answers it depends on which of these pictures one takes to be true. Notice that both of these skeptical pictures crucially depend on willing not being necessary for bodily movements to occur because the brain events at $t_1$, or the brain events at both $t_1$ and $t_2$, are *sufficient* by themselves to cause those bodily movements. Al Mele nicely documents how much of the neuroscientific literature seems to omit this crucial assumption, regarding it as enough to show that willings succeed in time those brain events initiating action.[22] As Mele points out, temporal order is no argument to all that the intermediary events are merely epiphenomenal: "After all, when the lighting of a fuse precedes the burning of the fuse, which in turn precedes a firecracker's exploding, we do not infer that the burning of the fuse plays no causal role in producing the explosion."[23] For the epiphenomenal view of the will to be inferred, we need the readiness potentials at $t_1$ to be sufficient for the bodily movements at $t_3$ without need for the subject to will such bodily movements. If negative shifts in readiness potentials sometimes occur without the usual bodily movements, that will suggest that the brain states evidenced by such potentials are not sufficient for such movements; if such brain states result in bodily movements only when there is also a willing of such movements, that will evidence the necessity of willing along with those brain states to cause such movements. In which case the evidence would be perfectly compatible with the hypothesis that willings are co-causers of bodily movements along with certain brain events. Such co-caused relationships could either be as depicted in Figure 18.2, where brain events operate entirely through such willings; or as depicted in a modification of Figure 18.4 above, where willings are simultaneous co-causers along with certain brain events, as in Figure 18.5:

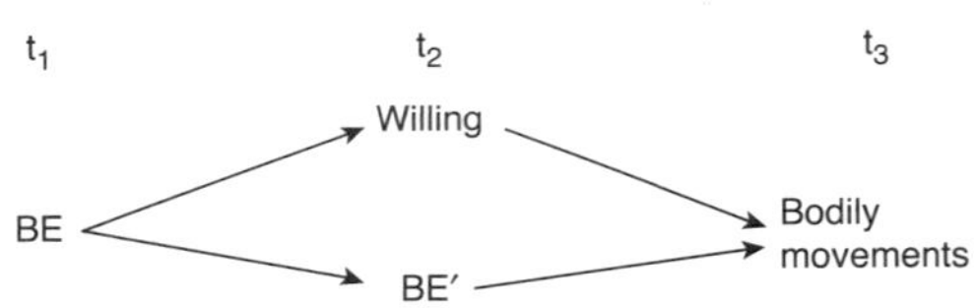


**Figure 18.5**

### C. Persons Are Not Conscious of the Processes Producing Actions Early Enough to Be in Control of Those Actions

For a long time (even antedating Freud) many have thought that one can *unconsciously* intend or will things. If so, then one response to the epiphenomenal skepticism above is to identify the brain events at $t_1$ as being nothing other than a willing, albeit an unconscious willing, and thus preserve the causal efficacy of willings. It is this possibility that brings the third aspect of Libetan skepticism into focus. For even if willings are the brain events at $t_1$ that cause bodily movements, still these are not *conscious* willings, and only *conscious* willings make one responsible, is the idea. We can only control that of which we are aware, this thought continues, so that even if the will is both free and causally efficacious, that would be without implications for responsibility because the willings that initiate movements are unconscious.

One should conceive of this as a second kind of epiphenomenal objection, pictured thusly:

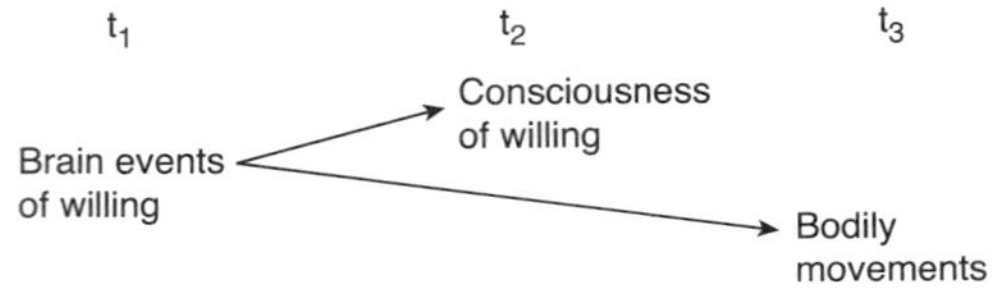


**Figure 18.6**

Consciousness of willing is now pictured in the "dangler" position, an effect of the willing/brain events at $t_1$ but without effect itself on the movements it doesn't control.

It is easy to miss the separation of this skepticism about responsibility from the first two skepticisms, if one thinks that intentions and willings must be conscious if they are to be intentions or willings at all. For if this last were the case, then the subject can will or intend the movement of his finger only when he is conscious of that fact, which on Libet's evidence seems to be at $t_2$; this means that *both* consciousness and intending are in the "dangler" position in the epiphenomenal chart, and so this third skepticism collapses into the second skepticism already considered. For reasons I go into in section 4, I do not share the supposition that willings and intendings must be conscious. There is in that case this separable skepticism to be considered.

### D. Two Queries about the Three Skeptical Challenges

There are two questions to ask of each of these three skeptical challenges to responsibility coming from neuroscience. The most obvious question is whether the scientific claims are true. Are willings caused by brain events? Are willings merely epiphenomenal of the bodily movements they putatively cause? Is consciousness of willing merely epiphenomenal with those bodily movements that are willed? These sound like empirical questions for the best science to answer, which they are, but as we will see they also involve a good deal of "philosophizing," that is, conceptual work in the philosophy of mind.

The second question to ask is whether it matters to moral responsibility whether any of these claims is true. Does responsibility require freedom of the will? Does it require that willings cause actions? Is consciousness of the willings that cause actions required for responsibility for those actions? These are more obviously philosophical questions, although the relevant branch of philosophy is moral philosophy rather than the philosophy of mind.

I shall proceed by asking the second question first, with respect to all three challenges. I will then proceed to the first question.

## 4. THE MORAL/LEGAL RELEVANCE OF THESE THREE ALLEGED FACTS OF NEUROSCIENCE

I come then to the second of my two questions, the question of moral philosophy: is it relevant to blameworthiness and responsibility that: (1) our choices are caused and thus not "free"? (2) our choices do not cause the bodily movements that constitute our actions? or (3) our choices are often made "before we know it," i.e., before we are conscious of choosing? I shall address these three subquestions *seriatim* in this part.

### A. Free Will

Beginning a discussion on free will is a daunting project for me. This is not just because the literature is vast, which it is. It is more because of the difficulty I have in motivating the discussion. As a lifelong compatibilist,[24] the answer is too obvious to me to motivate a detailed defense. As Nietzsche said somewhere in one of *The Untimely Meditations*, we can only meaningfully argue against positions that are plausible enough to tempt us.

A striking fact that nonetheless starts the engines here is that intelligent, educated people regard the incompatibilist answer as obvious too.[25] They think that *of course* if we are caused to choose what we do by factors themselves unchosen, then we couldn't have helped doing what we did, we had no real control, and we cannot fairly be blamed for our actions. Such people see the lawyers and the moralists as clinging desperately (poor devils!) to a libertarian metaphysics that even they at some level know is wildly implausible; when science rips off the mask of illusion by showing such desperate metaphysics to be false, much will have to change in the blaming and punishment practices of such moralists and lawyers. So I will endeavor in this section to take seriously a position I in fact think to be pretty obviously false, even if widely held.

Let me begin with a species of causation known to us long before there was a neuroscience. I refer to the causation of choice by beliefs and desires. As Aristotle charted over 2000 years ago, what we do is a function of what we want to achieve and what we believe the world is like making possible the achievement of these things.

Because I will later use Newcombe's Paradox as a contrast case to the cases discussed in the next succeeding section, imagine a simple-minded variation of this well-known paradox that goes like this: We are to suppose that there is a Great Predictor who is very, very good at predicting what someone will decide before they have decided it. The following game is set up: there are two boxes and you have a two-valued choice. You can pick both boxes, or you can pick only box number one. Whatever you pick determines how much money you get, because you receive the contents of the box(es) chosen. In box number two there is $1000, placed there by the Great Predictor no matter what you choose. However, in box number one the contents depend on your choice. If you choose the first box only, the Great Predictor after your choice but before you open the box will place one million dollars in that box; if you pick both boxes, the Great Predictor will leave box one empty.

The Great Predictor will predict your choice before you make it, but his prediction has nothing to do with what is placed in box one. That is determined solely by your choice.

The Great Predictor is not a magician. Rather, he is a very able scientist. He issues his predictions by noting certain facts (call them collectively, "F") about you, human nature, and the situation. This makes his prediction epiphenomenal of your decision because F determines both what he will predict and what you will decide. On a time line the structure is that depicted in Figure 18.7.

On this simple-minded version of Newcombe's Paradox we are all the Great Predictor: we predict, do we not, that you will choose box one only, because it pays much much better? (Indeed, Hume got here first: leave a pot of gold at Charing Cross Station in London, Hume said, and then come back in an hour. Hume's prediction: it will not be there, because someone will have made off with it.)[26] Yet is not the predictability of the choice—a predictability based on certain causally relevant facts—just beside the point when it comes to your making the decision and to our assessing it? That there is such a prediction, and that there are the causes that make such a prediction so reliable, is irrelevant to your reasoning about what to choose. Even if you know the prediction, and indeed, even if you too can make the prediction by knowing facts F yourself, these will not be your reasons for deciding on box number one. You will reason to your decision just as you would in ignorance of these predictions and the facts on which they are based. Moreover, these facts are also irrelevant to our assessment of the rationality of what you choose. And they are irrelevant to our assessment of your deserts with respect to the money: if the money was offered under the terms above described, and you chose the first box in reliance on that offer, you deserve the million dollars irrespective of how determined was your choice.

Many hard determinists and libertarian incompatibilists will respond that *this* kind of causation is not a challenge to responsibility. After all, it is because we know that almost everyone including you wants $1 million more than they want $1000, and because we know that you understand the instructions and thus have the requisite means/end belief about how to get $1 million rather than $1000, that we can predict your choice. The objection is that such belief/desire causation does not challenge our agency, control, or responsibility. But why not? A cause is a cause, as Stephen Morse says.[27] Our beliefs and our desires are often unchosen by us, being caused by factors over which we had no choice. So causation of our choices by what we most want and believe should challenge our sense of agency, control, and responsibility as much as any other form of causation. That it manifestly doesn't, counts against incompatibilist views, both determinist and libertarian.

To be sure, there was once a group of philosophers who denied that belief/desire sets were causes of the choices that they rationalized.[28] They were motivated to the view precisely by the insight that causation of the will by belief/desire sets challenged the libertarian idea of free will. Yet, as forty (plus) years of consensus in the philosophy of mind has shown, "reasons" (belief/desire sets) have to play causal roles vis-à-vis choice and behavior.[29] After all, we have many things we want, and we have numerous beliefs about the world and about the ability of various

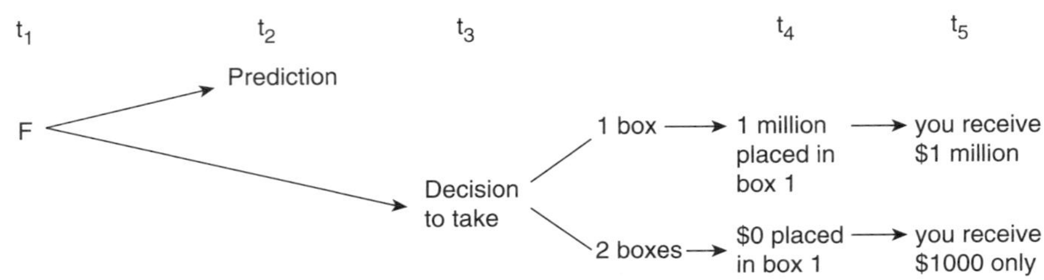


Figure 18.7

potential actions to get us what we want. Yet such pairs of beliefs and desires constitute the reason(s) for which we acted only if they caused the action in question. What *in the world* could be meant by the "because" in "I did it *because* I wanted X," other than that there is a causal connection between doing the action that achieves X, and wanting X?

Another logically possible wiggle here open to the incompatibilist, is to deny that we are responsible for those of our actions and choices that are caused by our reasons. Yet this would be a heroic denial, leaving us responsible only for those intrinsically motivated actions ("acts gratui") so favored in existentialist fiction. Yet "acts for no reason" are exceptional; most of what we do is choose to act, and act, *because* of what we desire and what we believe, even though those mental states are often unwilled by us.

Notice that our responsibility for actions done for reasons remains even when others manipulate us because they know our motivational structure. I once had a senior colleague whose proudest professional achievement had been a staff position with President Truman. He had a limited repertoire of stories about Truman, which all of his colleagues had heard many times. It was easy to elicit a retelling of one of these stories by weaving some allusion to Truman into one's conversation. In a perfectly straightforward sense of the word, when we did this we *caused* him to tell the story.[30] Equally clearly, however, he wanted to tell the story, he chose to do so, he did so intentionally, and (in the moral arena where it is an offense to bore your faculty colleagues at lunch) he was fully responsible for his retelling of the story. (That we also were responsible in no wise diminishes his responsibility in this regard—in criminal law ours would be but an accomplice liability, principal liability being reserved for he who retold the story.)

The only remaining arrow in the quiver of the incompatibilist here is to become what is sometimes called a "selective determinist."[31] Such a person is selective in terms of what kinds of causes are incompatible with responsibility. A common example is the liberal selective determinist:[32] even if the wealth of Loeb and Leopold caused them to kill Bobby Franks fully as much as the poverty of common thieves causes them to steal, only the latter but not the former is incompatible with responsibility for the wrongs done, for the liberal selective determinist. To be sure, the selectivity needed by the incompatibilist here is different: even if reasons cause behavior as fully as does the environment, genetics, or brain activity, still only the latter are incompatible with responsibility. Yet despite this difference, the damning question to selective determinism remains the same. If incompatibilism is generally motivated by the thought that choices that are caused by factors themselves unchosen are not choices giving the actor control over his actions—he "couldn't have done otherwise"—then that thought should be as applicable to reasons as causes as well as environmental, genetic, or brain factors as causes. If causation as such erodes the control needed for responsibility, the *kinds* of causes should be irrelevant.

Let me now leave my beachhead and move inland. I now want to show that just as causation of choice and action by belief/desire sets does not erode responsibility, so also causation of the will by brain states does not do so either. Although it ultimately will make little difference, it is helpful at this stage to introduce a temporal distinction. I shall distinguish causally efficacious brain states that occur at the time of willing or intending, from those that precede any such willings or intendings (and which are also causally efficacious of such willings and intendings). In introducing this distinction I here leave open the question of *when* such willings and intendings occur. If such willings and intendings occur prior to our awareness of them (see section 5 below), then the brain states occurring at the time of willing and intending may include those brain states evidenced by Libet's shift in readiness potential.

First consider the brain states occurring at the time of willing and intending. Putting aside the construal of the relationship between willings and voluntary bodily movements as being epiphenomenal, we might think that such brain states must be the most immediate, or direct causes of willing/intending. Under this last construal, the will is (*arguendo*) conceded to cause voluntary bodily movement, but (being itself caused by such simultaneous brain states) the will is not free. From which conclusion a lack of responsibility is supposed to follow.

Overlooked by this last chain of inference are some general questions of reference and identity. Perhaps when we say, "I willed the movement of my finger" or "I intended to shoot the gun by moving my finger," we are referring to just those brain states Libet and company regard as the putative causes of willing/intending. In which case the relationship between the mental states of willing and intending, on the one hand, and these simultaneous brain states, on the other, is one of identity and not of causation. In which case the discovery of such brain states should make us optimistic, not pessimistic, about the existence of the willings and intendings on which responsibility depends. After all, on this construal what Libet and company have verified is that there really are the mental states on which responsibility depends, and they have done this by discovering more about the nature of such states. Hitherto we only knew of such states by their phenomenal and behavioral properties; now we know the physical nature of such states too. Voila!

Whether this happy optimism (about willing, intending, and responsibility) is warranted depends on two kinds of facts.[33] One is a linguistic or language-usage fact: are the semantic intentions with which we use the vocabulary of willing and intending such that we can be referring to things we know very little about, such as the brain states in question? The second is an ontological or scientific fact: are the brain states in question in fact identical to the mental states of willing and intending? Let us call the first the question of reference, the second, the question of identity.

As to the question of reference, a common reaction to the hypothesis that we use words like "willing" and "intending" to refer to brain states that we know little about, is to object that we can't mean more than we know when we speak.[34] As applied here, the objection is that we only knew of willing and intending via their phenomenal and behavioral indications; we knew nothing (and even now know little) about the brain states in question, so we couldn't be referring to such brain states when we use the vocabulary of willing/intending. This objection can be voiced as to either individual speakers, or as to whole linguistic communities.

Framed either individually or collectively, the objection is a toothless one. Consider by way of example usage of the word, "dreaming." Prior to the Dement and Kleitman research of 1950s psychology, the only criterion we had that a person had dreamt something was that person's waking remembrance. Yet surely such phenomenological evidence does not exhaust the nature of dreaming. Surely there can be unremembered dreams, and surely there can be misremembered dreams. In which case "dreaming" refers to a process that is not exhausted, nor even universally evidenced, by waking remembrances. Behavioral evidence such as REM patterns, brain activity evidence such as EEG patterns, joins waking remembrances as evidencing a process whose full nature is hardly known. *That* process was what we were referring to when we spoke of dreaming pre-1950, and that is what we still mean when we speak of "dreaming" now that we know a little more about the nature of that process.

To go the other way here, and to think that words like "dreaming," "willing," or "intending" have their reference fixed exclusively by the way we first came to know of their existence—viz, by phenomenology—would render science discontinuous with ordinary thought in a way that is very counterintuitive.[35] It would mean, for example, that Dement and Kleitman's REM/EEG studies couldn't have been about dreaming; given the imperfect congruence of REM/EEG patterns with waking remembrances, if the latter fix the reference of the word then their studies must have been about something else—"schmeaming," perhaps, but not dreaming.[36] They were thus not discovering more about dreaming with their research. Rather, they were changing the subject and thus were talking past the folk psychological notion of dreaming. Scientific progress would become impossible under this view of semantics and reference.

We thus mean more than we know when we use words like "willing" and "intending."

We mean to refer to states that have a deeper nature than that we yet know. Our best bet is that that nature is to be found in just those brain states Libet and company typically think of as the causes of willing/intending.

What we mean with our words cannot of course make the world be the way we think it is. Whether willings and intendings have a sufficiently unitary physical structure that our phenomenologically and functionally derived concepts of those states can refer to that structure, is a scientific question (of identity) on which all the evidence is hardly in. Yet I find the neuroscientific evidence thus far encouraging.[37] However construed, such evidence hardly rules out the hypothesis that Libet's "immediate causes" of willings and intendings are nothing of the sort. Rather, such brain states may well *be* such intendings and willings, giving rise to the optimism about responsibility described earlier.

Some believe themselves possessed of an Alexandrian sword with which to cut through the knotty problem of identity here. That sword is the thought that choice, willing, intending, deciding, etc., cannot be identical with any brain states and still be mental states of choice, etc. For, this thought continues, if choice *is* a brain state, then it must be caused by earlier brain states, themselves caused by genetic and environmental factors in a continuous chain—and *choice*, the argument is, necessarily cannot be caused. The thought is that freedom from causation is an essential attribute of choice, willing, intending, etc.

The first thing to see is what an extraordinary thesis this is. When we explain phenomena like the presence of Lake Michigan in terms of that phenomena's causes—glaciation, rainfall patterns, etc.—the lake does not cease being a lake or even being Lake Michigan. To explain is not (usually, or perhaps ever) to explain away. Choice, the thought has to be, is different.

Perhaps, but how is this difference to be established? My armchair sociology of the beliefs of those who would wield the sword above described, tells me that they think the linking of choice to contra-causal freedom is *analytic*, that what we mean by "choice" is, in part, "uncaused." Yet even if ordinary usage patterns could yield analytic truths, the usage facts are against this claim. We speak of causing choices all the time. My earlier example of causing my colleague's choice to tell the Truman story is but one of many examples.

In any case, claims of analyticity in general are in poor repute. Even if it is true that the Big Bang, God, and the energy shifts of electrons are uncaused, it is hardly analytically necessary that this be so. If these be truths, it will not be because the meaning of "Big Bang," "God," and "electron," makes it true. Yet if we put aside the (unsustainable) claim that the very meaning of "choice," "willing," etc., requires that the states named be uncaused, how else does one justify the thought that contra-causal freedom is an essential attribute of these states?

Granting all of this will not allay the incompatibilist intuitions of many persons. After all, even if there are real states of willing and intending, states identical to certain brain states, surely those willing/intending brain states are themselves caused by earlier brain states that are *not* identical to such willings and intendings. And surely those earlier brain states are not subject to our wills, so that we can't and don't control them; and surely this means that our wills are not free and not (ultimately) in control. Man is indeed, as Freud once said, "not master in his own house."[38]

Here we reach the second kind of brain states I earlier distinguished, those that are not simultaneous with willings and intendings but which precede those latter states and cause them to exist. Here we also reach the very general question of the incompatibility of determinism with responsibility. Much to some neuroscientists' surprise, they have nothing new to offer at this stage of the argument, nothing that we haven't heard many times before, ever since Hobbesian materialism challenged traditional notions of responsibility. True, neuroscientists talk about early brain states and processes, whereas their predecessors talked about environmental stimuli, psychic energy, developmental stages, genetic makeup, instinctual drives, the repressed unconscious, etc. etc. True also, neuroscience is better science than the behaviorisms, sociobiologies, dynamic psychiatrics, etc., that came before.

But that is by-the-by. Whether advanced by a Freud or a Skinner, or by contemporary neuroscience, the point being advanced is the same: some state we didn't will causes our willings and intendings, so that we don't control them and can't be responsible and blameworthy. In assessing this incompatibilist claim, it doesn't matter a whit how one fills in the "state we didn't will that causes our willings." The incompatibilist intuition is unaffected by how the nature of such a state is fleshed out.

This is not the place to take on incompatibilism in general. This has been done too often and too successfully to justify a rehearsal of the compatibilist moves here.[39] I will allow myself these few observations. It is surprising, distressing, and even irritating: (1) to hear neuroscientists confidently proclaim their incompatibilist intuitions as if such intuitions were in the domain of their scientific expertise; (2) to ignore a deep, sophisticated, and long-running philosophical literature on this topic as if it didn't exist or as if it is disqualified because it isn't "scientific";[40] (3) to make proclamations about the truth of incompatibilism that would make undergraduate philosophy sophomores blush, in light of the compatibilism dominant in philosophy since World War II; and (4) to plunge headlong into the most outrageous doctrines—Cartesian dualism,[41] the Upanishads, Schoedinger's single consciousness, Idealism, etc.[42]—in order to escape the incompatibilism they think so obviously to be true.

All of this is an embarrassment for neuroscience, and an unnecessary embarrassment at that. The fact is that we will voluntary motor movements, intend and choose to do what we do intentionally, control our choices and our actions, are agents that perform voluntary actions, have the ability to have done other than we did do, act freely—all of the foregoing, even if our actions, choices, willings, and intendings are all caused by factors themselves unchosen. See this clearly, and one can put away entirely the free will branch of Libetan skepticism about responsibility.

Libet himself treated such compatibilist views as though they would be a *revision* of the ordinary understanding of the conditions of responsibility.[43] But that isn't the claim of the compatibilist. Compatibilism is not a revision of ordinary thought here; it is an explication of that thought, a rational reconstruction showing the true nature of that thought. Ability, for example, is not a concept that is incompatible with determinism. That I have the ability to run a mile in under five minutes only means I can do so in certain conditions if I so choose; it is not incompatible with thinking that every occasion on which I do or do not run a mile in under five minutes is fully determined by sufficient causes. Capacity, control, agency, intention, will, and the like all have similarly compatibilist readings.

Notice that this last issue is one of sociology—about the parameters of ordinary thought—and not about the moral truth of the matter. Yet it is important that the compatibilist win this issue too. The advance of neuroscience in discovering the causes of human behavior does not herald some needed change in ordinary thought, a change in the direction of compatibilism.[44] Ordinary thought (and the legal system built upon it) already presupposes such compatibilism. Neuroscience thus brings no relevant news to the sociology of ordinary belief, no more than to moral philosophy.

So why is the mistake (of incompatibilism) so commonly made, by laypersons and lawyers no less than by neuroscientists? Why do people *think* they think that causal accounts of human choice and behavior are incompatible with responsibility and blameworthiness for that behavior? My own long-held hypothesis is that sometimes causal accounts of human behavior tell us *more* than that behavior is caused by factors themselves unchosen.[45] Moreover, the something more that is implied sometimes is truly excusing, that is, truly diminishing of responsibility and blameworthiness. When we are given causal accounts of epileptic movements or of reflex reactions, for example, we are often told more than that such behaviors are caused; we learn in addition that the causes of such behaviors do not include the volitions/willings/choices that are required for responsibility. When we are given causal accounts of behavior responsive to coercive threats, to take another example, we are again told more than that such behaviors are caused by the threats in question; we learn in addition that the choices were made, and intentions formed, when the normal capacities or opportunities to make such choices was severely diminished.

An extended illustration (of this confusion of simple causal accounts with incapacitation accounts) was provided at a recent MacArthur Foundation Law and Neuroscience Project meeting.[46] Suppose, one of our members said, there was a 40-year-old man with no history of abnormal sexual activity. Suddenly, however, he reported both an interest in child pornography and urges to have sexual contact with children; indeed, he made sexual advances to his prepubescent stepdaughter. It turned out he had a right orbitofrontal tumor. When it was removed, the interest, the urges, and the inappropriate advances, all ceased; when it returned some time later, all these reappeared; when it was again removed, the three symptoms again disappeared. The case elicited sympathy for the view that the man is not responsible for his inappropriate (and illegal) sexual contacts with his stepdaughter.

There are two things to be learned from this story. One is that, *as stated*, there is nothing to excuse this man for his criminal misconduct.[47] True, we know a dominant cause of his urges and his behavior, namely, the tumor; true, he would not have done what he did but for the tumor; true, he would not have had the urges he did but for the tumor; and true, he had no control of—he did not choose or cause—the tumor that caused his urges and his behavior. Yet as stated, this man differs in no relevant way from everyone of us. We do not control the factors that produce our desires and the behavior which results from those desires. That we do not *know* what those factors are with the precision with which we know about the tumor of this 40-year-old man, is neither here nor there. When we, like the 40-year-old man, choose to act on such desires, we do actions that make us responsible and blameworthy if they are wrongful. Causation of our desires, our choices, and the behavior that emanates from both, excuses neither us nor him.

But . . . (and this is the second thing to be learned here) it is tempting to read something more into the causal story behind the 40-year-old man's behavior that we are not tempted to read into the causal story behind our own behavior. It is tempting to think that the tumor not only causes his urges and his behavior, but that it does so via causing changes within the 40-year-old man in ways that incapacitate him. The tumor, for example, may give him migraine headaches and hypertension; impairment of both free and copy drawing; delayed recall abilities; inability to write in long hand; change of gait and impaired ability to walk; impaired bladder control.[48] These, in turn, may be evidence of more relevant incapacitations: the brain area affected may generate "a loss of impulse control,"[49] such that there is an impairment "in behavior self-regulation and response inhibition, including the conscious regulation of sexual urges,"[50] and a change in his "decision-making that emphasizes immediate reward rather than long-term gain, impairing the subject's ability to appropriately navigate social situations."[51] Whether these more relevant incapacities actually resulted from the brain dysfunction marked by the earlier symptoms, is not here my concern. Rather, it is the assumption that some such relevant incapacities are part of the causal story for the 40-year-old man that explains why we might be tempted to excuse him while holding the rest of us fully responsible for our equally caused behaviors.

Lack of any choice at all, lack of an uncoerced choice, and lack of choice made by one of diminished capacity, are all indeed incompatible with responsibility. The mistake is to suppose that there is such lack whenever a sufficient causal account is given. As compatibilists have long asserted, nothing could be further from the truth.

### B. The Epiphenomenal Will

I turn now to the second form of skepticism, the epiphenomenal form. Suppose (for now) that the will is indeed epiphenomenal with the bodily movements that it putatively causes. Would that erode our sense of responsibility for the bad states of affairs that those bodily movements cause? Unlike the previous supposition about free will, the seeming implications of the epiphenomenal form of skepticism seems devastating of our sense of responsibility. Yet perhaps this is not so. To see the possibilities here, let me repair again to Newcombe's Paradox.

This time we need the real version of the paradox,[52] not the simple-minded version I used in the previous section. On the real version, as before, $1000 will be put into box two no matter what. Now, however, the decision of the subject is not what determines what is put into box one. Rather, it is what the Great Predictor predicts the decision will be that determines what will be put into box one: if the Predictor predicts a one-box decision, he will put one million dollars into box one before the subject makes his decision; if the Predictor predicts a both-boxes decision, the Predictor will place nothing in box one. The decision of the subject thus determines only that he receives whatever is in the box(es) he chooses; the decision does not determine what is in the boxes.

The structure is again epiphenomenal in nature, as depicted in Figure 18.8.

Now the "one box" solution is much more controversial. Nonetheless, I will confess to being a "one-boxer." Even though rational choice theorists have to choose both boxes—notice the pay off is greater if they so choose, no matter what the Predictor predicts—I think one-box is the rational choice here. There are two bases for thinking this, one of potential relevance to the epiphenomenal skepticism here discussed.

The first basis for defending the one-box decision lies in the probabilistic dependence that exists between a one-box decision and a one-box prediction. Just as it is more likely that there was a one-box decision if there was a one-box prediction, so it is more likely that there was a one-box prediction if there was a one-box decision. (Remember, the Great Predictor is really good at this!) Probabilistic dependence, unlike causation, is not temporally ordered: the existence of a later event can make more probable the existence of an earlier event as much as vice versa. So, on grounds of making the evidence as good as possible that there was a one-box prediction (and thus, a million dollars in box 1), the subject should decide on box one only.

As it stands, this justification of a one-box decision is unsatisfying. This is because the decision at $t_4$ cannot affect the prediction at $t_2$ without backward causation, and that is impossible if not incoherent. The evidential relation of probabilistic dependence does indeed work backward through time but seemingly one cannot manufacture evidence at $t_4$ that can make more likely some event at $t_2$. Suppose all boxes with the million dollars in them in all previous trials have been red boxes; surely painting box one red at $t_4$ while one makes the one-box decision would not up the probability of there being one million dollars in box one at $t_4$.

This brings in the second justification for the one-box solution, bolstering the first. Unlike the redness of the box at $t_4$, the decision made at $t_4$ is probabilistically connected to the prediction at $t_2$ *because of the common cause F*. It is this epiphenomenal structure that sometimes allows us to bring about one thing *by* doing something else at a later time. A time-honored example is getting a square hit on a golf ball.[53] It is said that we do this *by* getting a good follow-through on the swing. Yet the follow-through that is our means

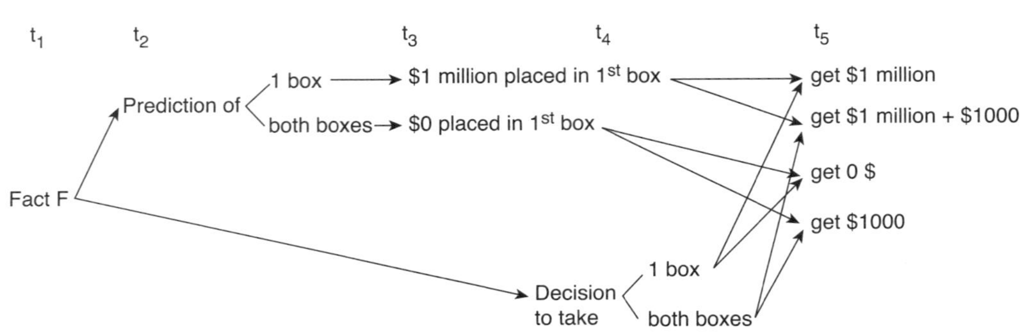


**Figure 18.8**

succeeds in time the square hit that is our end. So it looks like the later event caused the earlier event.

This last of course cannot be right but there are two things to learn from such examples. One is that the "by" relation of means to ends does not always follow causal direction. Usually, to be sure, when we do A in order to get B, A precedes B and not vice versa. But not always. When the thing we know how to do succeeds in time the thing we want to achieve, we sometimes can achieve the earlier thing by doing the later thing. Another time-honored example: when we have not been trained to flex isolated muscles, we can nonetheless move those muscles in our arms *by* moving our arms—even though the arm movement succeeds in time the muscle movements.[54]

Of course, these causally backward means-end relations are possible only if: (1) there is some earlier event preparatory to the later "means" event that is geared up at the earlier time by doing the later means event; and (2) this earlier preparatory event is also a cause of the "end" event. In the golfing example, to get a good follow-through at $t_3$ requires a mental focus at $t_1$, and this focus (on a good follow-through) causes a square hit on the ball at $t_2$ (as well as causing a good follow-through at $t_3$). One may well be unaware of the preparatory focus, and this is what gives the appearance that a more temporally remote effect of that focus (the actual follow through) causes the more immediate, epiphenomenal effect of that focus (the square hit on the ball).

Now return to the Newcombe problem. You can use your one-box decision at $t_4$ as your means to getting a one-box prediction at $t_2$ (and to getting one million dollars placed in box one at $t_3$) because of the control determinism gives you of facts F at $t_1$. We are assuming deterministically that F causes your decision. Although (as I have argued at length elsewhere) the singular causal relationship between F and your decision is not reducible either to counterfactual necessity or nomic sufficiency, either by themselves or in any combination, it nonetheless remains true that: (1) there are causal *laws* connecting facts of some type F to decisions of some type D; and (2) that those laws, if deterministic rather than probabilistic, do give conditions sufficient for decisions of the type.[55] Moreover, except in overdetermination cases (where there are redundancy mechanisms at work),[56] sufficient conditions like F are necessary for decisions of type D. F is necessary for D, then (logically) D is sufficient for F.[57] In Newcombe's problem, your decision is sufficient for the existence of the facts making up F. Put equivalently, you couldn't make your one-box decision at $t_4$ without certain facts within F being true at $t_1$; and these facts are the ones causing the great Predictor to predict a one-box decision by you. So long as F fully determines both the decision and the prediction of the decision, then you should make the decision at $t_4$ in such a way that it reflects facts existing in F at $t_1$ that have guaranteed the prediction you want at $t_2$. You have gotten yourself one million dollars *by* deciding for box one, even though that decision did not *cause* the million dollars to be placed in the box. Congratulations!

Notice that it is a full-blown determinism that makes this solution work. This is what allows the back-tracking sufficiency from $t_4$ to $t_1$, and then allows the causal sufficiency from $t_1$ to $t_2$ to $t_3$. Paradoxically, the very thesis that tempts some to the first skepticism about responsibility based on free will, is the same thesis that might allay the second skepticism about responsibility based on the epiphenomenal challenge.

To see whether this is indeed so requires that we leave this (quite controversial) defense of a one-box solution to Newcombe's Paradox and return to the epiphenomenal relationship alleged to exist between willings and bodily movements. A good transition vehicle is provided by a thought experiment concocted by V. S. Ramachandran,[58] who supposes that we perform the Libet experiment with one modification: we set up a screen on which the subject can see a signal indicating a shift in readiness potential, and this shift predicts that the subject is about to flex his finger. We thus have an epiphenomenal fork similar to that involved in Newcombe's Paradox, as depicted in Figure 18.9a.

Ramachandran supposes that we can get the timing so that the subject is aware of the signal before he is aware of his intention to flex his finger.

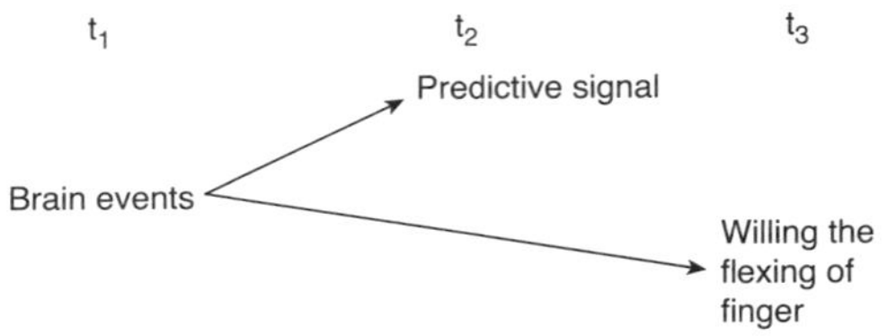


**Figure 18.9a**

In such a case Ramachandran concludes that you might well "experience a sudden loss of will, feeling that the machine is controlling you."[59] You might, but this is because we are communicating the predictive signal to the subject before he consciously makes his decision. Since the *by* relation depends on the knowledge (of how to do things) of the actor, adding this bit of knowledge may well change how he reasons and how he thinks about his reasoning processes. This would be like telling the box-chooser in the Newcombe problem what the Predictor has placed into the second box before the choice is made about selecting boxes. A better analogy would therefore be a slight amendment of Ramachandran's hypothetical: suppose at $t_2$ the subject has no awareness of the signal but that after he wills the flexing of his finger at $t_3$ he learns of the signal because of one of its effects, e.g., the signal at $t_2$ causes a light to go on at $t_4$, which the subject then sees. The structure then is as depicted in Figure 18.9b:

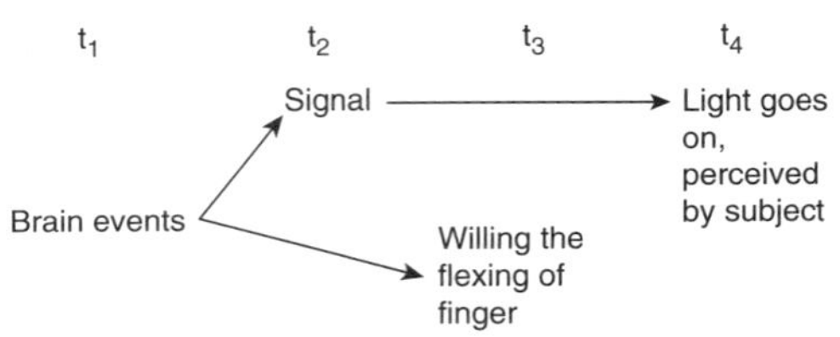


**Figure 18.9b**

Now won't the subject come to see what in fact is true: *by* willing the flexing of the finger at $t_3$, he can control whether the light goes off at $t_4$? My supposition is that you would see that you are controlling the light going on. You would understand what in fact is true: you are making the light appear at $t_4$ *by* intending at $t_3$ to flex your finger. That your means (willing) is epiphenomenal with your end (the light going on), in no way erodes your *control* over that end's occurrence.

With control comes responsibility. Suppose (this will be fanciful but bear with me, the point is serious) Paul Revere is so badly wounded that all he can do is flex his index finger in his right hand. Suppose further that flexing his finger has no chance of alerting his fellow rebels whether the British are coming by land or by sea, but this is what he wants to do. Suppose he is hooked up to my modified Ramachandran device in such a way that the light at $t_4$ can be seen by his fellow rebels. When Revere wills one flex or two, the light blinks once or twice, and the rebels know whether the British are coming by land or by sea, I take it that Revere has performed the action of *alerting* the rebels. Moreover, is there any doubt that he is morally responsible for this state of affairs, if it is a bad one, and that he could be fairly hung by the British for treason?

Now return to the Libet experiment without the supposed predictive signal showing upon some screen. Even if our willings are epiphenomenal of the actions they putatively cause, that would not mean that we don't control such actions. Our willings at $t_2$ cannot cause the brain events at $t_1$ (which brain events cause our bodily movements at $t_3$) if Figure 18.3 above is correct. But these willings could nonetheless give us control of those bodily movements, in the sense that what we will is back-trackingly sufficient for the brain events in question and those brain events are causally sufficient for the bodily movements at $t_3$. Put differently, if at $t_2$ we will a certain bodily movement, then it must be true that at $t_1$ certain brain events occurred, which brain events are sufficient to cause the bodily movements that were willed.[60]

This is all rather hypothetical for me because it is premised on a conclusion with which I do not agree, viz, that our willings are epiphenomenal with our actions and not the cause of those actions. The argument of this subsection is thus hypothetical: conceding *arguendo* the psychological conclusion, does lack of moral responsibility follow? As with free will, the answer may well be no, although it is perhaps not so obvious as with freedom of the will. But in any case, in the last section of this chapter I lay out why I think the psychological premise to be false and why things are in fact as they seem: our willings are indeed the direct cause of those bodily movements that are those willings' object, despite everything established in the Libet and Libet-inspired experiments.

### C. Does Responsibility Require Consciousness of One's Causally Efficacious Willings?

I come now to the third skepticism latent in Libet's work. This is the skepticism that can concede (*arguendo* at least) that (1): our wills are free in any sense that they need to be free, and (2) that our wills cause the behaviors that are their objects. Yet, the skepticism proceeds, we are not *conscious* of our willings at the time they do their causings, and (consciousness being required for responsibility) we are not therefore responsible and blameworthy for the actions we intentionally bring about.

As was said earlier with respect to Figure 18.6 above, the right way to see this skepticism is as a second epiphenomenal skepticism. As Figure 18.6 depicts, consciousness of willing is only epiphenomenal of the behavior willed; such consciousness does not cause that behavior to be done; only a willing of which the actor is unaware causes that behavior. This is supposed to show (again in Freud's words) that "man is not master of his own house." The heart of this skepticism lies in the view that consciousness is the true touchstone of responsibility, not willing or intending as such; the moral agent is the conscious agent, on this view, not just the causally efficacious agent. Put more starkly: *we*—the persons who are moral agents and can fairly be blamed—*are* consciousness more than anything else.

The connection(s) of consciousness to moral agency and to responsibility is a complicated business that I have addressed in detail before.[61] Briefly, the relevant conclusions are: (1) that "conscious" and "unconscious" are ambiguous between their phenomenological sense (the experiential, Joycean sense) and their dispositional sense (the ability to direct attention and to state that of which one is conscious);[62] (2) that consciousness in either sense is sufficient for responsibility, as is evidenced by the example of habitual or skilled performances where phenomenological but not dispositional consciousness has receded;[63] (3) that one cannot answer the skepticism about responsibility stemming from lack of consciousness, by claiming that Libet's subjects were only unconscious of their willings phenomenologically but not dispositionally, since that does not seem to be the case;[64] (4) that action initiation caused for forever unconscious intentions does constitute a kind of agency and can be the basic of a kind of aretaic responsibility, but this is not to be confused with the deontic or hypological responsibility that follows from culpable choice;[65] (5) that the only slightly deferred consciousness of intention of Libet's acting subjects constitutes an even stronger form of agency but is still insufficient on which to ground responsibility for culpable choice.[66]

I thus affirm what I argued in detail long ago,[67] that generally speaking consciousness of acting is required for responsibility for culpable wrongdoing; unconscious intentions, even when they cause the acts intended, do not make for such responsibility because there is no conscious execution of such intentions into action. I come then to my own reason for rejecting skepticism about responsibility based on the unconsciousness of the acting subject at $t_1$, when he first begins to intend to move. This reason begins with the thought that the intentions of Libet's subjects were conscious (in both senses) within 400 milliseconds of the willings initiating movement. We are thus *not* dealing with what I shall now call the issue of truly unconscious intentions. Truly unconscious intentions raise the issue of whether intentions that are never conscious can nonetheless be the basis for responsibility and blameworthiness. In assessing this issue many years ago with respect to Freud, my own conclusion was in the negative.[68] Although there can be truly unconscious agency that is nonetheless the agency of a person, that person's responsibility is not increased by virtue of such truly unconscious actions, intentions, or tryings.

In Libet's subjects the intention to initiate movement precedes awareness of that intention only by 400 milliseconds. It thus becomes possible to use a response analogous to the response I used to the other epiphenomenal skepticism in the preceding section of this paper: our consciousness at $t_2$ may well control our voluntary movements at $t_3$ because that consciousness controls the intention to move at $t_1$. One doesn't need causation of the intention by consciousness of it. We control our intention to move at $t_1$ *by* consciously willing that movement at $t_2$ even though consciously willing at $t_2$ does not *cause* the not-yet-conscious intention to occur at $t_1$.

The essential idea is that for these (not truly unconscious) intentions, consciousness is part and parcel of them, in the sense that unless we consciously willed movement at $t_2$ we would not have formed the intent to move at $t_1$ and in the sense that forming the intent to move at $t_1$ guaranteed that we would consciously will that movement at $t_2$. We thus can control the not-yet-conscious willing at $t_1$ by controlling the fully conscious willing at $t_2$. Put another way, in getting ready to consciously will a certain movement we inevitably unconsciously form the intention to make that movement. By controlling the former, we also are in control of the latter.[69]

## 5. THE TRUTH OF THESE THREE ALLEGED FACTS OF NEUROSCIENCE

I come now to the other of my two questions about the three skeptical challenges coming out of the Libet experiments. This is the question of scientific truth: is it the case that our wills are caused, that our wills are merely epiphenomenal with the behavior that they putatively cause, or that our consciousness comes too late to give us awareness that we are causing the bodily movements at the time we are doing such causing? I shall again consider the skeptical challenges one at a time.

### A. Free Will

Most neuroscientists are certain that our wills are not exempt from the causal laws that govern everything else we know about. They are certain, that is, that what we choose, decide, intend, and will is as caused as is anything else. I agree with them.

Libet is an exception. While the initiation of action is caused for Libet, the choice whether or not to veto that action was for Libet uncaused. Libet thus illustrates the kind of freedom some people think they want, because they think that if the will is not free in this sense, no one can be responsible.

Yet is the existence of such contra-causal freedom not an incredible idea, whether in Libet's hands or those of others? As Arthur Danto pointed out long ago about Libet's veto idea,[70] such an idea is "a kind of metaphysical hysteria" that literally puts a ghost in the machine. Like the ghosts depicted in cartoons, the uncaused ghost of a Libetan will can cause things to happen in the world, but is itself immune to causal influence. It can initiate causal processes, but when those very same processes are directed against it they are without effect. Ghosts can throw bricks, but when those bricks are thrown at them the bricks pass right through them, for example.

There is no science that can make sense of this. Even if one becomes a metaphysical dualist, positing a "mind stuff" that is not of this, the physical, world, that helps not at all. For in such desperate attempts to immunize mental states from causation one also renders those mental states impotent. Alternatively, if it is intuitive to think that mental states are not causally impotent, then it seems no less intuitive to think that our mental states of belief and will are also caused by events in the physical world.

Some believers in free will seek solace in the apparent indeterminism of modern physics. Yet as has been pointed out many times, the apparent indeterminism of quantum mechanics is as incompatible with responsibility as determinism is thought to be. If our choices are reflective of irreducibly probabilistic relations to unwilled events, that surely is no more comforting than those choices being reflective of causal relations to unwilled events. In either case, we don't control the events that (probabilistically or causally) "control" us.

I thus can make no sense of libertarian metaphysics. Such metaphysics is a holdover from the superstitions of a religious worldview, one according to which man achieves the capacity of a moral agent only when he becomes like God. God, if she existed, would have free will, being Aquinas' *causa prima*. It is a bit of megalomania to think we have to be godlike in this way to be responsible for choosing a matching pair of socks in the morning!

## B. The Alleged Epiphenomenal Status of the Will

I turn now to a more serious issue. I turn, that is, from the issue of whether the will is caused, to the issue of whether the will does any causing. This sounds like a strictly scientific question, and indeed it is. Only what is disputed here is by-and-large not the scientific facts. Rather, it is the interpretation of those facts that is up for grabs.

The main bones of contention are: (1) Whether we can identify willing with certain brain events; and (2) if so, with which brain events willing is to be identified. I have said my piece on the first of these questions in the earlier part of this paper. The neuroscientific evidence thus far adduced seems quite supportive of some kind of mind/brain identification here.

It is thus the second question that determines the truth of the epiphenomenal skepticism. There are two possibilities worth separately considering here, both of which would constitute an adequate answer to the epiphenomenal skeptic. The first is the possibility that a person's willing is to be identified as beginning with the brain events at $t_1$ in Figure 18.3, and not at $t_2$, as Figure 18.3 depicts. Such brain events causative of bodily movements would then not be the *cause* of one's willing (which itself then would be a causal dangler as depicted in Fig. 18.3). Rather, those brain events would *be* willings, and willings would thus be causes of voluntary bodily movement (because the brain events they are, are causes of such movements).

The second possibility is to date the brain events (that willings are) as beginning later, at $t_2$, which is when the subject becomes aware of willing. Although caused by earlier brain events at $t_1$, these willing brain events at $t_2$ could in turn be causes of voluntary bodily movements (as Fig. 18.2 depicts) and no mere danglers in an epiphenomenal fork (as depicted in Fig. 18.4).

In the literature critical of epiphenomenal skepticism about willings, these two possibilities correspond to the views of T. Bittner[71] and Gilberto Gomes,[72] respectively. Notice that the second, Gomes's view, is a possibility only if the epiphenomenal skepticism is based on the supposition that the brain events measured by RP at $t_1$ caused voluntary movement at $t_3$ only through other brain events (BE' in Fig. 18.4) at $t_2$. If there are no such brain events at $t_2$ operating as causal intermediaries between the RP onset brain events at $t_1$ and movement at $t_3$, then there would be no causally relevant brain events with which to identify willings at $t_2$; in which event willings, even if identical to some brain events, would be mere causal danglers as depicted in Figure 18.4.

The second possible reply, that of Gomes, is thus a possible reply only if there are the causal intermediary brain events as depicted on Figure 18.4. Yet surely this is a plausible supposition. True, in the 550 milliseconds between the RP onset brain events at $t_1$ and movement at $t_3$, there could be no causally intermediary brain events occurring, and still there would be no suspicious "action at a distance." This, because the persistence of states and objects are themselves causal processes capable of transmitting causal influence across substantial times.[73] Yet here, in light of the constant neural activity of the brain, it seems much more likely that there is a chain of causally intermediary events occurring between $t_1$ and $t_3$ and these transmit causal influence from the RP onset brain events at $t_1$ to bodily movements at $t_3$. In which event Gomes's answer to epiphenomenal skepticism (in terms of identifying willings at $t_2$) is as open as is Bittner's earlier identification.

Which of these two possible responses one adopts will be determined largely by one's view of the relation of consciousness of willing, to willing. Anyone who thinks that willings by their nature cannot be unconscious, will favor Gomes's answer to epiphenomenal skepticism; anyone who thinks that willings can be "purely unconscious" (never conscious), or at least unconscious for a time before becoming conscious later ("deferred privileged access"), will regard Bittner's response as a real possibility. I turn then to a question with a long history: must willings (intendings, choosing, deciding, etc.) be conscious? Is it, in other words, an essential property of these mental states that the holder of them be conscious of them at the time he holds them?

As I once examined at some length,[74] the philosophical reaction to Freud in the early part of the twentieth century was hostile to the idea of mental states being unconscious pretty much across the board. One could no more sensibly be said to have unconscious wishes, unconscious fears or hopes, unconscious beliefs, any more than one could sensibly be said to have unconscious intentions or willings. The mind, on this view, is conscious experience:

> When I reflect on what I mean by a wish or an emotion or a feeling, I can only find that I know and think of them simply as different forms of consciousness. I cannot find any distinguishable element in these experiences which can be called consciousness and separated from the other elements even in thought so as to leave anything determinate behind. And to ask us to think of something which has all the characteristics of a wish or a feeling except that it is not conscious seems to me like asking us to think of something which has all the attributes of red or green except that it is not a colour.[75]

Notice how implausible is this older rejection of there being unconscious mental states, for it uses "conscious" in what I earlier called its phenomenological sense. Surely there are many mental states which are unconscious in this sense, the sense that one is not now directing one's attention to them. Freud called these "preconscious" mental states;[76] my own terminology classifies them as conscious in what I called the dispositional sense of the word.

A more recent philosophy of mind more relevantly uses "conscious/unconscious" in their dispositional sense and rejects the idea that mental states can be unconscious, that is, that their subject lacks the abilities both to state what they intend and to direct their attention to that intention if necessary. This rejection is based on a cluster of ideas centered on the notion that each person has a "privileged access" to his or her own mental states.[77]

Privileged access consists of three central claims: (1) that we each have a noninferential, immediate way of coming to know our own mental states, when we know them; (2) that our beliefs in this regard are incorrigible, meaning that if we consciously believe we intend p, necessarily we intend p; and (3) that our mental states are transparent to us, so that if we do intend p, necessarily we are (dispositionally) aware that we intend p. The last two of these claims would debar there being unconscious mental states, if true. But such claims are widely regarded as false. I can have intentions, desires, beliefs, moods, emotions, and even sensations without being aware that I have them and I can be mistaken in my beliefs about being in such states.[78]

In any case, a 400-millisecond delay in becoming conscious of one's intentions can be accommodated by about any view one wants to hold about the privileged access we each have to our own mental states, so long as one allows sense to the idea of "deferred privileged access." That is, we can have the same noninferential way of coming to know our own mental states, the same incorrigibility, and the same transparency, only delayed by 400 milliseconds. That is all that is needed to make possible Bittner's kind of response to epiphenomenal skepticism.

Both responses thus being open, which should we prefer? My own bets are on Bittner, identifying willing as beginning at $t_1$, RP onset 550 milliseconds prior to movement, and continuing on through those brain events in the casual chain to $t_3$, the beginning of motor movement. Such an identification best corresponds to the functional characterization of willings as being the causal product of more distal intentions and the immediate cause of the voluntary bodily movements that execute such distal intentions. This is of course only a provisional bet. If, for example, it turns out that the causally relevant brain events occurring at $t_1$ occur irrespective of whether the bodily movements being initiated are voluntary or involuntary, then perhaps the beginning of willing as a state is either earlier or later than $t_1$. When precisely willing begins is a matter about which we can here be somewhat indifferent; so long as willings are in the causal chain of brain events producing voluntary motor movements, the epiphenomenal objection to responsibility is without bite.

Gomes argues that the intention to move now—what I call a willing—must begin closer to $t_2$ than to $t_1$.[79] This, because ordinarily it does not take 400 milliseconds for consciousness of a mental state to come into existence. To become conscious of the beginning of motor movements, for example, the time interval is considerably shorter. Since consciousness of willing occurs at $t_2$, Gomes reasons that the willing of which one becomes conscious should occur only at some shorter interval prior to $t_2$. This is why Gomes prefers the second possible reply distinguished earlier to the first.

Similarly, Al Mele has recently urged that willings must begin closer to $t_2$ than to $t_1$.[80] Mele's conclusion is based on the thought that willings are the last intentions in the hierarchy of intentions before motor movement. He therefore likens the time it should take such intentions to initiate motor movements, to the time it takes to react to an external signal, as in reaction time experiments. Surveying those experiments, Mele places that time between 93 and 231 milliseconds, much less than the 550 milliseconds separating RP onset from movement. Since $t_2$ is 150–200 milliseconds before movement initiation, this strikes him as the more likely locus of willings.

While not a lot turns on which temporal location for willings one affirms here, my bets are still on the earlier dating of the onset of willing. Nothing precludes the latency period for consciousness to be longer for willing than it is for movement, perception, or other mental states. Nor are the "quick-draw" reaction time experiments relied on by Mele necessarily a good proxy for ordinary willings, willings done where the subjects are not preset to move as fast as they possibly can. And it would be convenient if all of the causal process beginning with the RP onset were included as *willing*. Then one is not forced to resort to self-conscious metaphors, such as "the brain 'decides' to initiate . . . the act,"[81] the scare quotes indicating that we know that persons decide things, not brains without persons. Then one is not forced to cash out such metaphors by distinguishing "a process of preparation of the decisions that causes the movement"[82] from processes of decision itself, as does Gomes.

However these niceties are worked out, it will remain true that willings, being identical to some swatch of the chain of brain events that cause voluntary bodily movement, will be the initiators of action, just as the folk psychology and morality supposes.

### C. Is Consciousness of Willing Epiphenomenal with Voluntary Bodily Movements?

It may seem that we jump out of the proverbial frying pan and into the fire once we conceive of willings as occurring prior to consciousness of willings. For as we saw in section 3, this simply flips the epiphenomenal objection away from willings being epiphenomenal, to consciousness being so. And if consciousness of willing is the touchstone of our responsibility, the conclusion still is that we are not responsible for our bodily movements and all that they can cause. The objection is that for such responsibility, we need consciousness of willings *when those willings are causing movement*; even if willings cause movements at $t_1$, there is no consciousness of those willings until it is too late ($t_2$) for control and responsibility.

Often this form of the objection is implicit in the phrasings of neuroscientists. When John-Dylan Haynes, for example, describes his remarkable findings (of certain decisions having been made 7–10 seconds prior to awareness that they have been made), he like Libet often describes the situation in terms of the brain having decided what to do before the person whose brain it is does so.[83] Implicit in this phrasing is the view that persons are to be identified with their (phenomenological and dispositional) consciousness, and until a person is conscious of a decision or an intention it is not his/her decision or intention.

I also think that this is the best sense to be made of a view common among some philosophers of mind of a generation ago. Even though generally sympathetic to the idea that there can be unconscious desires, unconscious beliefs, unconscious emotions, moods, sensations, etc., such philosophers were unsympathetic to *intentions/decisions* being unconscious.[84] Implicit here too is the idea that intention/decision is the locus where all the things over which we have less than full control (such as our wishes, beliefs, and our emotions, which can come unbidden) get resolved by us as we decide. *We* need to do this consciously, or it isn't *our* resolution. Thus, although phrased as a denial of there being unconscious intentions, the motivating thought really is the one here to be examined: without consciousness of an intention, there is no control by the person of his intentions or his actions, and thus no responsibility can be generated by such unconsciously intentional actions.

My first response to this form of skepticism was in moral theory. In section 4 I urged that we could be in control of our intentions even if they "get started without us" (i.e., they exist before we are aware of them). Now I want to dispute that our intentions do their causings prior to our consciousness of them.

There are two ways to modify the epiphenomenal relationship depicted earlier in Figure 18.6 so as to get consciousness of willing to be contemporaneous with the causing of bodily movements by willing: we can move willings back to $t_2$, or we can move consciousness of willings forward to $t_1$. I shall explore both options, starting with the first.

As an example of the first option, consider Al Mele's suggestion that Libet's onset of RP at $t_1$ measures an *urge* to move, not an intention (or willing) to move.[85] One sees the general motivation for Mele's suggestion: it is to get the willing back to $t_2$ when consciousness of willing also exists. Yet this suggestion, by itself, accomplishes little. All Mele's suggestion by itself accomplishes is a modification of the relationships depicted in Figure 18.6 to the relationships depicted in Figure, 18.10:

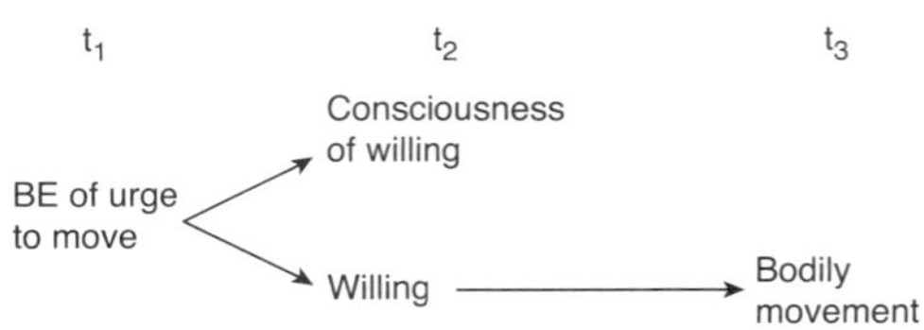


**Figure 18.10**

Getting willings simultaneous with consciousness of willings isn't helpful; what is needed is to show how consciousness of willings can have a causal role in the production of bodily movements.

As indicated earlier against Gomes, I find it more plausible to identify willings as beginning at least as early as $t_1$, 550 milliseconds prior to movement, and continuing as a causal process right up to the Rubicon Point, beyond which movement cannot be stopped; as measured by contemporary stop-action experiments, that averages out at about 50 milliseconds prior to movement. Consciousness of willing appears at $t_2$, 150 milliseconds prior to movement, and is also a cause of the movement. The relationships then could be as depicted in Figure, 18.11:

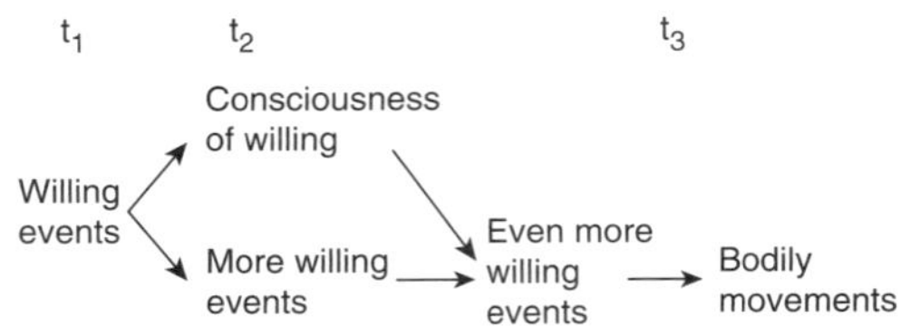


**Figure 18.11**

If these are the relationships, then consciousness of willing is not epiphenomenal; rather, it causes bodily movements by causing the continuation of willing between $t_2$ and the Rubicon Point, which is $t_2$ plus 100 milliseconds. If the later part of the willing process causes bodily movements, then so does consciousness of willing, and we consciously control our movements just as morality and the folk psychology suppose.

Note that consciousness of willing is not depicted as a mere *preventer* of willings and of bodily movements.[86] That is Libet's veto function, and that relation exists also. Rather, the claimed relationship is causal: there is a causal process connecting consciousness of willing to the 100 milliseconds of willing occurring on and after $t_2$, and a causal process connecting those states of willing to bodily movements. Consciousness of willings thus *causes* both the willings and the bodily movements willed; such consciousness is thus not merely a possible preventer of willings and movements. (It is a possible preventer, but only because it is more basically an active causer; all causers are possible preventers in this sense, because a failure to cause will prevent.)

Whether consciousness of willing enters into the causal process of willing is a scientific question. Are the brain events that are constitutive of consciousness of willing causative of bodily movement, with the brain events that are willings? Nothing in Libet's findings, or of post-Libet experiments, rules out that they are.

The second option distinguished earlier is to move consciousness earlier, at $t_1$ when willing begins. Then consciousness of willing could join willings as the cause of bodily movements, as depicted in Figure, 18.12:

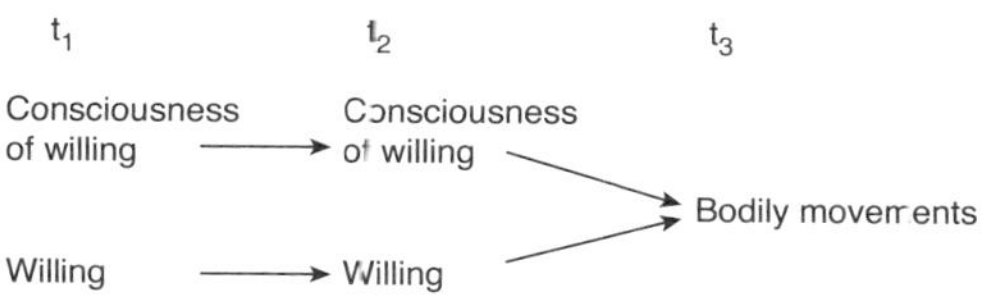


**Figure 18.12**

This sounds like it contradicts Libet's evidence: his subjects report awareness 350 milliseconds after the readiness potential appears, not when RP (willing) first occurs. Yet consciousness too surely is a brain process, and one that takes real time to occur. It should be no surprise that this process takes time to gear up before phenomenal awareness (or the dispositional ability) appears. Perhaps $t_1$ is when the "consciousness potential" appears, along with the readiness potential.

There are three things to worry about in exploring this option. One is terminological. The worry is that we have to make sense of there being an unconscious consciousness between $t_1$ and $t_2$. Yet this terminological hurdle is easily overcome. The deep nature of consciousness that we refer to is in terms of brain events; these can occur before the phenomenal/dispositional properties of consciousness come into being. Consciousness (the brain process) thus can be said to be (dispositionally and phenomenologically) unconscious.[87]

Second, there is the worry voiced before by Gomes: the start-up time for awareness/dispositional ability consciousness may be shorter than 350–400 milliseconds that separates $t_1$ and $t_2$, in which event consciousness of willing as a brain process would come later then the onset of willing at $t_1$. Yet even if this turns out to be true, that would only mean that consciousness of willing would enter the causal stream leading to movement later than does willing; it would not mean that consciousness of willing was only epiphenomenal.

The third worry is a moral worry. It is that the consciousness needed for responsibility is phenomenal awareness/dispositional ability, not the brain process that (eventually) gives rise to these properties. The worry is that the thing we need for control is the phenomenal/dispositional property of consciousness, and that this occurs only at $t_2$, well after willing has commenced causing bodily movement.

This is a nonworry for two reasons. One is that we can control the consciousness brain events at $t_1$ by controlling the phenomenal/dispositional properties at $t_2$, as was argued in section 4. The other is that the later phenomenal/dispositional consciousness of willing can still be part of the cause of willing in the 100 milliseconds after $t_2$, giving us control then even if not earlier (this is to return to the first option above.)

In exploring these two options for showing that consciousness of willing is not epiphenomenal, I have assumed the relationship between consciousness of willing, and willing, to be causal. This requires that the brain events of the one be distinct from the brain events of the other (for nothing is the cause of itself.) It is possible that the relationship is not that of cause and effect, but is rather one of partial identity. Then consciousness of willing would still be a cause of voluntary movement but only as an aspect or part of willing (which is the cause of such movements). Depending on which of the two possible temporal locations of willings described above is adopted, the relationships are then slight modifications of Figure 18.2, either:

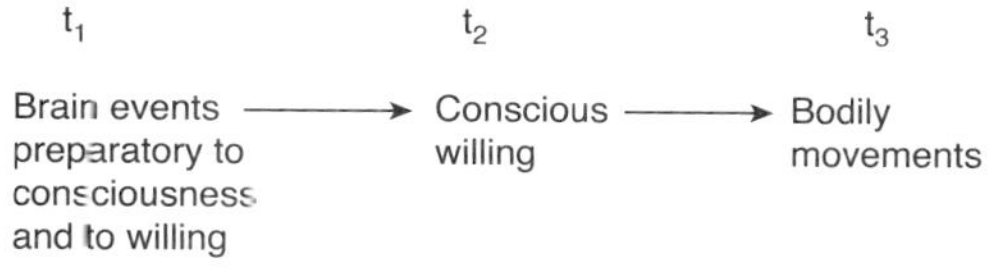


**Figure 18.13**

Or

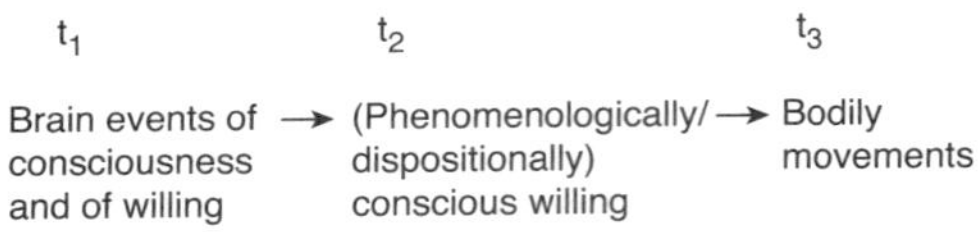


**Figure 18.14**

Whether consciousness of willing should be seen as a part of willing-type events (Figs. 18.13–18.14), or rather as part of separate consciousness type events (Figs. 18.11–18.12), depends on the integrity of consciousness as a brain process.[88] If consciousness as such is the type, of which consciousness of willing is an instance, then the relationship between it and willing is causal and not constitutive.

In any case, however this last issue comes out, we have good reason to be optimistic in preserving the folk psychology's view that conscious willings are not mere epiphenomena to bodily movements but are indeed the direct, immediate cause of the movements. We thus are secure in having a second reason (in addition to control of the relevant epiphenomenal forks) for thinking we are indeed morally responsible for our voluntary actions: neither willings nor consciousness of willings are merely epiphenomenal with the bodily movements that they do indeed cause.

## ACKNOWLEDGMENTS

This paper was written under the aegis of the MacArthur Foundation's Project in Law and Neuroscience, the support of which is gratefully acknowledged. The comments of Walter Sinnot-Armstrong and Gideon Yaffe on an earlier draft of this paper are greatly appreciated.

## NOTES

1. Oliver Wendell Holmes Jr., *The Common Law* (Boston: Little, Brown, 1881), 7.
2. *Morissette v. United States*, 342 U.S. 246 (1952).
3. I explore this thesis at length in Moore, *Act and Crime: The Implications of the Philosophy of Action for the Criminal Law* (Oxford: Oxford University Press, 1993), chapter 6.
4. *Edington v. Fitzmaurice*, L.R. 29 Ch. Div. 459, 483 (1882).
5. Defended in Moore, *Objectivity in Law and Ethics* (Aldershot, UK: Ashgate Press, 2004), chapter 6.
6. I have adopted Michael Bratman's version of practical rationality in separating intention from desire. See Bratman, *Intention, Plans, and Practical Reason* (Cambridge, MA: Harvard University Press, 1987). The older view is to lump intentions in with desires as a general "pro attitude." See, e.g., Donald Davidson, "Intention," in his *Essays on Actions and Events* (Oxford: Oxford University Press, 1980).
7. The Davidson/Bratman debate referenced in footnote 6 above. I align myself on the Bratman side in Moore, *Act and Crime*, chapter 6.
8. A prominent current form is the Bratman/Vellerman debate. An older form is William James's ideomotor theory of action. For discussion, see Moore, *Act and Crime*, 145–149.
9. Bratman, *Intentions, Plans, and Practical Reason*.
10. See, e.g., Alvin Goldman, *A Theory of Human Action* (Englewood Cliffs, NJ: Prentice Hall, 1970), 55–63.
11. Goldman, *A Theory of Human Action*, 61.
12. See, e.g., Frederick Siegler, "Unconscious Intentions," *Inquiry* 10 (1967): 51–67.
13. I defend a version of this thesis in Moore, "Responsibility and the Unconscious," *Southern California Law Review* 53 (1980): 1563–1675, rewritten as chapters 7, 9, 10 of *Law and Psychiatry: Rethinking the Relationship* (Cambridge: Cambridge University Press, 1984). (The original title of this book is more descriptive of its contents: *Persons and the Unconscious*.) The essential idea is that we need mental states of persons to have some connection to consciousness in some sense if we are to distinguish such states from the subpersonal states of brain functioning that are not at all accessible to consciousness.
14. B. Libet, C. A. Gleason, E. W. Wright, and D. K. Pearl, "Time of Conscious Intention to Act in Relation to Onset of Cerebral Activities (Readiness Potential); The Unconscious Initiation of a Freely Voluntary Act," *Brain* 106 (1983): 623–642. These findings are restated in Libet, "Unconscious Cerebral Initiative and the Role of Conscious Will in Voluntary Action," *Behavioral and Brain Sciences* 8 (1985): 529–539.
15. Libet, "Unconscious Cerebral Initiative," 532.

16. Patrick Haggard, Chris Newman, and Elena Magno, "On the Perceived Time of Voluntary Actions," *British Journal of Psychology* 90 (1999): 291–303, at p. 291.
17. Benjamin Libet, "Consciousness, Free Action and the Brain," *Journal of Consciousness Studies* 8 (2001): 59–65, at p. 61.
18. Benjamin Libet, "Do We Have Free Will?" *Journal of Consciousness Studies* 6 (1999): 47–57, reprinted in Benjamin Libet, Anthony Freeman, and Keith Sutherland, eds., *The Volitional Brain: Towards a Neuroscience of Free Will* (UK: Imprint Academic, 2004), 52.
19. Libet, "Unconscious Cerebral Initiative," 536–538.
20. Libet, "Do We Have Free Will?" 52–53.
21. On causal influence going across unchanging states as well as chains of events, see Michael Moore, "The Nature of Singularist Theories of Causation," *The Monist* 92 (2009): 3–23, reprinted in Moore, *Causation and Responsibility* (Oxford: Oxford University Press, 2009), 500–501, 510.
22. Alfred R. Mele, *Effective Intentions: The Power of the Conscious Will* (Oxford: Oxford University Press, 2009), pp. 70–76.
23. Mele, *Effective Intentions*, p. 71.
24. See, e.g., Michael Moore, "Causation and the Excuses," *California Law Review* 73 (1985): 1091–1149, reprinted in Moore, *Placing Blame: A General Theory of the Criminal Law* (Oxford: Oxford University Press, 1997).
25. The example that I have in mind was a lecture by Robert Sapolski, "Science will Eliminate Blame", given to the annual meeting of the McArthur Foundation Project on Law and Neuroscience, University of California-Santa-Barbara, May 29, 2008.
26. David Hume, *An Enquiry Concerning Human Understanding*, section 8.20 "Of Liberty and Necessity."
27. Stephen J. Morse, "Determinism and the Death of Folk Psychology: Two Challenges to Responsibility from Neuroscience," *Minnesota Journal of Law, Science, and Technology* 9 (2008): 1–35, at p. 14.
28. See the extensive list in Moore, *Law and Psychiatry*, 427 n. 5.
29. Beginning with Donald Davidson's seminal article, "Actions, Reasons and Causes," in his *Essays on Actions and Events* (Oxford: Oxford University Press, 1980).
30. A like anecdote (and more besides) is given by Joel Feinberg, "Causing Voluntary Actions," in his *Doing and Deserving* (Princeton, NJ: Princeton University Press, 1970), 157–158.
31. The selective determinist strategy is discussed in Moore, *Law and Psychiatry*, 358–360.
32. The kind of selective determinism discussed by Paul Hollander, who I believe coined the phrase. Hollander, "Sociology, Selective Determinism, and the Rise of Expectations," *American Sociologist* 8 (1973): 147–153.
33. That theories of direct reference require these two kinds of facts is defended in Michael Moore, "Can Objectivity Be Grounded in Semantics?" *Social, Political, and Legal Philosophy* 2 (2007): 235–260; and in Michael Moore, "Semantics, Metaphysics, and the Objectivity of Law," a paper given to the Conference on Objectivity in the Law, University of Texas Philosophy Department, April 5, 2008.
34. See, e.g., Eddy Zemach, "Putnam's Theory on the Reference of Substance Terms," *Journal of Philosophy* 73 (1976): 116–127.
35. Argued for originally in Hilary Putnam, "The Meaning of 'Meaning,'" in his *Mind, Language, and Reality* (Cambridge: Cambridge University Press, 1985).
36. The counterintuitive conclusion of Norman Malcolm, *Dreaming* (London: Routledge and Kegan-Paul, 1959).
37. See, e.g., Susan Pockett, "The Neuroscience of Movement," in Susan Pockett, William Banks, and Shaun Gallagher, eds., *Does Consciousness Cause Behavior?* (Cambridge, MA: MIT Press, 2006).
38. Sigmund Freud, *Introductory Lectures on Psycho-analysis*, in *The Standard Edition of the Works of Sigmund Freud* (London: Hogarth Press, 1966–1974), vol. 15, p. 285.
39. Standard compatibilist texts include John Bishop, *Natural Agency* (Cambridge: Cambridge University Press, 1989); John Martin Fisher and Mark Ravizza, *Responsibility and Control* (Cambridge: Cambridge University Press, 1998); Stephen Morse, "Culpability and Control," *University of Pennsylvania Law Review* 142 (1994): 1587–1660; D. C. Dennett, *Elbow Room: The Varieties of Free Will Worth Wanting* (Cambridge, MA: MIT Press, 1984).
40. Thus Libet shrugs off much of the criticism his views have received as being from "philosophers and others with no significant experience in experimental neuroscience of the brain." These nonscientific ignoramuses are

contrasted with "many of the world's leading neuroscientists" who "have not only accepted our findings and interpretations, but have even enthusiastically praised these achievements" B. Libet, "The Timing of Mental Events: Libet's Experimental Findings and Their Implications," *Consciousness and Cognition*, Vol. 11 (2002), p. 292. My, how little distance we have come! Recall that Freud used to write off the logical criticisms offered up by *his* philosophical critics with his right as a true scientist to make brute empirical discoveries no matter what the armchair types might say, Freud, *Introductory Lectures*, *Standard Edition*, vol. 16, p. 277.

41. E.g., John Eccles, *How the Self Controls Its Brain* (Berlin: Springer-Verlag, 1994).
42. E.g., Libet, Freeman, and Sutherland, "Editor's Introduction: The Volitional Brain," in Libet, Freeman, and Sutherland, eds., *The Volitional Brain*, xvii–xix.
43. Libet, Freeman, and Sutherland, "Editor's Introduction," xiii–xv.
44. Compare Joshua Greene and Jonathan Cohen, "For the Law, Neuroscience Changes Nothing and Everything," *Philosophical Transcript of the Royal Society of London* 359 (2004): 1775–1785. Greene and Cohen believe that the insights of an advancing neuroscience will erode the criteria we currently use to ascribe responsibility, and that no degree of philosophically correct compatibilism can stop this erosional process.
45. See Moore, *Placing Blame*, 531–534.
46 Lecture of James Q. Wilson, "Neuroscience and Morality," Meeting of the Network on Responsibility, MacArthur Foundation Law and Neuroscience Project, Santa Monica, California, January 8, 2009.
47. As Wilson rightly concluded.
48. The "hypothetical" was based on a real case, reported in Jeffrey Burns and Russell Swerdlow, "Right Orbitofrontal Tumor with Pedophilia Symptom and Constructional Apraxia Sign," *Archives of Neurology* 60 (2003): 437–440. The actual patient suffered all of the impairments listed in the text.
49. Burns and Swerdlow, "Right Orbitofrontal Tumor," p. 440.
50. Burns and Swerdlow, "Right Orbitofrontal Tumor," p. 440.
51. Burns and Swerdlow, "Right Orbitofrontal Tumor," p. 440.
52. The real paradox is described and analyzed in Robert Nozick, *Socratic Puzzles* (Cambridge, MA: Harvard University Press, 1997), chapters 2–3.
53. Jennifer Hornsby, *Actions* (London: Routledge, 1980), 76 n. 1.
54. Hornsby, *Actions*, 25. Such examples were earlier discussed in A. I. Melden, *Free Action* (London: Routledge, 1961). These kinds of examples of the *by* relation are discussed by me in Moore, *Act and Crime*, 100–101.
55. I defend such suppositions in Moore, *Causation and Responsibility*, chapters 15 and 19.
56. I discuss the overdetermination cases at length in Moore, *Causation and Responsibility*, chapter 17.
57. A symmetry noted long ago as a puzzle about causation, in Richard Taylor, *Action and Purpose* (Englewood Cliffs, NJ: Prentice-Hall, 1965), chapters 1–3.
58. Vilayanur S. Ramachandran, *A Brief Tour of Human Consciousness* (New York: Pi Press, 2004), p. 87.
59. Ramachandran, *A Brief Tour of Human Consciousness*, p. 87.
60. One might go further than this in analogizing our epiphenomenal willings to Newcombe's problem. Revert to the simple-minded version of Newcombe's Paradox discussed in the previous section. Our willings at $t_2$ may not just be in the same position as the Great Predictor's prediction in the simple-minded version of Newcombe. On some philosophies of mind our willings are a prediction just like that of the Great Predictor. Given our privileged epistemic position vis-à-vis our own future actions, these views make each of us our own Great Predictor. Some such as David Velleman argue that privileged predictions is all our willings ever amount to anyway. J. David Velleman, *Practical Reflection* (Princeton, NJ: Princeton University Press, 1989); Velleman, *The Possibility of Practical Reason* (Oxford: Oxford University Press, 2001). In which case we control our actions by making predictions at $t_2$ responsive to facts F at $t_1$, the prediction being a backtrackingly sufficient condition for those facts to exist. F in turn is causally sufficient for the bodily movements at $t_3$. Our control on this picture is less direct than we imagine, is not causal, and is not even based on our forming a mental state distinct from

predictive belief. Yet we could be responsible nonetheless on some such basis, even if our willings are epiphenomenal with our actions.

61. Moore, "Responsibility and the Unconscious"; Moore, *Law and Psychiatry*, 337–348. I review in more detail the arguments supporting the five conclusions summarized in the text, in Moore, "Intention, Responsibility and the Challenges of Recent Neuroscience," *Stanford Technology Law Review*, www.stanford.stlr.edu (February 2009).
62. See the discussion in Moore, *Law and Psychiatry*, 126–129.
63. The American Law Institute's Model Penal Code recognizes this moral fact in its definition of voluntary action as being the product of "the effort or determination of the actor, either conscious or habitual." (What the Code calls "habitual" is just "conscious" in my dispositional sense when one is unconscious in the phenomenological sense.) American Law Institute, *Model Penal Code* '2.01(2)(d) (Proposed Official Draft, 1962).
64. I take it this is why Libet (rightly) rejects one of his critic's reformulation of Libet's findings, *viz*, the one classifying Libet's experimental subjects as being only *preconscious* (rather than unconscious) of their intent to move. See Libet, "Can Conscious Experience Affect Brain Activity?" *Journal of Consciousness Studies* 10 (2003): 24–28.
65. Freud's moral philosophy would make us responsible for whatever we intend, however unconscious may be the intention in question. Freud derided the law's requirement of consciousness for responsibility, saying that "the physician will leave it to the jurist to construct for social purposes a responsibility that is artificially limited to the metapsychological ego." Freud, "Moral Responsibility for the Content of Dreams," in *The Standard Edition*, vol. 19., p. 134.
66. My general reconstrual of Freud in Moore, *Law and Psychiatry*, 130–134, 254–265, is that unconscious intentions exhibit "deferred privileged access" on the part of the subject whose intentions they are. The idea is that when we become aware of such unconscious intentions, we also become aware of having experienced them earlier. We come to know them in the same noninferential way that we know our conscious mental states, except that there is a temporal separation between the existence of such mental states and our coming to know them in this way. We have, in other words, a first-person *memory* of having had such states rather than the more usual perception of them while we have them.
67. Moore, *Law and Psychiatry*, 337–348.
68. Moore, *Law and Psychiatry*, 337–348.
69. This response may sound a bit like Libet's own mode of reconciling his findings with holding persons responsible via the supposed "veto function." There are two fundamental differences however. One is that Libet's "veto" conceptualization is passive: at $t_2$, on Libet's view, we merely *allow* the action to proceed. My way of conceptualizing this, by contrast, is active: by consciously willing at $t_2$, we have actively begun (at $t_1$) the processes of action-initiation. Secondly, Libet requires the actor's veto/nonveto decision at $t_2$ to be uncaused; on the contrary, I assume that our conscious willings at $t_2$ are caused by the $t_1$ brain events that are our unconscious willings, and these in turn are fully caused by even earlier events. There is no magic in my account, whereas there is in Libet's.
70. Arthur Danto, "Consciousness and Motor Control," *Behavioral and Brain Sciences* 8 (1985): 540–541.
71. T. Bittner, "Consciousness and the Act of the Will," *Philosophical Studies* 81 (1996): 331–341.
72. Gilberto Gomes, "Volition and the Readiness Potential," *Journal of Consciousness Studies* 6 (1999): 59–76.
73. Moore, *Causation and Responsibility*, 500–501, 510.
74. Moore, *Law and Psychiatry*, 252–254.
75. G. C. Field, "Is the Conception of the Unconscious of Value in Psychology?" *Mind* 31 (1922): 413–423, at pp. 413–414. As another contemporary critic also put it, Freud's claim that unconscious mental states are just like ordinary mental states except that they lack consciousness, "is just like Mr. Churchill's 'cannibals in all respects except the act of devouring the flesh of victims.'" J. Laird, "Is the Conception of the Unconscious of Value in Psychology?" *Mind* 31 (1922): 433–442, at pp. 434–435.
76. On Freud's usages of "preconscious," "unconscious," and "conscious," see Moore, *Law and Psychiatry*, 129–140. As I noted earlier, one of Libet's critics, M. Velmans, "How Could

Conscious Experience Affect Brains?" *Journal of Consciousness Studies* 9 (2002): 3–29, would construe Libet's subjects' intentions as only being preconscious at RP onset at $t_1$, a view Libet rejected.

77. For an introduction to the extensive literature on the privileged access we are each thought to have to our own mental states, see Moore, *Law and Psychiatry*, 254–265.
78. Moore, *Law and Psychiatry*, 254–265.
79. Gomes, "Volition and the Readiness Potential," 71–72.
80. Mele, *Effective Intention*, 70–75.
81. Libet's sometimes wording. Libet, "Unconscious Cerebral Initiative," 536.
82. Gomes, "Volition and Readiness Potential," 72.
83. Chun Siong Soon, Marcel Brass, Hans-Jochen Heinze, and John-Dylan Haynes, "Unconscious Determinants of Free Decisions in the Human Brain," *Nature Neuroscience* 11 (2008): 543–545, at p. 543 ("Because brain activity in the SMA consistently preceded the conscious decision, it has been argued that the brain had already unconsciously made a decision").
84. See, e.g., Frederick Siegler, "Unconscious Intentions," *Inquiry* 10 (1967): 51–67. Al Mele's more contemporary book, *Effective Intentions: The Power of Conscious Will*, shows some of this reluctance, insofar as Mele distinguishes decisions from intentions and is sympathetic to the view that decisions must be conscious (at least in the dispositional sense).
85. Alfred Mele, *Free Will and Luck* (Oxford: Oxford University Press, 2006), 36.
86. On the notions of *prevention* and of *failure to prevent* (omission), and how these are distinct from but are related to causal relationships, see Moore, *Causation and Responsibility*, 435–459.
87. Here we also tread on old ground. Freud too was driven to conclude that there can be an unconscious consciousness. What he meant by the phrase was that part of that functionally characterized (and ultimately brain realized) system termed the "System Csc" could be phenomenologically and dispositionally unconscious. On Freud's theory construction in this regard, see Michael Moore, "Mind, Brain, and Unconscious," in Peter Clark and Crispin Wright, eds., *Mind, Psychoanalysis and Science* (Oxford: Basil Blackwell, 1988).
88. On this, see the discussion by Daniel Dennett and Marcel Kinsbourne, "Time and the Observer: The Where and When of Consciousness in the Brain," *Behavioral and Brain Sciences* 15 (1992), pp. 183–247.

# CHAPTER 19

## Lessons from Libet

*Walter Sinnott-Armstrong*

Libet's followers sometimes claim that his famous experiments undermine all freedom and responsibility. Libet's critics often respond that his experiments are completely irrelevant to freedom and responsibility. When intelligent people disagree so starkly and accuse their opponents of simple mistakes, I suspect that each side misunderstands their apparent opponents.

One common mistake is to think that Libet's experiments are about determinism and free will. They are not. Libet's experiments do not even pretend to show that our wills are or are not determined by prior causes or that we can or cannot control our wills. Libet himself often talks as if his experiments address the traditional issue of free will and determinism, but that only shows how badly people can misinterpret their own work.

The real question that Libet's experiments raise is whether our conscious wills cause the willed actions. What is at issue is the effects rather than the causes of conscious will. The question is whether conscious will is impotent, not whether it is free. If conscious will is impotent, then we cannot control our actions by means of conscious will, and this disability might reduce our freedom of action. Nonetheless, this challenge to freedom of action is separate from the traditional challenge to freedom of will that comes from determinism, since our wills might be impotent even if they are not determined, and even if determinism is compatible with free will.

A major contribution of Libet's experiments is to raise or sharpen this new question. Of course, many predecessors denied that conscious will causes action,[1] but they rarely, if ever, gave enough reason to make people take that apparently outrageous denial seriously. And none of these predecessors focused on the issue of timing that was central to Libet's research. By raising a new issue in a new way, Libet's work made (and continues to make) many people rethink their assumptions. That accomplishment is a mark of good philosophy as well as good science.

The assumptions at stake are both normative and descriptive. The relevant normative assumption is, roughly, that causation by conscious will is necessary for responsibility. The descriptive assumption that Libet questions is, again roughly, that conscious will causes the willed action. This chapter will address these assumptions in turn. My conclusion will be that Libet's experiments do not undermine responsibility in general, but they do illuminate some particular cases as well as common standards of responsibility.

### 1. IS CAUSATION BY CONSCIOUS WILL NECESSARY FOR LEGAL RESPONSIBILITY?

Let's begin with legal responsibility, because the standards of responsibility in law are stated explicitly in legal statutes and decisions. Although consciousness and will are crucial to law at several points,[2] the most direct connection between conscious will and legal responsibility is in the voluntary act requirement. The dominant formulation of this requirement is in the Model Penal Code (MPC) Section 2.01:

> (1) A person is not guilty of an offense unless his liability is based on conduct that includes a voluntary act or the omission to perform an act of which he is physically capable. (2) The following are not voluntary acts within the meaning of this Section: (a) a reflex or convulsion; (b) a bodily movement during unconsciousness or sleep; (c) conduct during hypnosis or resulting from hypnotic suggestion; (d) a bodily movement that otherwise is not a product of the effort or determination of the actor, either conscious or habitual.

This formulation does not require that the offense itself is a voluntary act. All it requires is that the conduct "includes" a voluntary act. In one case, a driver had an epileptic seizure while driving, and the resulting accident killed four people.[3] The epileptic seizure was not a voluntary act, but the driver was held liable on the grounds that a larger slice of his conduct included starting to drive while knowing that he was susceptible to epileptic seizures. Profound time-framing problems arise regarding how far back the law reaches in order to find a voluntary act.[4] Still, if no act within an appropriate scope counts as a voluntary act, then the defendant is not liable at all, according to MPC 2.01.

The Model Penal Code does not define what voluntary acts are, but it does give examples of what voluntary acts are not. The crucial example here is "a bodily movement that otherwise is not a product of the effort or determination of the actor, either conscious or habitual." An act is not habitual unless it has been repeated on several occasions in the past. Thus, when an act has not been done repeatedly, clause (2)(d) in MPC 2.01 implies that a voluntary act must be "a product of effort or determination" that is "conscious." The word "product" requires a causal relation. The phrase "effort or determination" suggests will. Hence, this clause directly implies that a nonhabitual act is not voluntary unless it is caused by conscious will.

The same requirement is also suggested less directly by other parts of MPC 2.01. Clause (2)(a) says that a reflex or convulsion is not a voluntary act. When doctors probe for reflexes, their patients are usually conscious of the resulting reflex movements, and they also usually desire that those movements occur, since something is wrong with them if no reflex movements occur. Nonetheless, the patients are not held responsible for those reflex movements or for their effects (such as kicking the doctor). Thus, consciousness of movement and desire to move are not enough for responsibility. Why not? Because conscious will does not cause the willed action in reflexes and convulsions. Thus, the rationale for clause (2)(a) seems to be that causation by conscious will is required for responsibility.

These requirements are not idiosyncratic. As of 2002, twenty states in the United States adopted an explicit voluntary act requirement. Most of these states explicitly based their requirement on the Model Penal Code. Most of the other states followed the Model Penal Code requirement implicitly. In one way or another, almost all jurisdictions in the United States require causation by conscious will for responsibility.[5]

Critics might deny that the voluntary act requirement really requires causation by conscious will for responsibility. After all, if scientists showed that conscious will does not cause the willed action, judges would still never interpret the voluntary act requirement (or any other clause) so as to imply that nobody is ever responsible for any act. That is correct. No matter what scientists find, judges are likely to stretch the law so that normal acts count as voluntary acts. Otherwise, all criminals would be released, and mayhem would result. However, except in the minds of legal realists, judges do not make the law and do not alone determine what the law is. Insofar as law is at least partly determined by the plain meaning of what is written in black and white on the pages of statutes,[6] the law (or, at least, Model Penal Code section 2.01) seems to hold on its face that legal responsibility requires causation by conscious will.

## 2. IS CAUSATION BY CONSCIOUS WILL NECESSARY FOR MORAL RESPONSIBILITY?

What about morality? Standards for legal responsibility need not always reflect standards for moral responsibility. However, when the law deviates from common morality, it is most often for practical reasons. It is hard to imagine any practical reason for the law to add a requirement of causation by conscious will. To the contrary, there seem to be practical reasons *against* requiring prosecutors to prove causation by conscious will within the evidential and temporal limits of actual legal trials. Hence, when the law does require causation by conscious will for legal responsibility, this legal requirement seems to be based on moral assumptions.

The fact that this legal standard is so widespread provides additional evidence that common morality includes this requirement. It is also relevant that this standard is a central part of criminal law. Criminal laws—or at least those involving *mala in se* crimes—usually reflect common moral judgments. Thus, the fact that causation by conscious will is so widely seen as necessary for legal responsibility in cases of (*mala in se*) crimes suggests that this requirement for responsibility is part of not just law but also common morality.

This moral claim receives further support by comparing cases. Consider someone who is asleep but grabs a knife, walks into an adjoining bedroom, stabs her daughter, walks back to her own bedroom, and is completely surprised in the morning to find her daughter dead.[7] Of course, it is often hard to know what is happening in real cases like this. Perhaps some are faking. But suppose the facts are just as claimed. Since this person grabs a knife rather than a pencil and stabs into a body rather than randomly, she might seem partially conscious, and her action looks intentional at some level. Still, most people would say that the agent is not responsible or, at least, not fully responsible.[8] This intuition is confirmed when the MPC section 2.01 (2)(b) as well as various courts[9] excuse acts during sleep, presumably because many people would view it as morally unfair to hold real sleepwalkers responsible. Why? The answer seems to be that they are seen as lacking consciousness and, hence, control.

Now modify just one fact: A different sleepwalker is conscious of what he is doing, but his conscious will does not initiate his bodily movements and cannot control them. He simply observes what is happening. Despite being conscious of his act, he does not seem any more responsible than in the previous case when the sleepwalker was not conscious. Why not? Because this new sleepwalker's consciousness does not play any causal role in his act. Impotent consciousness does not increase his control over what he does, so adding impotent consciousness cannot make him responsible for his action. This comparison thus suggests that and why conscious will without causation is not enough for full moral responsibility.

Contrasts like these suggest to many people that a person is fully responsible for an act only when the act results from the agent's conscious thought or choice in some way. Of course, many details need to be spelled out, and qualifications need to be added. Still, the point for now is simply that causation by conscious will seems necessary for complete moral responsibility, at least in many circumstances.

We still need to narrow the issue. Sleepwalkers are abnormal and unconscious of most features of their surroundings and movements. In contrast, other abnormal agents are conscious of almost all aspects of their surroundings and movements, but they are not conscious of any intention to make their movements. Examples include Tourette's syndrome and alien hand syndrome.[10] Such cases suggest that general consciousness is not enough for responsibility if the agent lacks consciousness of any intention related to that bodily movement. But what about cases where an agent is both normal and conscious of a specific intent to do the act? Full responsibility still seems to be lacking if that conscious intention does not cause the action.

To see why, imagine that someone plans to kill a rival by running him over at 9:00 as the rival jogs by his house. It is 9:00 now, but the driver thinks it is 8:00, since he forgot daylight saving time, so the driver decides to go buy breakfast. As he drives carefully out of his driveway, the jogger appears unexpectedly and is run over and killed by accident. The driver did will to kill the jogger, had that will at the time when he killed the jogger, and killed him in the intended way at the intended place and time. The driver's will was presumably free in any way that any will is ever free. Nonetheless, the driver's will did not cause the accident or the death, because only his intention to buy breakfast caused him to leave then. Hence, this particular act of killing was not done *from* free will, and the driver is neither morally nor legally responsible for first-degree murder. He might not even be guilty of reckless driving or attempted murder. Thus, full responsibility for an act requires more than a free will to do the act. It also requires that the will causes the act.

Fine, critics say, but what if the will is unconscious? Imagine that a cook makes soup for a friend. The cook's only conscious goal is to please the friend. Unfortunately, the soup contains nuts to which the friend is allergic. The allergy is unforeseeable, so the cook is neither negligent nor morally or legally responsible for harming the friend. Now suppose the cook has a totally unconscious desire to hurt his friend. The cook envies his friend's success and wants to punish his friend for succeeding, but the cook is totally unaware of any envy or any plan to punish. Even if such an unconscious intention could be established, it would not be enough to make the cook responsible.[11] After all, if the cook is totally unconscious of any plan to hurt his friend, how can he control whether or not he hurts his friend? Without this kind of conscious control, how can the cook be responsible?

The jogger example suggests that *causation* by will is required. The cook case suggests that *consciousness* of will is required. Nonetheless, it is still possible that consciousness need not play any role in the causation. However, it would be hard to understand why both elements—causation by will and consciousness of will—are necessary if they need not work together so that consciousness plays a role in the causation. Hence, despite possible responses, I conclude that causation by consciousness or by conscious will is necessary for full moral responsibility.

## 3. DO CONSCIOUS WILLS CAUSE ACTS?

The reason why law and common sense can feel free to impose the above requirement on moral responsibility is that conscious will normally seems to cause the acts for which people are responsible. A challenge arises only if there is some reason to believe that conscious will does not really cause the willed act.

Such a reason might come from the dualistic view that mind and body are separate substances plus an account of causation that rules out causal relations between such separate substances.[12] Another reason could come from the claim that all of our actions have mechanistic causes (that is, causes that do not depend on any mental property) plus the claim that mechanistic causes exclude causation by conscious will (possibly along with other kinds of mental causation).[13] Although these other challenges are interesting as well, I will focus here on separate challenges raised by Benjamin Libet.

Libet's experiments are discussed in several places in this volume, but it is worthwhile to describe them briefly in my own terms. Libet asked his subjects to flex their wrists at any time they wanted and then report the location of a dot moving quickly around a clock face when they first felt the urge or intention to flex their wrists. Throughout this process, he recorded their neural activity (with EEG) as well as their wrist movements (with EMG). By averaging forty trials, Libet found a pattern in the brain electrical activity recorded by the vertex electrode. That activity ramped up slowly, reaching its pinnacle at the time when bodily movement began, and then fell quickly after movement. This ramp-shaped activity—called a readiness potential or RP—was not found in trials where subjects were asked to time stimuli but not to move, so this pattern seemed to be connected either to will or to movement. It cannot be due simply to watching the clock or trying to time a mental event.

What was surprising was the order: The readiness potential with unplanned actions (type II RP) began around 550 ms before the hand movement (M) began, and the reported time of conscious will (W) was around 150–200 ms before the hand movement (M) began, so the readiness potential (type II RP) began around 350–400 ms before the reported time of conscious will (W). This order suggests that conscious will does not initiate the readiness potential, assuming that causation cannot run backward in time.[14] This implication is surprising, because most people think that their conscious choice is what begins the process that makes their body move in such cases.

These results have engendered an avalanche of scientific and philosophical commentary, including the essays in this volume, but there remains tremendous confusion about what exactly Libet's findings show and what they are supposed to show. To cut through this fog, we first need to specify what Libet does *not* show or try to show.

First, Libet's experiments do not show or pretend to show that our actions or wills are not determined. His results have nothing to do with determinism. Hence, they also do not have anything to do with any kind of free will that is equivalent to a denial of determinism. As I said before, the old issue of free will versus determinism is quite distinct from the new challenge to responsibility that Libet raises.

Second, Libet's experiments do not show or try to show that agents do not have intentions or wills or that their intentions or wills do not cause their actions (despite what he sometimes seems to say). Physicalists claim that intentions and wills (or choices) are constituted by, realized in, or identical with certain brain states or events. That brain activity might just be the readiness potential or RP that Libet measured. The readiness potential started before any consciousness of an intention or will, but it still might be an intention or will as long as wills or intentions can be unconscious. Moreover, if that readiness potential is or constitutes an intention or will, and if the readiness potential causes the bodily movement, then the intention or will causes the bodily movement, just as it seems. The issues that Libet's results raise are not about will in general but only about conscious will and consciousness of will.

Third, Libet's experiments do not support epiphenomenalism about all conscious mental states or even all conscious intentions or willings. Libet's subjects were conscious of general distal intentions to follow the instructions. Libet's results do not pretend to show that those general distal intentions did not affect what his subjects did. They would not have sat still and flexed their wrists if they had not intended to comply with his instructions. Hence, Libet's results do not support epiphenomenalism in general about all consciousness or even about all conscious intentions.

Fourth, even if we focus on proximal (not distal) conscious (not unconscious) intentions or wills, Libet does not show that this specific kind of intention has no effects at all. After all, we might feel more guilt at a later time if we had a proximal conscious intention to do the action than if we lacked such an intention.[15] What matters to Libet is not such later side-effects. His concern is whether our wills cause the willed acts in particular.

Fifth, Libet does not claim to show that conscious proximal wills do not play any role at all in action. He seems to hypothesize that consciousness of our will (at about 150–200 ms before movement) makes us aware of what we are about to do, and this enables us to veto the movement if we decide to veto it.[16] This is how he reinstates free will (or free won't—as Ramachandran dubbed it), despite his findings. Thus, Libet grants that consciousness of intention can affect what we do, at least in those cases where we veto an action (and maybe also when we could but do not veto our actions). His results are not about whether conscious proximal will plays any role at all in action. They are, instead, about which role conscious proximal will does play in action and, in particular, whether conscious proximal will initiates bodily movement.

Sixth, Libet's results do not show that conscious proximal will never initiates any action process (including the bodily movement and the brain activity that causes it). After all, his experiments tested only one kind of action, and it was a strange kind. We do not normally consciously intend to move a body part for no reason. Hence, it would be way too hasty to generalize from the few actions that he tested to all actions in general.

So, what do Libet's results show? He showed that, in *some* cases, a *conscious proximal* will to move now does *not initiate* the brain activity (or RP) that begins the process that produces the bodily movement or action. This modest conclusion might seem disappointing, but it still might have important implications for responsibility.

Whether it does have important implications depends on which interpretation is correct. Like all experiments, Libet's results rule out some possibilities but leave others open.

On one interpretation, the brain activity (or RP) causes the conscious will or consciousness of will, which then in turn causes the bodily movement.

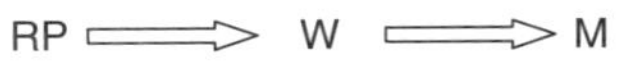


**Figure 19.1**

I will call this the *commonsense interpretation*, because it does not challenge common views about action and responsibility. It fits right into what most people think about themselves and others.

On other interpretations, the brain activity (readiness potential, or RP) causes the bodily movement directly without involving consciousness or conscious will as an intermediate step in the causal chain. I will call these interpretations revolutionary because they do undermine what most people think about their actions. Revolutionary interpretations come in three versions, depending on what is supposed to cause conscious will.

On one version, the brain activity (RP) is a common cause of both the conscious will (W) and also the bodily movement (M):

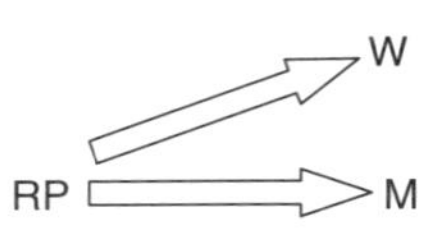


**Figure 19.2**

I will call this the *common cause interpretation.*

On another version, the brain activity (RP) causes the bodily movement (M), but some other brain activity (B2—not detected by Libet and not caused by RP) causes the conscious will (W).

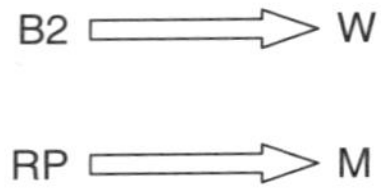


**Figure 19.3**

I will call this the *distinct process interpretation.*

On a third version, the brain activity (RP) causes the bodily movement (M), and, when we notice our body moving, then later we ascribe a conscious will (W) to ourselves in certain circumstances.

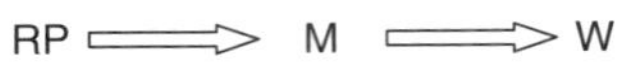


**Figure 19.4**

I will call this the *reconstruction interpretation.*[17]

These last three interpretations are revolutionary, because they all imply that conscious will does not initiate action in the way that it seems to. Even on these revolutionary interpretations, agents might have conscious access to the initiating causes of their acts, but this conscious access occurs later, not at the time of initiation. Consciousness also still might affect prior planning, sustaining of effort, and even guiding the act after it starts. All that consciousness does not do is initiate the action, on these views. Hence, agents still might have some conscious control, such as by vetoing acts or stopping an action after it has started, but they cannot control their acts by means of refusing to initiate the acts.

What's so revolutionary about that? To many people, their actions seem to be initiated and caused by a conscious proximal will to act. When I decide not to raise my hand to ask a question after a lecture, sometimes I feel the urge and have to stop myself, but often I just decide not to ask my question, and I feel no urge that I need to resist. And when I do raise my hand, it feels as if my conscious proximal will to raise my hand now to attract attention so that I can ask a question is what causes the physical process that includes my hand going up. Thus, the revolutionary interpretations suggest that the phenomenology of action is illusory in this respect.[18]

Most importantly, if responsibility requires causation by conscious will (as I argued in sections 1–2), and if Libet's results show that conscious intention does not cause action (as the revolutionary interpretations suggest), then the revolutionary interpretations of Libet's results seem to undermine some common views of responsibility.

These unnerving implications of the revolutionary interpretation make it crucial to determine which interpretation of Libet's results is correct. Does RP cause W, which causes M? Or is RP a common cause of W and M? Or does RP cause M and something else causes W? Or does RP cause M, which causes W?

Several recent experiments have tried to shed light on this issue. Haggard and Eimer[19] used the fact that Libet needed to average 40 trials in each run for each subject. Within the averaged set, there was a great deal of variation in timing. Haggard and Eimer replicated Libet's method, but then split the cases where the RP began early from the cases where the RP began late. They also split the cases where W was reported early from the cases where W was reported late. They found no correlation between early RPs and early Ws or between late RPs and late Ws. They did, however, find a correlation between early versus late Ws and early versus late LRPs (lateralized readiness potentials).

Correlation does not prove causation, of course, but lack of correlation is still evidence against causation. When one event causes another, the timing of the effect should vary with the timing of the cause. This point is an instance of John Stuart Mill's method of concomitant variation.[20] Applying that method to our case, if RP did cause W, then there should be a correlation between early RPs and early Ws as well as between late RPs and late Ws. Haggard and Eimer's failure to find any such correlation between RP and W thus suggests that RP does not cause W. Their finding then provides some evidence against the commonsense interpretation as well as the common cause interpretation of Libet's results. In contrast, Haggard and Eimer's findings are consistent with both the distinct process interpretation (where LRP might be that distinct process that causes W) and possibly the reconstruction interpretation (if the time between M and W can vary independently of RP).

Another way to test these causal models is to manipulate various events. Lau and colleagues[21] replicated the crucial parts of Libet's set-up but applied TMS (transcranial magnetic stimulation) to preSMA (presupplemenatary motor area) shortly *after* the bodily movement began. They found that TMS at this later time affected the reported time of W, even though consciousness of will (W) seems to occur before movement (M). Banks and Isham[22] similarly found that an auditory beep 5–60 ms *after* movement (M) affected reported time of conscious will (W). With later TMS and beeps, some subjects reported a time of conscious will even *after* the movement began. The point is that, if conscious will (W) causes movement (M), then W must occur before M, but then it is hard to see how TMS or a beep after M could affect the time at which subjects report first feeling or detecting W. These manipulation findings thus create trouble for the claim that W causes M and, thereby, for the commonsense interpretation. In contrast, these manipulation results are perfectly consistent with the other three interpretations (common cause, separate process, and reconstruction).

A group at Dartmouth College is planning to use a different method of manipulation: hypnosis. Subjects will be hypnotized so that their hands will move without them being conscious of willing to move (M without W) and also so that, when they consciously will to move, their hands will not move (W without M). If we find the distinctive RP shape (ramp up then fall quickly) in cases of M without W but not in cases of W without M, then that result will suggest that RP causes M but does not cause W. This finding would be contrary to the commonsense and common cause interpretations but consistent with the distinct process interpretation and possibly the reconstruction interpretation (though the latter would need to explain how we can have W without M). And if we find the distinctive RP shape in cases of W without M but not in cases of M without W, that finding will suggest that RP causes W but does not directly cause M. That finding would be contrary to the common cause interpretation and the reconstruction interpretation but consistent with the commonsense interpretation and the distinct process interpretation. Unfortunately, this experiment is still being planned, so no results are available yet.

Of course, none of these experiments is (or will be) conclusive. Each needs to be replicated (or finished!), and other techniques need to be tried. It is not yet clear which interpretation is best. The commonsense interpretation is under some pressure from the results so far, but we do not yet know whether the revolution will succeed in the end.

## 4. IMPLICATIONS?

Nonetheless, it is not too early to ask what would follow *if* the commonsense view were refuted. In particular, would all responsibility be undermined if scientists found that conscious will did not cause bodily movements? No.

One reason is that conscious will and intention *does* cause action in Libet's experiments. As mentioned before, Libet's subjects chose to participate and intended to follow his instructions. These distal wills and intentions occurred minutes before they flexed their wrists. Nothing in Libet's findings throws any doubt on the natural assumption that his subjects would not have sat there and moved their hands as they did if they had not had those distal wills and intentions.[23] Thus, Libet did not show or try to show that no kind of conscious will ever causes actions (or at least it would be uncharitable to interpret him as trying to show that).

Nonetheless, although subjects decided in advance *what* to do, they did not decide in advance *when* to do it. Their distal wills did not cause the subjects to move their hands at the precise time when they did move. They could follow the instructions as they intended whether they moved their hands at time t or at time t plus one second or at time t minus one second or at many other times.[24] Thus, even if their distal intentions caused them to move at one time or another within a certain time period, that distal intention did not cause them to move at the particular time when they did move rather than at some other time during that period. It caused them to make some movement of a general kind, but it did not cause the particular movement that actually occurred.

Which is necessary for responsibility: the general distal intention or the particular proximal intention or both? Suppose that Bill makes a conscious plan to push Carl in front of a subway car. When the time arrives, somebody else, Andy, pushes Bill into Carl, and the impact makes Carl fall in front of the subway car where he is killed. Bill does not seem guilty of murder, because Bill's general distal plan or intention did not cause his impact with Carl. Cases like this suggest that a general distal intention is not enough for responsibility when an agent's particular proximal intention does not cause the movement or the harm for which the agent might be responsible. Hence, an efficacious proximal intention seems necessary for full responsibility.

The proximal intention still might not have to be conscious. If a conscious distal intention or plan causes an agent to develop a brain state that later causes a proximal intention along with the act, then it is not clear why the proximal intention also needs to be conscious in order for the agent to be responsible for the planned act.

Whether a conscious proximal will is crucial for responsibility might depend on the kind of act in question. In some cases, it does not matter exactly when an action is done. Then responsibility seems to depend only on a distal will to do some act of the general kind and not on a conscious proximal will to do the particular act at the particular time. For example, if I plan to poison someone or rob a bank, it usually does not matter exactly when I do it, so I can be held responsible for doing some act of that general kind (poisoning or bank robbery), even if I was not conscious of choosing the exact time to pour poison in the victim's cup or to enter the bank. In contrast, there are other cases where the precise timing of a bodily movement does makes all the difference to whether the movement causes harm or violates a rule or law. For example, the precise time when a driver swerves a car to avoid an obstacle can determine whether that driver hits and kills a pedestrian. In that subclass of cases, responsibility seems to depend not only on a general intention to do an act of the kind but also on the proximal intention to act at that particular time.

Even when we focus on proximal will or intention to act right now as opposed to slightly earlier or later, the actions, intentions, and wills in Libet's experiments are too odd in several ways to support any general conclusion about all of human action where proximal will matters. First, Libet's subject had no reason to act at one time instead of somewhat earlier or later. It seems possible that conscious proximal will does *not* cause bodily movement when an agent has no reason to move at a particular time, but conscious proximal will still *does* cause bodily movement when the agent does have a reason to move at a particular time.

Second, the proximal will or intention of Libet's subjects was simply to move a certain body part. They had no goal beyond that movement, other than to comply with the instructions or to finish the experiment quickly. It was not as if their finger was on the trigger of a gun, and they wanted to achieve a goal of harming someone by pulling the trigger. It is rare in everyday life to move a body part with no intention other than to move it (or just in order to fulfill instructions to move it). Again, it seems possible that conscious will does *not* cause bodily movement when an agent has no intention other than to move a certain body part, but conscious will still *does* cause bodily movement when the agent does have a goal or intention beyond mere bodily movement.

Third, Libet asked his subjects to move the same body part many times. He spent a full day training his subjects, and, even after the experiment began, he needed forty trials to average in each run. It seems plausible that Libet's subjects quickly developed a habit, so later trials (perhaps after the first ten or so) were done unthinkingly by habit. It is common sense, supported by psychological experimentation, that habitual actions are done with less consciousness than nonhabitual actions. This is recognized by the reference to habit in MPC 2.10 (2)(d), quoted above. Hence, it seems plausible that conscious will does *not* cause bodily movements that are habitual but still *does* cause bodily movements that are not habitual.

All of these differences dictate against hastily generalizing from Libet's research to human action in general. Still, it is not completely clear which generalizations are too hasty. After all, much science begins with simple cases and then hypothesizes a general rule to be tested in other cases. That is what Libet does. Defenders of Libet's generalizations can respond that we have no compelling evidence that other acts differ in relevant ways. It might seem plausible that conscious will precedes and causes bodily movements in other cases, but those other cases have not been tested in careful experiments.[25] If we have tested only a sample of a larger class, and if all of that sample shows a certain property, and if there is no reason to think that the rest of the class differs from the sample, then that finding is at least some reason to expect that the property generalizes to the whole class or most of that class. Still, the differences listed above do give at least some reason to think that the sample tested by Libet is not representative of the wider class of human actions.

Another response is that complex actions for reasons and goals are made up of little bits of bodily movement like those that Libet studied. It is not clear how the larger actions can be free or controlled if their smaller parts are not. It is also not clear how an agent can be responsible for the larger action when the agent is not responsible for any of its smallest parts. This puzzle is an instance of a more general puzzle of emergent properties of wholes that are not properties of any parts. (Compare: How can water be liquid when none of its molecules is liquid?) If this puzzle cannot be solved, then there might potentially be some route to argue from Libet's results to a general conclusion about all human actions, including the larger actions done for reasons and goals. However, it really should not be surprising that humans can be responsible for larger complex actions without being responsible for the parts of which those larger actions are constituted. A city council with ten members can be responsible for voting a tax increase, even if that vote is constituted by ten individual votes, and the council is not responsible for any of those individual votes. I can be responsible for making noise by drumming my fingers, even if I am not aware of the movement of any particular finger. And so on. Although it is not completely clear how this works, it does seem to work, so we do seem to be able to be responsible for a complex action without being responsible for any of its individual parts.

Does this make Libet's experiments completely irrelevant to responsibility? No. Just as we should not infer from the actions Libet studied to all actions, so we should not infer that, since Libet's experiments do not apply to all actions, they show nothing about any action. Libet's findings are limited in scope, but they can still illuminate action, the role of consciousness, and responsibility in a special set of cases.

In particular, Libet's results still might suggest that specific requirements for responsibility are not met in a subclass of actions. Consider what I will call minimal actions—actions done quickly without awareness of what one is doing until after it is too late to stop. Minimal acts come in many varieties, but examples should clarify the idea.

Imagine that Sally was driving her car carefully under the speed limit down the main street of a town when a cat ran out in front of her car. She automatically swerved to the right in order to miss the cat. Unfortunately, she hit and killed a pedestrian on the sidewalk, whom she had seen only peripherally. It seems to me that Sally was reckless and, hence, responsible for the pedestrian's death if she was conscious of forming a plan to swerve in order to save the cat, and if she was also conscious that swerving to the right would create a risk of serious injury to people on the sidewalk. In contrast, Sally was not responsible if the whole incident happened so quickly that she was never conscious of turning the car, much less of any risk to anyone, before it was too late to avoid the accident. The tricky case is in the middle, where Sally turned the car automatically without becoming conscious of any plan or risk, but she was conscious of turning and yet was not able to stop herself in time to avoid hitting the pedestrian. She essentially looked on as her body reacted. Some people might doubt that cases like this are possible. What Libet contributes is a better understanding of how they can happen. He shows how much can happen in our brains before we become conscious of willing anything. He also shows how short the window is when we are able to veto our automatic actions. Libet's research, thus, might make some people more willing to believe that Sally was not in conscious control, even if she was conscious.

Another case is *State v. Utter* (1971). Sadly, a father stabbed his young son when his son unexpectedly approached him from the rear:

> Defendant testified that as a result of his jungle warfare training and experiences in World War II he had on two occasions reacted violently toward people approaching him unexpectedly from the rear and that his act of stabbing his son was a conditioned response, which was defined by his psychiatrist as an act or pattern of activity occurring so rapidly, so uniformly as to be automatic in response to a certain stimulus.

This defendant was found guilty, largely because he had been drinking (though not heavily) so he was held responsible for slowing his own ability to inhibit or veto his actions. However, the court suggested that the defense might have worked if he had not been drinking, even though the act does look organized and directed in the same way as an intended act. Again, Libet helps us understand how a quick action that was not planned in advance could happen without consciousness, even though it looks fairly complex and intentional.

Agents like these might be responsible if their acts were habitual. Recall that MPC section 2.01(2)(d) denies responsibility for acts that are "not a product of the effort or determination of the actor, either conscious or habitual." This voluntary act requirement suggests that causation by conscious will is not required for responsibility in cases of habit. However, Sally's swerve and Utter's knifing are not habitual in any normal sense. Sally might have swerved before, and Utter did react violently "on two occasions," but neither of them did such acts regularly. Thus, if their acts were not the product of conscious will, they would seem not to be responsible for what they did. At least, Libet can help us understand how such people could have failed to meet the requirements of responsibility.

Other minimal actions might include a quick reaction to provocation or to being shot,[26] some acts during sleep or immediately upon awaking,[27] and some cases of succumbing to temptation.[28] Libet's research suggests that some cases like these (maybe more than we think) might be automatic rather than the product of conscious will. It is still often not at all clear what the role of consciousness in such quick reactions is, so it is also not clear which of these agents should be held responsible. Despite these unclarities, Libet's findings, along with the work of his followers, might make some people more sympathetic and willing to excuse some minimal actions. Of course, some of these acts might be excused even without relying on Libet or any science at all, but at least Libet and related research can help us to gain better understanding of why such agents do not meet the requirements for responsibility and should be excused.[29]

What, then, does the law need to do in light of our improved understanding of minimal or automatic actions? Perhaps nothing. Sometimes the law already handles such cases well enough. However, where the law of criminal responsibility requires causation by conscious will, we need to think about various kinds of automatic or minimal actions to see whether the law yields the correct results. Various moves are available if an act does not seem to result from conscious will: Either (a) we cannot hold the person responsible at all or (b) we need to remove consciousness from the requirements for responsibility or (c) we need to specify that only general consciousness is required or (d) we need to stretch the "action" to include a prior voluntary act or (e) we need to reduce the legal effects of minimal or automatic acts (e.g., by mitigation). Which legal response is proper is a policy decision for society rather than a scientific issue that could be settled by Libet, but what Libet adds is a better understanding of these fascinating cases.[30]

## NOTES

1. See the introduction to this volume for a brief discussion of some predecessors.
2. Although I focus on the voluntary act requirement, consciousness and will are also relevant to other legal standards for responsibility. One example is the defense of automatism, which some states define in terms of consciousness: e.g., "Automatism is the state of a person who, though capable of action, is not *conscious* of what he is doing." (*Fulcher v. State* 633 P.2d 142, 145 (Wyo. 1981)) Other examples are definitions of *mens rea* in Model Penal Code section 2.02, including: "A person acts purposely with respect to material element of an offense when: (i) if the element involves the nature of his conduct or a result thereof, it is his *conscious* object to engage in conduct of that nature or to cause such a result; and (ii) if the element involves the attendant circumstances, he is *aware* of the existence of such circumstances or he believes or hopes that they exist" (my emphasis). Awareness and consciousness are also required by the MPC definitions of acting knowingly and recklessly. And some formulations of the insanity defense (e.g., *Regina v. M'Naghten, Eng. Rep.* 718, 1843) require the agent to know (and, hence, be conscious of?) the nature and quality of his action order to be responsible. However, what is relevant according to these definitions is consciousness of elements other than will, and these definitions do not explicitly require causation by that consciousness. That is why I focus on the voluntary act requirement in the text.
3. *People v. Decina* 2 N.Y.2d 133, 157 N.Y.S.2d 558, 138 N.E.2d 799 (1956).
4. See Larry Alexander, "Reconsidering the Relationship among Voluntary Acts, Strict Liability, and Negligence in Criminal Law," *Social Philosophy and Policy* 7, no. 2 (1990): 84–104.
5. See Deborah Denno, "Crime and Consciousness: Science and Involuntary Acts," *Minnesota Law Review* 87 (2002–2003): 269–399.
6. See my "Word Meaning in Legal Interpretation," *San Diego Law Review* 42, no. 2 (2005): 465–492.
7. Compare the case of Cogdon discussed in Norval Morris, "Somnambulistic Homicide: Ghosts, Spiders, and North Koreans," *Res Judicatae* 29, no. 5 (1951): 29–30; and the case of *Regina v. Parks* 95 D.L.R.4th 27 (1992) discussed in R. Broughton et al., "Homicidal Somnambulism: A Case Report," *Sleep* 17 (1994): 253, 255.
8. Freedom and responsibility, like control, come in degrees. One person can be more responsible than another, even if neither is fully responsible.

When I discuss responsibility, I refer to full responsibility associated with acting purposely (see note 2), rather than minimal responsibility that is necessary for any person to be liable to any negative moral judgment or punishment. If Libet's work showed that agents are not fully responsible, that would be important and interesting even if his work did not undermine minimal responsibility.

9. See note 7 and the case of "sexsomnia" reported in http://news.bbc.co.uk/1/hi/england/north_yorkshire/4543340.stm
10. These cases are discussed in the introduction to this volume.
11. See Deborah Denno, "Crime and Consciousness," note 5.
12. This challenge is discussed briefly in the introduction to this volume.
13. I plan to address this challenge from mechanism in a future paper.
14. This assumption is questioned by Stuart Hameroff, among others, but I do not have space to discuss that alternative here.
15. The importance of such side-effects is stressed by Daniel Wegner, *The Illusion of Conscious Will* (Cambridge, MA: MIT Press, 2002), chapter 9.
16. Libet claims that this veto (or choice to veto) is uncaused, but he gives no reason for this claim, and it is not necessary, since the real issue here is not determinism. Libet also assumes that agents have enough time to veto, but that is not at all clear. In addition, Simone Kuhn and Marcel Brass, "Retrospective Construction of the Judgment of Free Choice," *Consciousness and Cognition* (2008) argue, "the act of vetoing cannot be consciously initiated." Nonetheless, the possibility of veto at least shows that Libet's results do not directly entail any lack of freedom or responsibility. Additional premises or assumptions are needed before any philosophical lessons can be drawn from Libet's scientific results.
17. See Ebert and Wegner as well as Wheatley and Looser in this volume (chapters 12 and 13).
18. Pace Horgan in this volume (chapter 14).
19. Patrick Haggard and Martin Eimer, "On the Relation between Brain Potentials and Awareness of Voluntary Movements," *Exp Brain Res* 126 (1999): 128–133.
20. John Stuart Mill, *A System of Logic* (1843), chapters 8–10.
21. This volume and H. C. Lau, R. D. Rogers, and R. E. Passingham, "Manipulating the Experienced Onset of Intention after Action Execution," *Journal of Cognitive Neuroscience* 19, no. 1 (2007): 81–90.
22. This volume and W. P. Banks and E. A. Isham, "We Infer Rather Than Perceive the Moment We Decided to Act," *Psychological Science* 20 (2009): 17–21.
23. See Mele, chapter 4, this volume.
24. In some experiments (such as Haggard and Eimer, "On the Relation between Brain Potentials and Awareness of Voluntary Movements"), subjects did decide what to do (such as which button to push) as well as when to do it, and similar results were found, but they still decided at the last moment for no reason. See also Pockett and Purdy, chapter 4 in this volume.
25. But see Pockett and Purdy, chapter 4 in this volume.
26. See the case of Huey Newton discussed by Gideon Yaffe in this volume, chapter 16.
27. *Fain v. Commonwealth* 1879: "a prosecution for murder of a defendant who had shot a hotel porter when the latter was attempting to awaken him . . . . he had been a sleepwalker since his infancy."
28. For example, imagine that a kleptomaniac finds his hand reaching out to take an item and then put in it his pocket before he can stop himself.
29. Of course, some such agents might be responsible because they should not have gotten themselves into the position where their unforeseen minimal acts could cause such harm, but that is a different issue that I will not address here. Here the point is only that, even if the agent is responsible indirectly by way of past acts, the agent is not responsible directly or fully.
30. Thanks to Adina Roskies for helpful comments on a draft and also to the audience at the University of Arizona.

# AUTHOR INDEX

Note: Page numbers followed by "*f*" denote figures.

# SUBJECT INDEX

Note: Page numbers followed by "*f*" and "*t*" denote figures and tables, respectively.